Textbook of Rheumatology: Volume I

Marylin Harter

AMERICAN
MEDICAL PUBLISHERS
www.americanmedicalpublishers.com

AMERICAN
MEDICAL PUBLISHERS
www.americanmedicalpublishers.com

Cataloging-in-publication Data

Textbook of rheumatology : volume I / Marylin Harter.
p. cm.
Includes bibliographical references and index.
ISBN 979-8-88740-490-5
1. Rheumatology. 2. Rheumatism. 3. Connective tissues--Diseases.
4. Joints--Diseases. I. Harter, Marylin.
RC927 .T49 2023
616.723--dc23

American Medical Publishers,
41 Flatbush Avenue,
1st Floor, New York,
NY 11217, USA

ISBN 979-8-88740-490-5 (Hardback)

Contents

Preface

Every book is a source of knowledge and this one is no exception. The idea that led to the conceptualization of this book was the fact that the world is advancing rapidly; which makes it crucial to document the progress in every field. I am aware that a lot of data is already available, yet, there is a lot more to learn. Hence, I accepted the responsibility of editing this book and contributing my knowledge to the community.

Rheumatology is a field of internal medicine that deals with the diagnosis and treatment of rheumatic diseases. These diseases are usually autoimmune or inflammatory disorders associated with arthritis, dermatomyositis, gout, lupus erythematosus, Lyme disease, mixed connective tissue disease, polychondritis, polymyositis, and vasculitis. Rheumatology focuses on diseases and conditions that affect joints, soft tissues, or connective tissues. Disorders of bones such as fluorosis, osteoporosis, osteomalacia, renal osteodystrophy, and rickets are also treated by rheumatologists. Treatment of rheumatic conditions may involve the use of one or more methods such as administering drugs, physical and occupational therapy, rehabilitation, and surgery, depending on the specifics of the case. Commonly prescribed drugs include anti-inflammatory medications, opioids and antidepressants. This textbook provides comprehensive insights into the basic concepts as well as recent developments in field of rheumatology. It is appropriate for students seeking detailed information in this area as well as for experts.

While editing this book, I had multiple visions for it. Then I finally narrowed down to make every chapter a sole standing text explaining a particular topic, so that they can be used independently. However, the umbrella subject sinews them into a common theme. This makes the book a unique platform of knowledge.

I would like to give the major credit of this book to the experts from every corner of the world, who took the time to share their expertise with us. Also, I owe the completion of this book to the never-ending support of my family, who supported me throughout the project.

Marylin Harter

Part I

Rheumatology Fundamentals

1

Rheumatology: Taking History of a Patient

Laila Alharbi and Hani Almoallim

1.1 Introduction

History taking in rheumatology is the most important skill needed for proper handling of a patient with a rheumatological complaint. Obtaining a good history will help you to reach almost 90% of your diagnosis. However, history taking is mostly depending on experience and practice rather than theoretical recall. Here in this section, we provide you with the most important points in history taking you should use while dealing with rheumatological patients. There is an approach to history taking in rheumatology started as with the classical approach in history taking like any other disease. There is much focus on rheumatological aspects related to the onset of joints pains, patterns, symmetry of joints involvement, number of joints involved, and ultimately rheumatology review of systems. We summarized the classic symptomatic correlations with certain rheumatological diseases. We present briefly a suggested approach to your presentation of the entire case.

L. Alharbi
Medical College, Umm Al Qura university, Makkah, Saudi Arabia

Department of Internal Medicine, Skåne University Hospital, Malmoe, Sweden

H. Almoallim (✉)
Medical College, Umm Al-Qura University (UQU), Makkah, Saudi Arabia
e-mail: hmmoallim@uqu.edu.sa

1.1.1 Objectives

1. To compose a comprehensive and organize history for patients with rheumatological problems.
2. To recall the most important points in eliciting history for certain rheumatological diseases.
3. To construct a differential diagnosis in rheumatology.
4. To develop an approach for monitoring patients with arthritis.

1.2 Approach to History Taking in Rheumatology

This approach is based on the assumption that majority of patients with rheumatological diseases present at the beginning with joint(s) pain. Rheumatological diseases are systemic diseases affecting almost all body systems with no system that is preserved. You may have patients with neurological complaints (like hemiplegia because of ischemic stroke) end up with the diagnosis of a rheumatological disease like systemic lupus erythematosus (SLE) and secondary antiphospholipid syndrome (APS). Here the initial presentation was not joints pain, but yet the final diagnosis was rheumatological. This concept emphasizes the point that good foundations in general internal medicine is essential to the rheumatology practice.

The approach to joints pain for any new patient should establish two basic issues: the personal data and then full analysis of the presenting illness. The latter includes the followings (Fig. 1.1).

1. Onset.
2. Duration.
3. Patterns of joints affected.
4. Symmetry.
5. Number of joints affected.
6. Associated symptoms.
7. Constitutional symptoms.
8. Functional impairment.
9. Relieving and aggravating factors.
10. Rheumatology review of systems.

This should be followed by the classical components in any history taking in internal medicine (past medical and surgical history, family history, drug and allergy, and social history).

Here is a brief description about each one of the above.

1. Onset: The patient should determine whether joint(s) pain have started suddenly or gradually. This is essential as the top differential diagnoses that should be ruled out for sudden

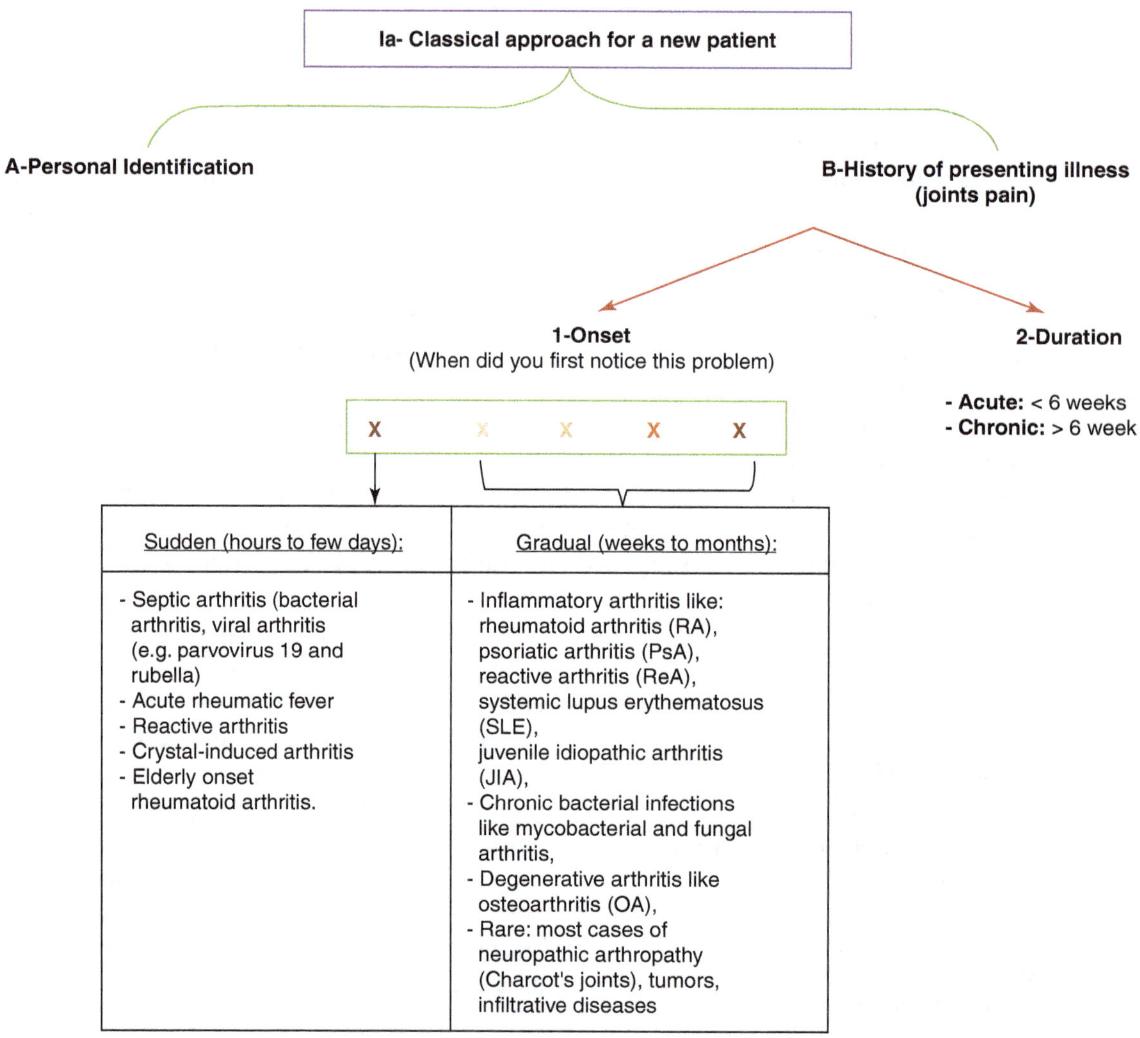

Fig. 1.1 Approach to history taking in rheumatology

onset of joints pains are septic arthritis and crystal-induced arthritis (after excluding trauma as a possible cause for joints pains) (Fig. 1.2). Gradual onset joint pains have long list of differential diagnoses including the classic rheumatological diseases like rheumatoid arthritis (RA) and SLE (see Fig. 1.2).

2. Duration: It is essential to determine whether the joint pains have been present for less or more than 6 weeks. Classically, arthritis caused by acute viral illnesses like parvovirus B19 infection can cause RA-like arthritis in distribution but with less than 6 weeks duration. Duration more than 6 weeks is an essential criteria to diagnose RA based on 2010 classification criteria of RA (see Chap. 25).
3. Patterns of joints affected: Each rheumatological disease has a pattern of presentation that should be recognized from this early stage. Each pattern has a differential diagnosis (Figs. 1.3 and 1.4).

   Predominant small joints involvement (like in pattern A) particularly the wrists, metacarpophalangeal (MCP), proximal interphalangeal (PIP), and metatarsophalangeal (MTP) joints is a classical presentation for RA. Other disorders like SLE, psoriatic arthritis (PsA), polyarticular gout, and reactive arthritis (ReA) can present in a similar way. The commonest joints involved in RA, for example, are wrists and MCP (2nd and 3rd). It has to be noted that distal interphalangeal (DIP) joints involvement is rarely ever involved in RA. These joints (DIP) are

> Make sure the origin of the pain is from the joint itself, NOT from the periarticular sructures. One tip is to ask the patient to point the site of the pain by his/her finger!

Fig. 1.2 Identifying the site of the pain

Fig. 1.3 Patterns of joints affected

Joints	Differential Diagnosis
Symmetrical polyarticular MCP PIP and MTP joints	RA, SLE, PsA, Polyarticular gout and ReA.
DIP joint(s)	PsA, OA
Bony swellings of DIPs or PIPs or 1st CMC joint (base of thumb)	OA
Proximal girdle joints	Polymyalgia rheumatica and RA
Asymmetrical large joint oligoarticular dIsease	ReA, PsA, ankylosing spondylitis {AS)
Acute monoarticular disease	Infection, gout, pseudogout
Chronic monoarticular	PsA, RA, AS, OA and chronic infection (e.g. tuberculosis (TB))
Axial, sacroiliac and girdle joints	AS
Axial joints	Lumbar & cervical spondylosis/OA
Dactylitis (sausage digit)	PsA, ReA, AS, TB, sarcoidosis, sickle cell disease.

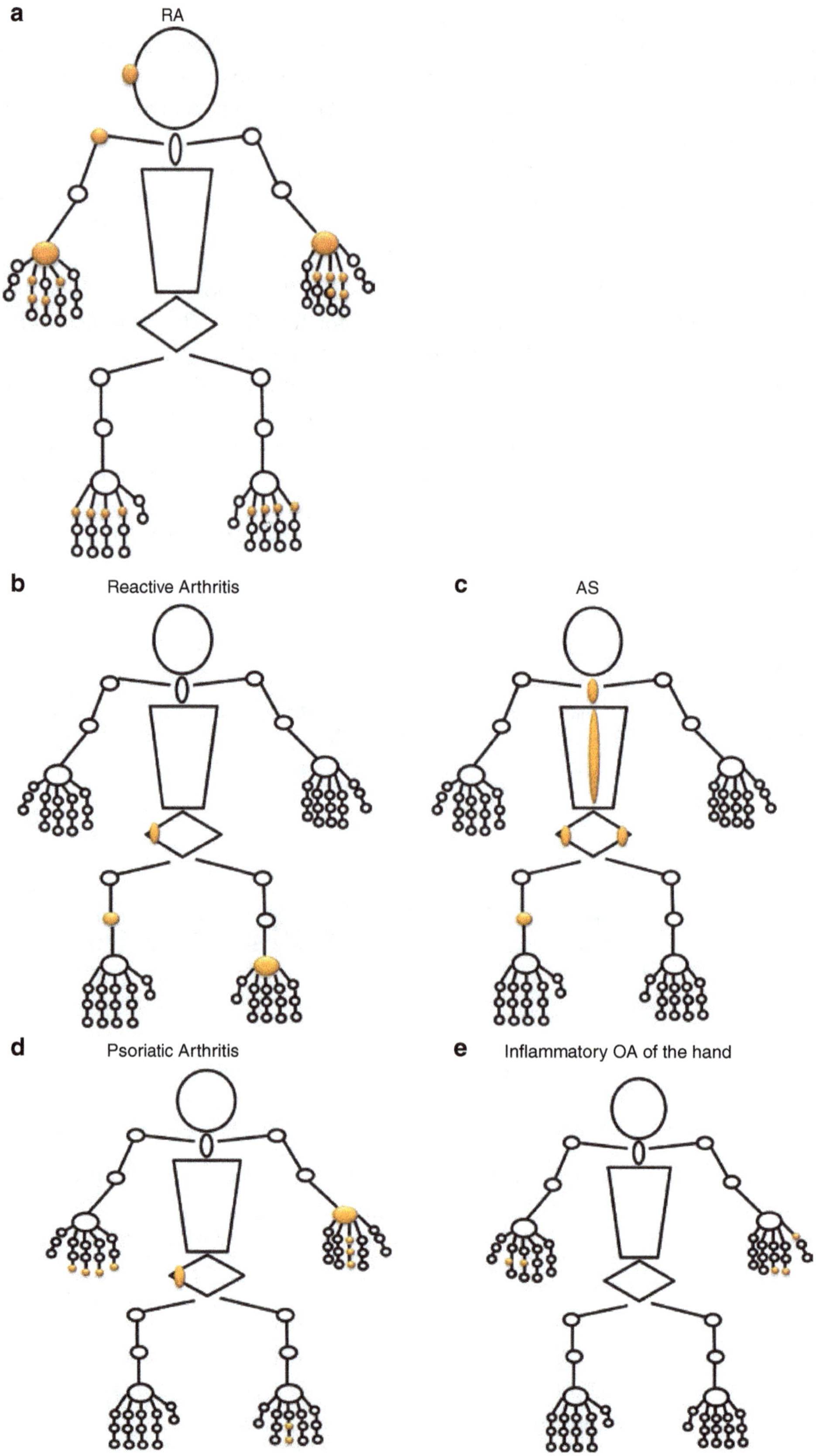

Fig. 1.4 Each rheumatological disease has a pattern. (**a**) Rheumatoid arthritis. (**b**) Reactive arthritis. (**c**) Ankylosing spondylitis. (**d**) Psoriatic arthritis. (**e**) Inflammatory osteoarthritis of the hand

predominantly involved in patients with PsA and inflammatory osteoarthritis (OA) of the hands. Classical presentation of inflammatory OA of the hands (pattern E) involves DIPs, PIPs, and first carpometacarpal joint just at the base of the anatomical snuff. It has to be noted as a physical examination caveat that the swellings of the joints in inflammatory OA of the hands are bony! It represents the degenerative changes happening in the cartilage with osteophyte formation. Predominant large joints involvement in the lower limbs (pattern B) is a classical presentation for ReA. A group of disorders called spondyloarthritis (SpA) (include ankylosing spondylitis (AS), PsA, ReA, and arthritis associated with inflammatory bowel diseases (IBD-related arthritis) and undifferentiated spondyloarthritis) (see Chap. 23 for detailed classification criteria) has particular predilection of large joints of the lower limb. Sacroiliac joints can be involved in an asymmetrical fashion (pattern B) in ReA or can be symmetrically involved (pattern C) with inflammation of all the insertions of tendons and ligaments to the bones of the back (this is called enthesitis, and such inflammatory process in the back is called spondylitis). Therefore, (pattern C) is a classical presentation for AS. Spondylitis per say can be a manifestation of any disease of the SpA group of disorders. Large joints like proximal girdle joints (shoulders and hips) can be involved predominantly in diseases like polymyalgia rheumatica and RA. There is one feature that is quite classical for PsA and crystal induced arthritis. It is the inflammation of all articular and periarticular structures in one digit (dactylitis). This is not a feature for RA. It has to be noted then, involvement of small joints like in (pattern D) with predominance of DIPs, dactylitis, and asymmetrical sacroiliac joint involvement is classical for PsA.

For acute sudden monoarticular joint involvement, a septic process and/or crystal-induced arthritis should be ruled out. The knee joint is the commonest joint involved in septic arthritis, while the first metatarsophalangeal joints are the commonest joint involved in gout. For chronic monoarticular joint involvement, a chronic infectious process should be ruled out like tuberculosis or brucellosis. However, systemic rheumatic diseases like RA can rarely present with a monoarticular joint only.

4. Symmetry: This might have been covered partly in the above section. It has been included here to help the evaluator remember it all the time and consider it while composing the differential diagnosis. There are diseases like PsA that can present in several different ways including symmetrical arthritis like RA and asymmetrical arthritis involving only few joints like the DIPs. Symmetrical arthritis does not include in the differential diagnosis only known rheumatological diseases like RA and SLE. There are less common diseases like sarcoidosis, and paraneoplastic syndromes can present with arthritis (Fig. 1.5).
5. Number of joints involvement (How many joints affected?): Again, this feature has been covered partially above (Figs. 1.6 and 1.7). The emphasis is on a monoarticular single joint involvement when it should be considered a medical emergency. If a septic monoarticular joint was not diagnosed and treated properly, it will lead unfortunately to irreversible damage and lifelong disability if not death from disseminated infection [1]. It is hard clinically to separate between oligoarticular and polyarticular in the initial workup as will be shown in Chap. 3. A list of possible differential diagnosis is provided for you just to give a knowledge background base to proceed further in the history from patients with joints pains.
6. Associated symptoms: Obtaining history of redness, swelling, and morning stiffness is essential in any patient with joints pains. Any severely inflamed joint will cause obvious swelling observed by the patient. Keep in mind that sometimes, swellings of the small joints can be detected by physical examination only as the patient did not notice any

Symmetry of the joints

Symmetrical arthritis

Inflammatory:	- RA, PsA, SLE, JIA (systemic and polyarticular types), adult onset Still's disease, Sjögren's syndrome - Other systemic rheumatic diseases: SLE, mixed connective tissue disease (MCTD), adult onset rheumatic fever, polymyalgia rheumatica, erosive inflammatory osteoarthritis, calcium pyrophosphate deposition disease (CPPD) (pseudo-RA type)
Infectious:	- Viral arthritis especially parvovirus arthritis - Lyme disease
Infiltrative:	- Sarcoid arthritis (acute type) - Amyloid arthropathy - Hemochromatosis arthropathy
Neoplastic:	- Primary infiltrative/paraneoplastic: Leukemia - Chemotherapy induced (classically post breast cancer therapy)
Endocrinal:	- Myxedematous arthropathy

Asymmetrical arthritis:

Inflammatory:	- ReA - PsA - Pauciarticular JIA - Oligoaricular or polyarticular gout - CPPD disease (pseudogout type)
Infectious:	- Bacterial arthritis - Bacterial endocarditis.

Fig. 1.5 Symmetry of the joints

Fig. 1.6 Number of joints involvement (How many joints affected)

MONOARTICULAR (Single joint)	**OLIOONUICULAR (2-4 joints)**	**POLYARTICULAR (More than 4 joints)**
DD	**DD**	**DD**
- Traumatic - Inflammatory: Pauciarticular JIA, crystal-induced - Infectious: bacterial, fungal, TB, viral (AIDS). - Neoplastic - Infiltrative: one type of chronic sarcoidosis - Miscellaneous: Acute coagulopathy, Hemoglobinopathy	- Oligoarticular JIA - Reactive Arthritis - Psoriatic arthropathy	- Inflammatory: RA, JIA (polyarticular and Still), adult Still, Sjögren's - SLE and other connective tissue diseases - Seronegative spondyloarthropathies - CPPD disease - Vasculitides - Neoplastic: Paraneoplastic syndromes, metastasis, leukemia, lymphoma - Infiltrative: Sarcoidosis

Single red hot joint in RA: It should be remembered that the uncommon occurrence of a red hot joint in the context of RA may be due to superimposed septic arthritis and not to the disease process itself.

Monoarthritis in SLE: The occurrence of monoarthritis in a patient with SLE suggests infection or osteonecrosis.

Fig. 1.7 Alarming presentation of arthritis in RA and SLE

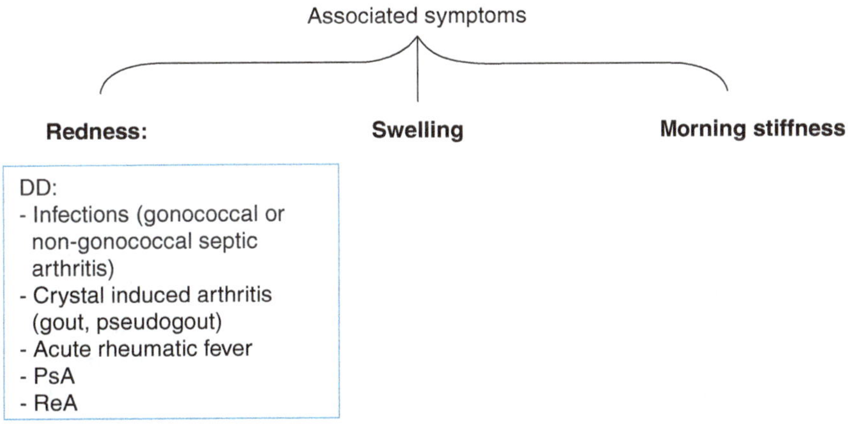

Fig. 1.8 Associated symptoms

because of its small size. Redness is one of the cardinal signs of inflammation. Active RA does not cause redness usually unless there is a superimposed infection in that joint that it is red. Therefore red and swollen joints are caused classically by septic arthritis and/or crystal induced arthritis (Fig. 1.8).

7. Constitutional symptoms: Obtaining these symptoms in any history obtained from patients for whatever symptoms presented is essential. Fever and arthritis are common clinical association. Again, septic arthritis whether in a monoarticular or polyarticular presentation should be ruled out. There is a full outline for this combination: fever and arthritis in Chap. 11. Apart from fever, the following symptoms should be obtained: weight loss, loss of appetite, night sweat, and fatigue. It has to be noted that patients with inflammatory arthritis often feel a general malaise. Fibromyalgia patients often report feeling ill (if I go shopping I am wiped out for the next 3 days). On the other hand, OA patients may be a bit tired but not really unwell.
8. Functional impairment: any inflamed joint will affect the functionality of the patient. The followings should be obtained:
   - How has the arthritis affected your daily ability to self-care?
   - How has the arthritis affected your ability to sleep well and to do things at home, work, and leisure?
9. Relieving and aggravating factors: Here the focus should be mainly on the effect of activity on the symptoms. Activity tends to aggravate joint pains caused by a degenerative process of the interarticular cartilage, i.e., OA, to be a reliving factor for inflammatory back pain as going to be shown in Chap. 6 about low-back pain. Use of nonsteroidal anti-inflammatory drugs (NSAIDs) tends to relive symptoms in a remarkable way in patients with inflammatory arthritis in comparison with patients with degenerative arthritis (OA) (Fig. 1.9).
10. Rheumatology review of systems: After your full analysis of the joints pain(s), now it is time to think which rheumatological diseases might be the top in your differential

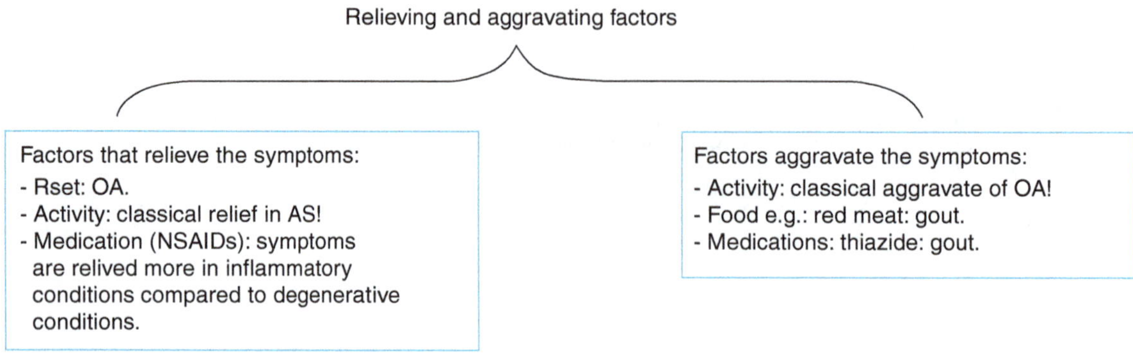

Fig. 1.9 Relieving and aggravating factors

diagnosis. All rheumatological diseases are systemic diseases with significant involvements of other body parts (Fig. 1.10). Some patients may not correlate the relationship between numbness, tingling sensations, and joints pain(s) (some patients may present with arthritis and mononeuritis multiplex like in vasculitis or RA). Others may not remember to mention history of skin disease like psoriasis. Obtaining obstetric history is extremely important for any childbearing female patient as there are many complications in pregnancy related to SLE and/or APS (see Chap. 17). For all of these reasons, it is your rule to review all possible symptoms that might be present and help you in composing your differential diagnosis. All possible symptoms are complied in an approach from head to toe just to help you mastering this part of the history.

- **Past medical history:**
  – History of any rheumatic disease (RA, SLE, gout, psoriasis, etc.).
  – History of recent infections (think of ReA!).
  – History of chronic diseases. There are some rheumatological associations with diabetes mellitus (see Chap. 21).
- **Family history:**
  – Ask if similar condition happened in the family.
  – Any family history of RA, SLE, psoriasis, etc.
- **Medications and allergy:**
  – Detailed medication history.
  – Any allergy from food and/or drugs?
- **Past surgical history:**
  – History of any previous operations.
  – History of blood transfusion.
- **Social history:**
  – Marital status and occupation (tendinitis in typist!). How many children? Where do they live?
  – History of contact with TB or jaundiced patients: essential prior to start of disease modifying anti-rheumatic drugs (DMARDs) and biological therapy.

1.3 Historical Correlation

Some patients may present initially with symptoms suspected for a certain disease. Then you need to check other symptoms related to this disease that might help you to make your diagnosis from historical grounds only! This is different than rheumatology review of systems mentioned above. Actually, as your skills in obtaining history from patients with joints pain grow, you will notice yourself combing this step with rheumatology review. For example, you are evaluating a young female patient with joint pains. You have a suspicion for SLE as you are proceeding in your history; then during your history taking, you should cover all common presentation of SLE!

SYSTEMS	SYMPTOMS SHOULD BE ASKED
1- Hair	Hair loss, alopecia, psoriatic rashes (in the hair line)
2- CNS:	History of stroke, weakness, seizure, psychosis: SLE. Mononeuritis multiplex, peripheral neuropathy: vasculitis, SLE Lymph node enlargement in the neck: SLE, lymphoma with sjögren syndrome
3- Eyes:	Dryness: sjögren syndrome. Redness (uveitis): AS Pallor: anemia from many causes in RA or SLE.
4- Face:	Cheek: Photosensitivity: SLE Red cheeks (butterfly rash): SLE Scaring hyperpigmentation: SLE Parotid gland enlargement: sjögren Telangectasia: scleroderma Mouth: Dryness: sjögren syndrome Ulcer: SLE (painless), inflammatory bowel disease (IBD), Behcet's, RA (from methotrexate use)
4- Chest (Respiratory & Cardiovascular systems):	SOB, chest pain, palpitation: SLE, RA History of PE/DVT: SLE, antiphospholipid antibody syndrome (APS) History of bronchial asthma: Eosinophilic granulomatosis with polyangitis (EGPA) (Churg- Straus)
5- Gastrointestinal tract (GIT):	Ask about all symptoms of GIT! History of jaundice: viral hepatitis. History of recent gastroenteritis or bloody diarrhea: ReA History of IBD: enteropathic arthritis. History of dysphagia: scleroderma History of HBV: vasculitis. History of HCV: chronic HCV can present as RA! Ask about risk factors of HBV, HCV and HIV prior to start any disease modifying antirheumatic drug (DMARDs).
6- Urinary system:	Frothy urine: lupus nephritis. Hematuria: lupus nephritis, anti-glomerular basement membrane disease (Goodpasture).
7- Sexual and obstetric history:	History of recent STD's: ReA. History of oral/genital ulcers: Behcet's disease. History of still birth at any age and/or history of three recurrent abortion: APS
8- Lower Limb:	History of non-palpable purpura, lower limb edema, nodules: vasculitis
9- Ask about Smoking and alcohol intake.	Smoking predisposes to RA, decrease response to DMARDs and biological therapy Adjust alcohol intake in patients recieveing methotrexate Alcohol is a risk factor for gout

Fig. 1.10 Rheumatological review of systems

The common symptoms for some diseases have been complied for you (Figure 1.11**a**, **b**, **c** historic correlation). Some of the questions may not be related to symptomatology! It might just address risk factors. If you are assessing a patient with pain in the first MTP and/or with a red swollen knee joint and you are suspecting gout as a possible diagnosis, then you need to check for risk factors for gout: prior history of uric acid renal stones, alcohol intake and use of diuretics, etc.

Diseases	Certain historical points
1- Patient with suspected SLE	Ask about the following symptoms: - Alopecia (hair loss) - Malar rash - Mouth ulcer - Photosensitivity - Discoid lupus - Raynauds phenomenon - Pleuritic chest pain - Headache - Hematuria - Psychosis, seizures - Vascuilitic rash - Urinary symptoms - Detailed obstetric history
2- Patient with suspected vasculitis	Ask about the following symptoms: - Claudication: Takayasu's arteritis - Fatigue, fever, myalgias, headache, diplopia, jaw claudication: giant cell arteritis - Wight loss, myalgias, peripheral neuropathy (numbness), abdominal pain, livedo retieularis: Polyarteritis nodosa (PAN) - Sinusitis, saddle nose deformity, hemoptysis, chest pain, hematuria, uveitis, history of DVT or PE, granulomatosis with polyangiitis (GPA) (Wegener's) or microscopic polyangiitis (MPA). - History of Asthma, granulomatous vasculitis, eosinophilia: EGPA. - Abdominal pain, palpable purpura, polyarthralgias, microscopic hematuria: IgA vasculitis (IgA V) (Henoch-Schonlein). - Oral/genital ulcer, uveitis, erythema nodosum: Behcet's syndrome. - Weakness: gradual, progressive, painless, symmetrical and proximal. It may involve shoulder, pelvic girdle and neck flexors, but no involvement of facial or ocular muscles! - Dermatologic: erythematous rash on sun exposed skin, heliotrope rash over upper eyelid, Gottron's papules over the dorsum of PIP and MCP joints.
3- Patient with suspected myositis	Ask about: - Myalgia and arthralgia. - Dysphagia and dysphonia. - Raynoud's phenomena. - Symptoms suspected of malignant conditions: weight loss, fatigue, bleeding per rectum, smoking and chronic cough .. etc. - Drugs.
4- Patient with suspected gout	- Pain in 1st MTP (sudden onset), may involve ankles, feet and knees, bursitis (olecranon, patellar). - History of previous attack of gout, chronic tophaciuos gout (deforming arthritis). - Risk factors: uric acid renal stones, history of hyperuricemia, chronic renal disease, myelo & lymphoproliferative diseases, increase meat, seafood and alcohol intake, use of diuretics and pyrazinamide. - Alcohol. - Family history of gout.
5- Patient with suspected Sjögren's syndrome	Ocular: dry eyes Mouth: dry mouth, decrease salivation, drinking fluid while swallowing, difficulties with speech, change in taste and parotid enlargement Ask about the following risk factors: - Head and neck radiation. - AIDS. - HCV. - Lymphoma. - Sarcoidosis. - Anticholenergic drugs. - GVHD (graft versus host disease)
6- Patient with suspected Spondyloarthritis	Ask about the following symptoms: - Red eye (uveitis) - Psoriasis - Recurrent/previous infections: gastroenteritis, STDs, tonsillitis - Dysphagia - IBD - Inflammatory back pain - Lower limb joints pain - Plantar fasciitis/Achilles tendinitis
7- Patient with suspected Septic Arthritis.	Ask about the following symptoms: - Joint pain, - Joint swelling or history of joint edema, - Fever, - Sweating and Rigors (I) - Role out any source of local or disseminated infections by asking about: - Headache - Sore throat - Productive cough - Urinary symptoms, GI symptoms. - History of wound infection or abscess.

Fig. 1.11 Historical correlation

1.4 Physical Examination

This is just to remind you about the particular approach of physical exam techniques that should be performed and then presented (Fig. 1.12). A comprehensive approach to joints examination is presented in Chap. 2.

1.5 How to Present your Case

You are ready now to present your case! You have built an organized approach to history taking from patients with joints pain(s). You have performed a comprehensive physical examination focusing on evaluation of these joints and whether there is true articular process like arthritis or periarticular process like tendinitis (see Chap. 22). Simply you need to present your history and physical examination in the same manner mentioned above with focusing on positive findings and important negatives. After your history and physical examination presentation, it is required from you to sum up all your information together. It is better to start with your impression (summary of the case) and then your problem list and differential diagnosis.

1.5.1 Impression

This (age) who is (known to have (chronic diseases)) presents with:

- History (usually presenting complain).
- Physical exam(mention obvious findings).
- Lab results (mention the important results related to the case) (if it is known to you).

1.5.2 Problem List

In this section you have to make a list with all your patient's problems or complains starting with the most serious and important one. This should guide you to reach the diagnosis easily.

This is a suggested approach on how to write a problem list:

Regarding the first problem:

1. Write your differential diagnosis for this issue and mention which diagnosis is more relevant with your case and why.
2. Write your management plan, if further investigations and/or referral are needed.

Fig. 1.12 Physical examination

Physical Examination	Details
1- General Appearance and Vitals sign	As usual.
2- General Exam	Eyes Scalp Mouth Parotid Neck lymph nodes Skin (redness, thickness) Nails (pitting, periangular erythema)
3- Specific exam for any joint	I- General appearance: Deformity , swelling II- Inspection: Skin: redness, sacrs and rash Ligaments and tendons Muscles Bones III- Screening Exam: Check for range of motion (ROM) IV- Palpation: Effusion, tenderness, warm and crepitus. V- Range of motion: Active and passive. VI- Special tests.
4- Examination of the other systems	CNS, CVS, Chest and Abdominal exam.

See the diagram below for more details (Fig. 1.13).

1.6 Follow-Up Patient

Established patients with rheumatological diseases have frequent visits to outpatient clinics. They come for routine visits for assessing the progress of their disease and review the management plan of their chronic disease. Here are suggested tips for you to help you deal with these patients.

You should ask about:

1. Pain (how he/she is doing since last visit).
2. Which joints are particularly affecting you today?
3. Associated symptoms (morning stiffens (mins), swelling).
4. How well controlled do you feel the arthritis is?
5. What drugs are you taking? Your adherence? Do you get any benefit?
6. Any functional impairment?

   You should not forget to:

7. Do not forget to examine his/her all joints.
8. Do not forget to review all his/her medications.
9. Do not forget to review his/her previous investigations (Fig. 1.14).

1.7 The 2011 ACR/EULAR Definitions of Remission in Rheumatoid Arthritis Clinical Trials

1.7.1 Boolean-Based Definition [2]

At any time point, patient must satisfy all of the following:

- Tender joint count ≤1⁺
- Swollen joint count ≤1⁺
- C-reactive protein ≤1 mg/dl
- Patient global assessment ≤1 (on a 0-10 scale)⁺.

1.7.2 Index-Based Definition

Simplified Disease Activity Index score of ≤3 [3].

Definitions for some of the outcome measures in rheumatology are compiled in Fig. 1.15. Further

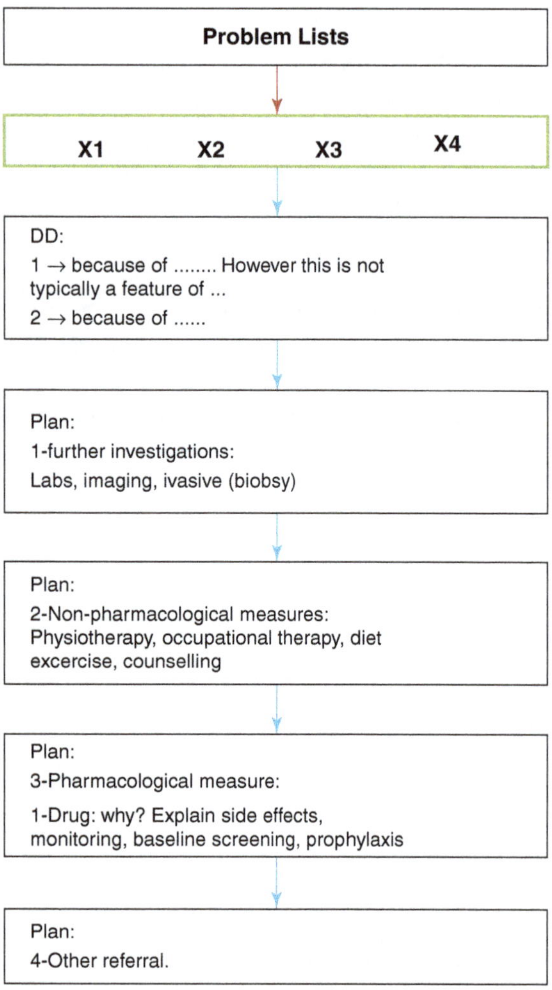

Fig. 1.13 Problem lists

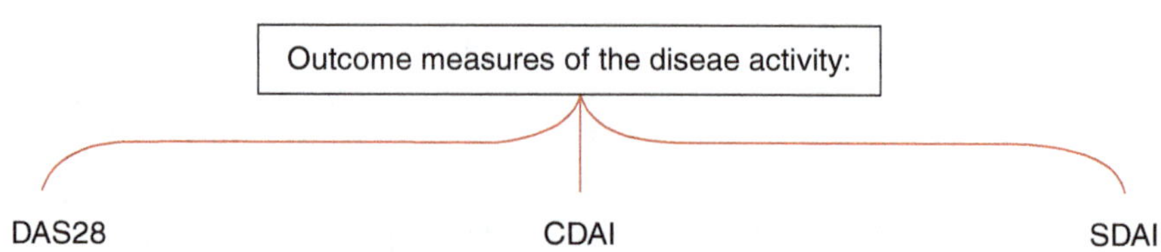

Fig. 1.14 Outcome measures of the disease activity

Outcome measures of the disease activity	Parameters	Interpretation
1-DAS28	a. How many Tender joints? b. How many Swollen joints? c. ESR or CRP level.	1- DAS28 <= 2.6: Remission 2- DAS28 > 2.6 and <= 3.2: Low disease Activity 3- DAS28 > 3.2 and <= 5.1: Moderate Disease Activity 4- DAS28 > 5.1: High Disease Activity
2-CDAI	a. How many Tender joints? b. How many Swollen joints? c. The PGA represents the patient's self-assessment of disease activity (0 to 10 scale) d. The EGA represents the evaluator's assessment of disease activity(0 to 10 scale)	1- CDAI <= 2.8: Remission 2- CDAI > 2.8 and <= 10: Low disease Activity 3- CDAI> 10 and <= 22: Moderate Disease Activity 4- CDAI > 22: High Disease Activity
3-SDAI	a. Tender joint count (using 28 joints) b. Swollen joint count (using 28 joints) c. PGA (0 to 10 scale) d. The EGA (0 to 10 scale) e. CRP level	1- SDAI <= 3.3: 2- SDAI > 3.3 and <= 11: Low Disease Activity 3- SDAI > 11 and <= 26: Moderate Disease Activity 4- SDAI > 26: High Disease Activity

Fig. 1.15 Outcome measures of disease activity in RA and their interpretation

reading is required from you to know more about the implications of its use in the management of patients with RA (Fig. 1.15 outcome measures of disease activity in RA and their interpretations).

Abbreviations

AIDS	Acquired immunodeficiency syndrome
AS	Ankylosing spondylitis
CDAI	Clinical Disease Activity Index
CMC	Carpometacarpal joints
CNS	Central nervous system
CPPD disease	Calcium pyrophosphate dihydrate *disease*
CVS	Cardiovascular system
DAS-28	Disease activity score
DIP	Distal interphalangeal
DVT	Deep venous thrombosis
EGA	Evaluator Global disease Activity
GVHD	Graft vs. host disease
HBV	Hepatitis B virus
HCV	Hepatitis C virus
IBD	Inflammatory bowel disease
JIA	Juvenile idiopathic arthritis
MCP	Metacarpophalangeal joints
MCTD	Mixed connective tissue disease
MTP	Metatarsophalangeal
NSAIDs	Nonsteroidal anti-inflammatory drugs
OA	Osteoarthritis
PAN	Polyarteritis nodosa
PE	Pulmonary embolism
PGA	Patient Global disease Activity
PIP	Proximal interphalangeal
RA	Rheumatoid arthritis
SDAI	Simplified Disease Activity Index
SLE	Systemic lupus erythematosus
STDs	Sexually transmitted diseases

References

1. Margaretten ME, Kohlwes J, Moore D, et al. Does this adult patient have septic arthritis? JAMA. 2007;297:1478–88.
2. Balsa A, Carmona L, González-Alvaro I, et al. Value of disease activity score 28 (DAS28) and DAS28-3 compared to American College of Rheumatology-defined remission in rheumatoid arthritis. J Rheumatol. 2004;31(1):40–6.
3. Aletaha D, Smolen J. The simplified disease activity index and clinical disease activity index to monitor patients in standard clinical care. Rheum Dis Clin N Am. 2009;35:759–72.

2

Epidemiology of MSK Disorders and Competency Skills

Hani Almoallim, Doaa Kalantan, Laila Alharbi, and Khaled Albazli

2.1 Introduction

Musculoskeletal (MSK) symptoms are one of the most common reasons for patients to seek medical attention. Despite the high prevalence of musculoskeletal disorders in all fields of clinical practice, doctors continue to describe poor confidence in their musculoskeletal clinical skills. Here in this chapter an overview of the epidemiology of MSK disorders and the current status of MSK competency skills among clinicians will be discussed. Then a general approach to MSK examination will be introduced. The rest of the chapter will address detailed approach to upper limb and lower and back joints examination. Each section will start with a brief approach to pains originating from each site. Good history is part of the MSK examination.

2.1.1 Objectives

1. To discuss the current status of musculoskeletal (MSK) examination competency skills among clinicians.
2. To construct a diagnostic approach to single joint pain.
3. To demonstrate a comprehensive approach to MSK examination of all body joints.

2.2 Epidemiology of Rheumatic Diseases

MSK symptoms are the most common health complications requiring medical attention and accounting to 20% of both primary care and emergency room visits. MSK conditions affect one in five adults [1]. In a health survey, MSK disorders were ranked first in prevalence as the cause of chronic health problems, long-term disabilities, and consultations with a health professional [2]. In Saudi Arabia, MSK disorders are the second major cause of outpatients visit in primary care centers and private clinics. This is corresponding to findings in several other reports from different parts of the

H. Almoallim (✉)
Professor of Medicine, College of Medicine, Umm Al-Qura University (UQU), Makkah, Saudi Arabia
e-mail: hmmoallim@uqu.edu.sa

D. Kalantan
Al-Noor Specialist Hospital, Makkah, Saudi Arabia

L. Alharbi
College of Medicine, Umm Al Qura University, Makkah, Saudi Arabia

College of Medicine, Skåne University Hospital, Malmoe, Sweden

K. Albazli
Department of Medicine, Faculty of Medicine in Al- Qunfudhah, AlUmm Al-Qura University, Makkah, Saudi Arabia

The George Washington University School of Medicine and Health Sciences, Washington, D.C., USA

world. Low back pain is the most prevalent of musculoskeletal conditions; it affects nearly everyone at some point in time and about 4–33% of the population at any given point [2].

MSK disorders are a very common cause of health problems. They result in limiting work in developed countries. Besides, up to 60% of people on early retirement or long-term sick leave claim a MSK problem as the reason [1].

2.3 Current Status of MSK Examination

A continuous neglect is observed in musculoskeletal examination skills in clinical practice. Thus problems of patients with complaints about bones and joints are often ignored and underestimated by doctors. Many studies suggest that training in MSK disorders is inadequate in both medical schools and most residency training programs. In Saudi Arabia and in many parts of the world, undergraduate and postgraduate medical teaching of MSK disorders is currently brief and not directly relevant to the knowledge and skills commonly required for management of these conditions in an outpatient setting [1, 3]. Educational deficiencies in MSK disorders have been reported extensively in undergraduate curricula and postgraduate training programs (Box 2.1) [3].

Box 2.1 Educational deficiencies in MSK examination skills

Causes of musculoskeletal (MSK) examination skills deficiencies [2]	Solution of MSK examination deficiency [2]
1. Vague training of MSK disorders in undergraduate programs. 2. Examination of the MSK system is often regarded to be complex in comparison with other organ systems. 3. Underestimation of the prevalence of MSK conditions and their impact on individuals and society. 4. MSK disorders are not considered to be main competencies of medical graduates because they are not life threatening conditions. 5. The lack of standardized approach to the clinical assessment of MSK problems, whether pertaining to primary care, rheumatology, or orthopedics. 6. Lack of proper standard teaching in MSK disorders results in the low competence in MSK examination skills. 7. Lack of summative evaluation of MSK examination skills contributes to low level of competency among medical graduates. 8. The disparity in the approach to examination between rheumatologists and orthopaedic surgeons mostly lead to poor performances in MSK examinations. 9. The lack of appropriate teaching and evaluation in MSK disorders; clinical teachers are not usually skilled in MSK examinations and thus bone and joint diseases are not screened.	1. To define competencies that should be mastered while dealing with MSK disorders. 2. To agree on what MSK skills should be mastered by medical students. 3. Standardized approach to the clinical assessment of MSK problems (Figs. 2.1 and 2.2). 4. Experts in various specialities work more closely together and look for the commonality of approach when treating a patient as they often treat the same patients but from separate angles. 5. Another solution would be an integrated MSK disease course for medical students, bringing together orthopedics, rheumatology, and physical medicine and rehabilitation. This approach has been found to be effective. 6. The method of teaching MSK examination skills should follow interactive approaches and hands-on teaching sessions where learners are involved in the teaching process.

As there is no standardized approach to the clinical assessment of MSK problems, one of the direct solutions for this is to have unified approach to MSK disorders. The approach should consist of screening examination (this is basically active range of motion testing (ROM)), inspection, palpation, ROM, and special tests (see below). The other direct solution is to have a clear objective from each MSK examination encounter based on historical facts obtained from patients. Each clinician should have then an objective for the MSK examination, whether signs of arthritis to be sought or signs of periarthritis with soft tissue inflammation (ligaments, tendons, bursae, cartilage, etc.). For example, a young female patient with small joints pain for 6 weeks should have a different objective for the MSK examination than a young male with knee joint pain following a football match. The objective for the MSK examination for the female patient with small joints pain should be to look for signs of arthritis, while the objective for the MSK examination of the male patient is to look for signs of periarthritis mainly ligamentous or meniscus injuries in his knee. This is not to underestimate the comprehensive approach to any joint with performing all steps (screening, inspection, palpation, ROM, special tests) but rather to get more focus on the techniques that should yield the signs suggestive of the preliminary diagnosis that was made initially based on the history obtained from the patient.

A number of different medical specialties are usually involved in treating patients with musculoskeletal complaints. This comprises general practitioners, family physicians, internists, orthopedic, and surgeons. However, the various practitioners may work in teams with other health professionals, but they often lack a multispecialty focus which results in treating the same patients in a segmented manner and from different inconsistent angles.

Based on a literature review published with details in reference [2], Box 2.1 shows some summarized causes of MSK examination skills deficiencies. Some suggested solutions were mentioned as well. One of these solutions is to have a standardized approach to MSK examination (see examination of the hand and wrist joints) (see Table 2.1.)

2.4 General Approach to MSK Examination

Clinicians have perceived the MSK examination across the world as complex and difficult to perform. This can be solved if the approach to MSK examination across different disciplines were unified. This approach starts by initiating the MSK examination using the following steps:

- Inspection: The basic anatomical structures overlying joints should be inspected for any changes. This includes inspection of the skin, tendons, muscles, and bones (joints). Skin changes like redness, rashes, and color changes should be noted. Loss of skin wrinkling may indicate swelling in underneath structures. Synovial sheaths covering tendons might be swollen. Muscles might be wasted. Bone and/or deformities might be obvious to observe.
- Screening exam: this is basically an active range of motion (ROM) testing to assess for gross pathology. The patient performs the full range of movement of the examined joint by own effort. If the active ROM was entirely normal without any limitation and/or pain, the joint examined can be considered normal. This step is introduced early on in this approach in order to focus the detailed MSK exam in joints with significant abnormal active ROM testing. The screening exam might be normal for arthritis affecting small joints of the hand and/or feet particularly in early stages of arthritis.
- Palpation: this is basically palpating for tenderness over different anatomical structures (bone, joint, tendons, bursae, fascia). Tenderness over the joint line (where two bones forming the joint are meeting) might indicate arthritis. There are special approaches to palpate small and large joints that will be explained in this chapter. Palpation for one of

the cardinal signs of inflammation, hotness (warmth), should be considered as well.

- Range of motion testing: there is active and passive ROM testing. If you have done the active ROM during the screening exam, you may now just perform the passive form or repeat it again. In cases of true intra-articular disease process (true inflammation of synovial membrane as in case of inflammatory arthritic disorders, for example, rheumatoid arthritis or psoriatic arthritis), the active and the passive ROM will be both restricted. While in cases of periarticular disease processes (affecting tendons, ligaments, bursae, fascia) the active ROM will be restricted and/or limited with tenderness, the passive ROM should be entirely normal. It is normal because you exclude the contribution of the affected tendon or ligament in the movement by doing it passively. However, there are exceptions to this general rule. Handling of the joints during MSK examination is essential. You should avoid assessing ROM while you are holding the joint itself. You should hold the assessed joint from distal and proximal areas trying also to hold other joints. You should mainly assess the ROM by holding bony structures forming the joint rather than the joint itself. This is not to cause pain over the joints from your holding. An issue might interfere with your ability to evaluate the origin of the pain; whether from the ROM or from your holding that causes stress over the joint results in pain.
- Special tests: these tests are conducted to examine for possible causes of the joint pain particularly soft tissue structures around the joint. As a general rule to examine for tendon- and/or ligament-related problems, you need to "stretch" the tendon to assess if this stretch can aggravate the symptoms and/or to "stress" it. If the function of tendon that you are assessing is extension, for example, to stress it you need to exert your force as an examiner in flexion while the patient is maintaining his joint in extension and resisting your flexion. If there is tenderness while performing this test, it might be due to tendinitis.
- Complete your exam: the MSK exam for any particular joint is not complete without evaluating other joints (above and below the joint being examined). In addition, a neurovascular evaluation is essential to exclude any possibility of neurological and/or vascular origins of the joint pain. Assessing peripheral pulses, examining the motor system, and evaluating for sensory loss are essential for comprehensive evaluation.

There are two important steps that should be addressed for any patient with joints pain. The first is determining in your history the location of the pain whether it is anterior, posterior, lateral, or medial pain. This could be achieved by simply asking the patient to point by his/her finger to the site that is causing pain at the joint. Each one of these sites has its differential diagnosis as a cause for pain. This should lead to the next step that is considering the anatomical structures at the site of the pain determined by the patient. You should continue taking your comprehensive history addressing the risk factors and trying to rule in or rule out the possible differential diagnosis you created by now from these steps.

After completing your history, you should determine now the objective of your MSK examination. Examining a young female who presents with small joints pains should have different objective than examining a young college student who presents with knee joint pain after a soccer game! For the young female patient, your objective should be looking for signs of arthritis: small joints pain swelling and/or tenderness. You may base on your history to look for signs of systemic lupus erythematosus, for example. While the objective of MSK examination for the college student should be to look primarily for signs of soft tissue injuries in his affected knee. This is not to underestimate the value of performing comprehensive MSK examination for the affected joint. It is rather a process to construct an approach to diagnosis utilizing historical findings and combining it with an objective-oriented MSK examination.

The following section is divided into three: the upper limb, the lower limb, and the back examination. Each section starts with a brief review of the anatomy and then a description on the approach to pain origination from that particular joint. This is followed by a stepwise approach to examination of that joint using the inspection, screening exam, palpation, ROM, and special tests approach. The reader should realize the importance of applying the knowledge learned from this chapter into practice. This continued practice is the assuring way to the mastery level in competency skills in MSK examination.

2.5 Musculoskeletal Examination of Upper Limb Joints (Fig. 2.1)

The joints included in upper limb are hand and wrist, elbow, and shoulder. There is a brief review of the important anatomical landmarks that should be mastered because it has clinical correlations. This will be referred to as the first step. Then an approach to pain originating from this joint will be discussed focusing on anatomical differential diagnosis. The second step will be to follow the stated approach in MSK examination with descriptions whenever it is necessary. Illustrations have been used sometimes as a self-explanatory toll.

2.5.1 The Hand and Wrist Joints

2.5.1.1 First Step: The Anatomy

Anatomy of the Hand Joints (Fig. 2.1)
Each hand consists of 27 bones: 8 carpals, 5 *metacarpals*, and each finger having three phalanges except the thumb which has only two phalanges (Fig. 2.1). The joint is the articulation between two bones, so between the two phalanges there is interphalangeal joints, proximal (PIP) and distal (DIP); between the phalanges and metacarpal bones, metacarpophalangeal joint (MCP); between the metacarpals and carpal bones, carpometacarpal joint (CMC); and between the carpals bones, the intercarpal joints.

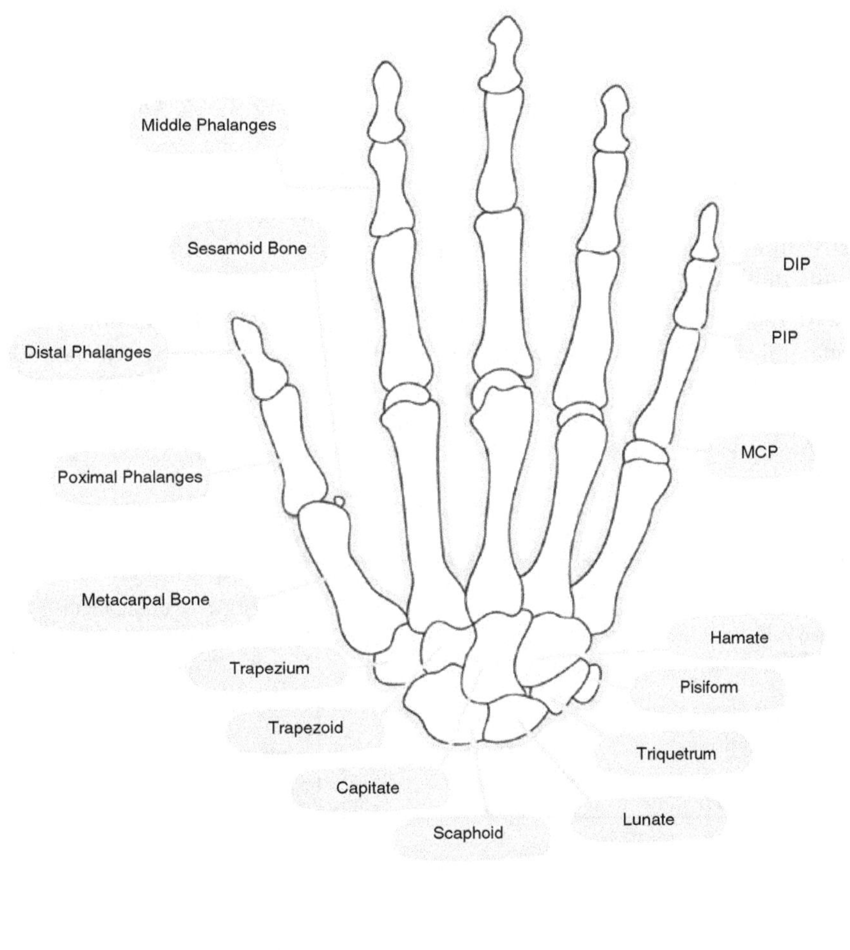

Fig. 2.1 Anatomy of the hand

There are around 62 muscles in the hand divided as intrinsic and extrinsic muscles. The intrinsic muscles are thenar, hypothenar, and interosseous muscles. The extrinsic muscles are flexors in the volar of the hand and extensors in the dorsum of the hand. There is also the synovial sheath, which is always involved in inflammatory arthritis.
The hand is innervated by three important nerves, which are radial nerve providing sensory supply to the dorsum of the hand, median nerve providing sensory supplies to three, and half finger and ulnar nerve sensory supplying the little finger and half of ring finger. All the small muscles of the hands are supplied by ulnar nerve except (LOAF) the lateral two lumbricals, opponens pollicis, the abductor pollicis brevis, and the flexor pollicis brevis. Be aware that the extensors of the thumb are supplied by radial nerve.

Approach to Hand Pain

The approach of any patient presenting with hand pain should include:

- History.
- Physical examination.
- Differential diagnosis.

In the history, you should ask about the location of the pain whether it is located in the dorsal, volar, radial, or ulnar sides of the hand (Table 2.1). Then you should think about the anatomical structures in each one of these sites and what possible diseases might cause the pain.

If the patient presents with dorsal pains, the anatomical structures that might be included are MCPs, PIPs, DIP joints, or wrist joint. The diseases that affect these joints are mainly arthritic disorders. Detailed approach to history taking should be undertaken as it was explained in Chap. 1. Tendons can be involved which result in tendinitis or, if the entire finger is swollen, dactylitis.

The anatomical structures included in patients presenting with volar pains are flexor tendons causing flexor tenosynovitis or what is known as trigger finger. Palmar fascia involvement results in Dupuytren's contracture. Median nerve compression as it passes below the flexor retinaculum causes a condition called carpal tunnel syndrome.

If the patient presents with radial pain (the thumb), the anatomical structure are snuffbox area. This is surrounded laterally by tendons of extensor pollicis brevis and abductor pollicis longus muscles, medially by tendon of extensor pollicis longus muscle and in the roof the scaphoid bone. The classical diseases affecting this area are de Quervain's tenosynovitis and first carpometacarpal osteoarthritis. Other diseases like thumb fracture and extensor carpi radials tendinitis are less commonly observed.

Ulnar pain is rare. Possible diseases affecting this site of the hand could be originated from ulnar nerve compression, tenosynovitis of flexor carpi ulnaris, and/or traumatic injuries.

2.5.1.2 Second Step: The Approach

It is always:
- Inspection.
- Screening exam.
- Palpation.
- Range of motion.
- Special tests.

Table 2.1 The differential diagnosis of wrist and hand pain according to the location of the pain

Dorsal	Volar	Ulnar	Radial
Arthritis • Wrist • MCP • PIP • DIP • Tendinitis – Dactylitis Trauma: – Scaphoid fracture	• Carpal tunnel syndrome • Dupuytren's disease • Trigger finger • Arthritis	• Trauma • Ulnar nerve entrapment • Tenosynovitis: Flexor carpi ulnaris	• Anatomical snuff box: – De Quervain's tenosynovitis – First carpometacarpal osteoarthritis • Tenosynovitis of extensor carpi radialis • Trauma: Thumb fracture

Inspection

Nails: evidence of psoriasis, vasculitis.
Skin: redness, scars, rashes.
Muscles: wasting, atrophy.
Bones and joints: swelling, deformities.

> Remember:
> - Always inspect dorsal and palmar aspects.
> - Start distally to proximally.

Screening Exam

The aim is to screen for gross pathology.

- It is basically active ROM testing.
- First, extend fingers and wrist (palmar aspect upward). Make a fist, and then extend again. Make a tuck position, and then extend again. Make a prayer sign and then wrist flexion with all fingers facing the ground opposite of the prayer sign. Lastly, assess grip strength (Fig. 2.2).

Palpation

The major aim is to look for evidence of arthritis in the form of warmth, effusion, and joint line tenderness.

Palpate: joints, bone, and soft tissue.

Start with dorsum of the hand for nodules; palpate MCPs with a scissor technique and PIPs and DIPs with four fingers technique, follow the third metacarpal bone to feel capitate and the joint line of the wrist; and then feel scaphoid in the anatomical snuff box and other bones for tenderness.

Make a scissor-like shape with your fingers, joining the index and middle fingers together and joining the ring and little finger together. Hold the patients hand from the sides at MCPs level. Flex the MCPs to 90° and with your two free thumbs from both hands, feel the joint line for every MCP joint to assess for effusion, swelling, and/or tenderness (Fig. 2.3) [3].

This technique is called four fingers because you should use your four fingers which are the thumb and index finger of each hand (Fig. 2.4). With your thumb and index fingers of one hand, hold each PIP from the side and press firmly. With your other hand's thumb and index fingers, hold the same PIP joint from an anteroposterior direction and push intermittently in and out, looking for effusion, swelling, and/or tenderness [3].

With your thumb, follow the third metacarpal bone on the dorsal aspect of the hand until reaching a dimple at the capitate level (Fig. 2.5). Your thumb should exert a firm, continuous pressure on this point with your other thumb pushing intermittently in and out, just half an inch away from the other thumb on the wrist joint line, looking for effusion, swelling, and/or tenderness [3].

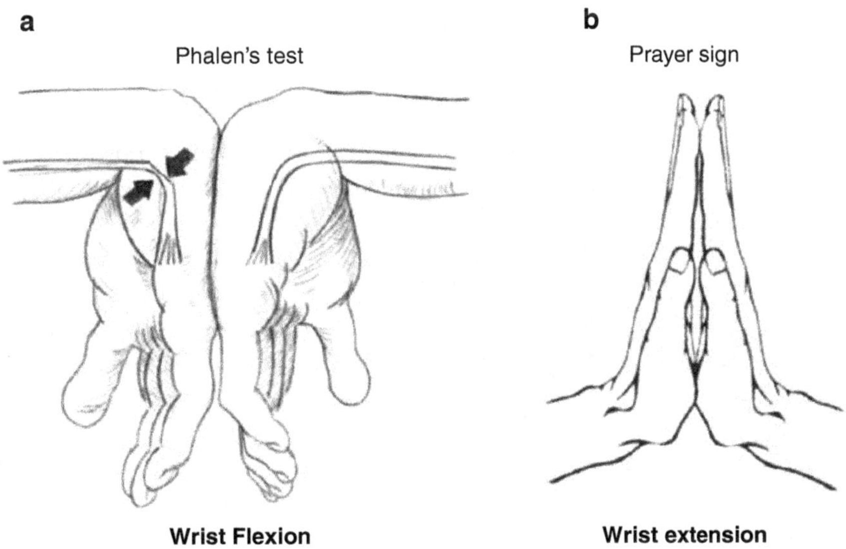

Fig. 2.2 (**a**) Wrist flexion and (**b**) wrist extension

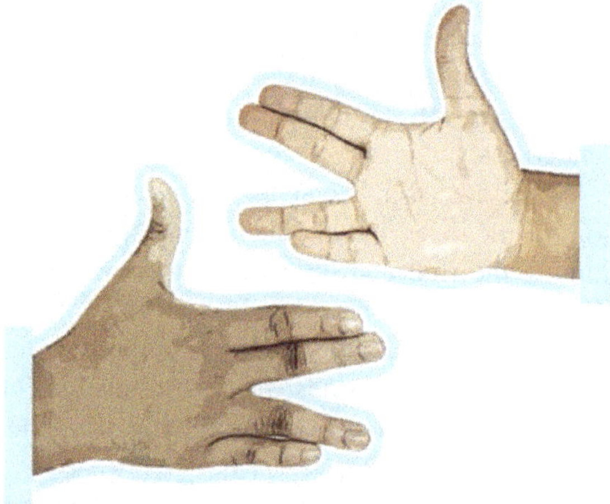

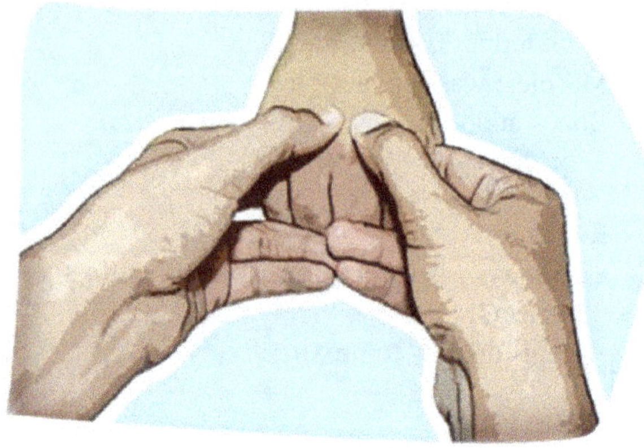

Fig. 2.3 Scissor technique

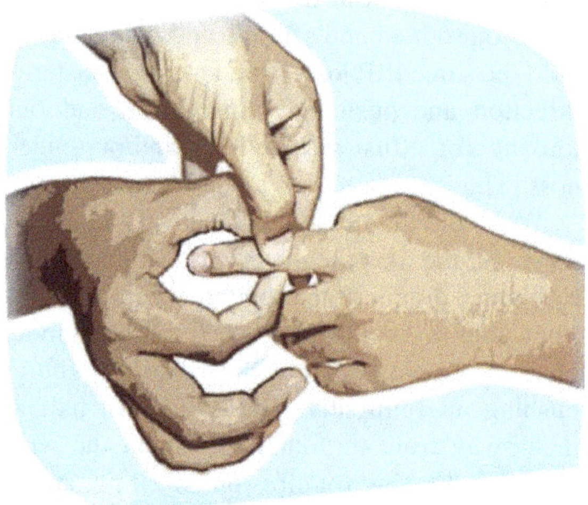

Fig. 2.4 Four fingers technique

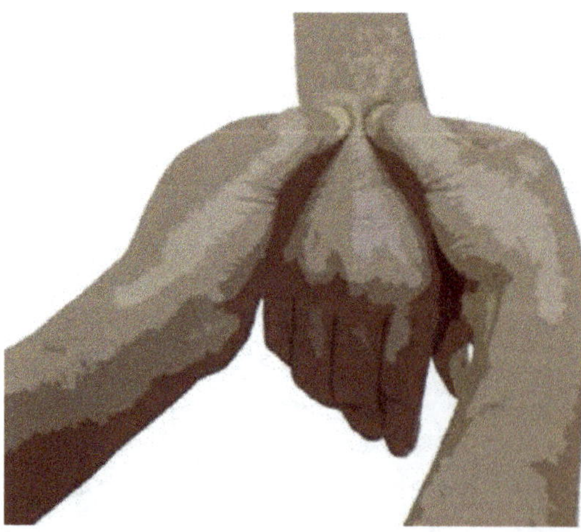

Fig. 2.5 Two thumbs technique

Range of motion

- You have done active ROM in your screening exam.
- Do it again for the wrist joint: extension, flexion, ulnar deviation, and radial deviation.
- For passive ROM of the wrist: hold the distal forearm with one hand, and grasp the palmar aspect with the other hand. Avoid holding the hand from the MCP site as this might be painful if there is arthritis.
- Now move the wrist passively to extension, flexion, ulnar deviation, and radial deviation.

You should observe and comment on tenderness, stiffness, and/or limitation of movement and end-range stiffness. All these are expected signs of arthritis.

Special tests

- This is to assess stability of the wrist joint. This is important particularly in pain in wrist joint following traumatic injuries.
- For de Quervain's tenosynovitis: do Finkelstein's test (Fig. 2.6). This is simply a trial to overstretch the tendon and examine for tenderness if it is elicited with this technique to suggest the diagnosis. To stress the tendon, push the extended thumb to flexion and ask the patient to resist your flexion. If there is pain, this would confirm the diagnosis.
- Carpal tunnel syndrome is reviewed thoroughly in "Diabetes and Rheumatology" Chap. 21.

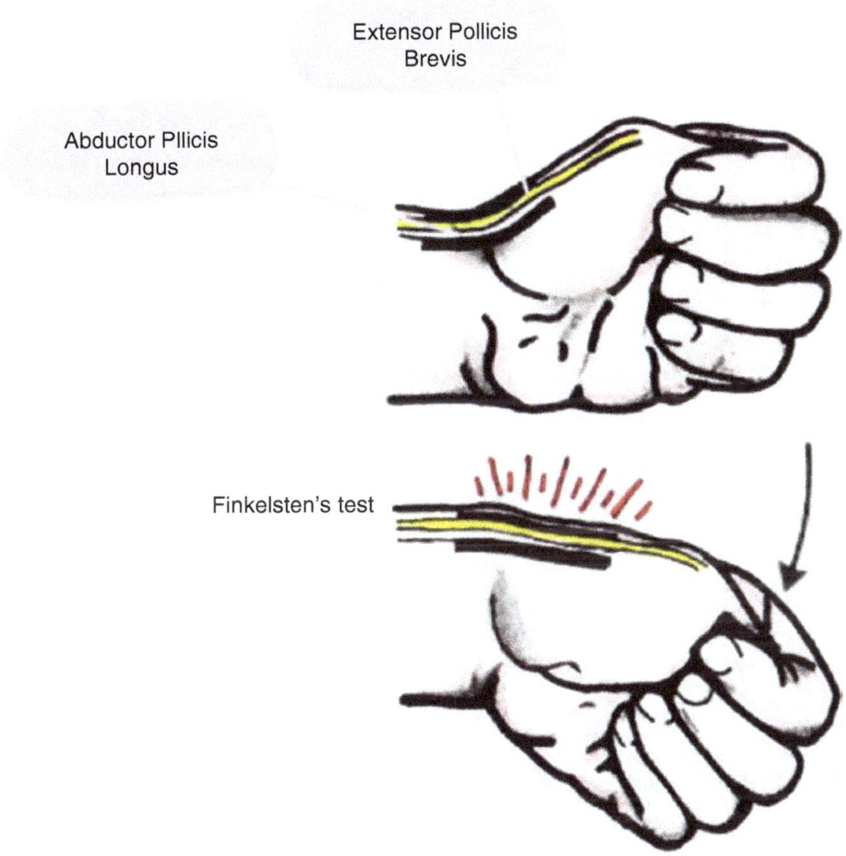

Fig. 2.6 Finkelstein's test

2.5.2 The Elbow Joint

2.5.2.1 First Step: The Anatomy (Figs. 2.7 and 2.8)

The elbow joint is composed of three bones, which articulate together to form three joints, three ligaments, and muscles. The bones that form the joints are the distal part of the humerus, the proximal part of the radius, and the ulna laterally and medially. They articulate together to form three joints, the humeroulnar joint, the radiohumeral joint, and the proximal radioulnar joint. These joints are held together through a network of ligaments; the major three ligaments are the medial collateral ligament, the lateral collateral ligament, and the annular ligament. What makes the elbow flex, extend, supinate, and pronate are the muscles of the elbow joint, such as the biceps muscles and its tendon, the triceps muscles, the brachioradialis, the flexor forearm muscles attached to medial epicondyle, and the extensor forearm muscles attached to lateral epicondyle. Branches from median, ulnar, musculocutaneous, and radial nerves supply this joint.

Approach to Elbow Pain

The approach to any patient presents with elbow pain should include:

- History.
- Physical examination.
- Differential diagnosis.

In the history you should determine the location of the pain by simply asking the patient to point to the tender spot in his elbow. Lateral elbow pain is the most common site for clinical presentation. Other sites are medical and posterior elbow pains. After determining the site, then a simple standard approach should be followed including the onset of the pain, its duration, severity, radiation, aggravating and reliving factors, and history of trauma. The occupation of the patient as well as detailed history of sports activities is essential to obtain.

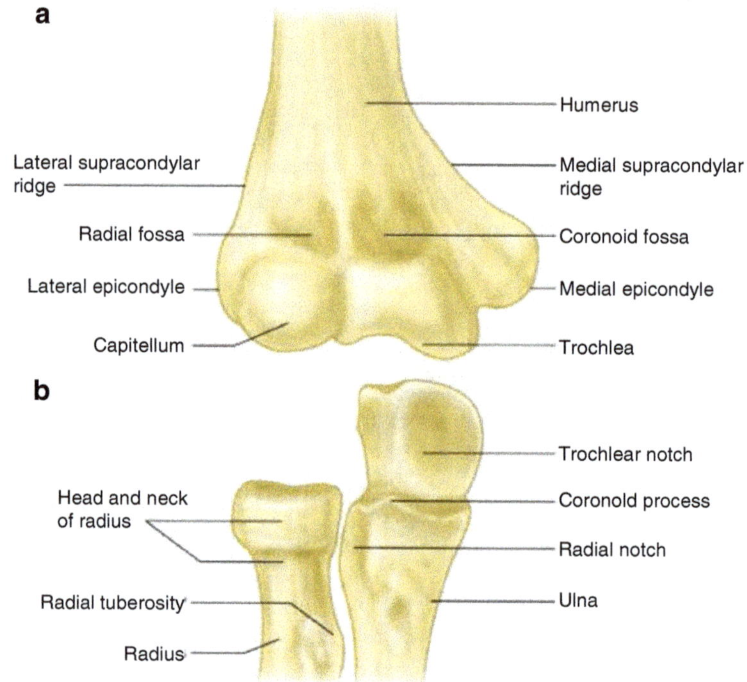

Fig. 2.7 Elbow Joint anatomy: bones

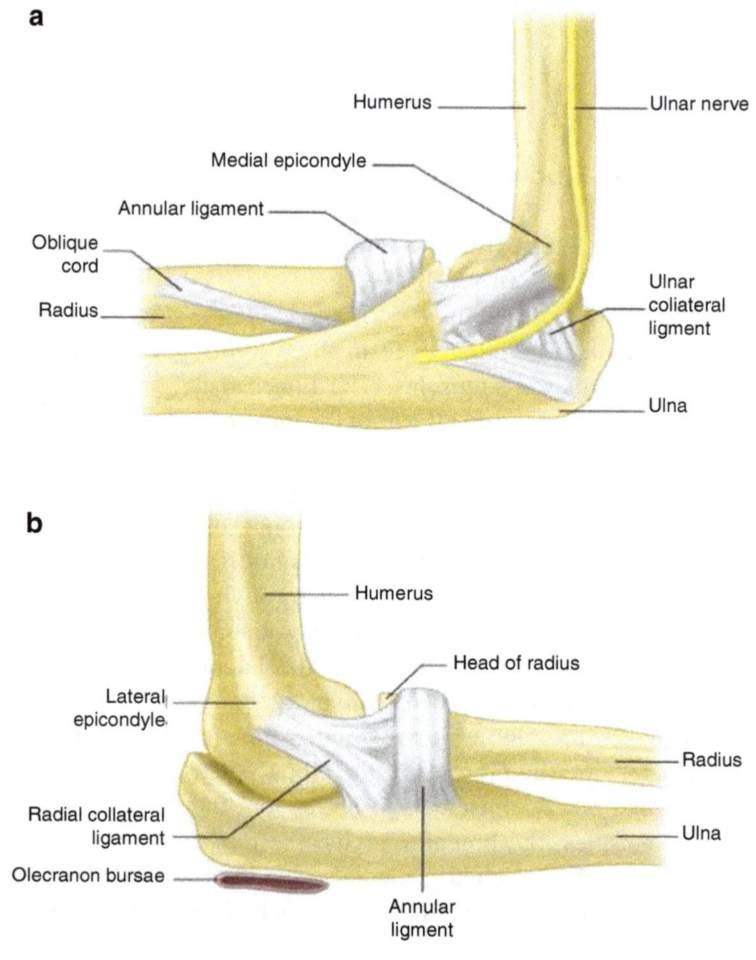

Fig. 2.8 Elbow Joint anatomy: nerves and ligaments

Box 2.2 Differential Diagnosis of Elbow Pain

Lateral elbow pain
Common: 1. Lateral epicondylitis 2. Referred pain (cervical, upper thoracic spine)
Less common: 1. Synovitis 2. Radiohumeral bursitis 3. Radial tunnel syndrome (posterior interosseous nerve entrapment)
Not to be missed: 1. Osteochondritis dissecans.
Medial elbow pain
Common: 1. Medial epicondylitis 2. Medial collateral ligament sprain
Less common: 1. Ulnar neuritis 2. In children: Avulsion fracture of the medial epicondyle
Not to be missed: 1. Referred pain
Posterior elbow pain
1. Olecranon bursitis 2. Triceps tendinopathy 3. Posterior impingement

Repetitive minor trauma from overuse might precipitate epicondylitis with micro tears affecting the common tendon insertion. You may ask also about functional limitation, swelling, and/or instability of the joint. A swollen elbow should lose its ability to be fully extended. History of shoulder and/or neck pain should be obtained as pain in the elbow may be simply a referred one from these sites.

Differential Diagnosis

Depends on the location of pain (Box 2.2).

2.5.2.2 Second Step: The Approach

It is always:

- Inspection.
- Screening exam.
- Palpation.
- Range of motion.
- Special tests.

Inspection

Examine both elbows for asymmetry

Expose the upper arm completely and examine:

- Skin: rashes, abrasions, erythema, redness, scars, subcutaneous nodule, subcutaneous psoriasis.
- Muscle: wasting, atrophy.
- Bones and joints:
  - Swelling: localize over olecranon bursae, e.g., olecranon bursitis or diffuse particularly in area between olecranon process and lateral or medial epicondyle, e.g., elbow arthritis.
  - Deformity: assess the carrying angle (Fig. 2.9):

Ask patient to extend arm in anatomical position (palm facing anteriorly), the longitudinal axes of upper arm and forearm from a lateral (valgus) angle at elbow joint known as the carrying angle (5°in male, 10°–15° in female).

Screening Exam

- The aim is to screen for gross pathology.
- It is basically active ROM testing (Fig. 2.10).
- A quick way to evaluate this is to ask patient to comb the hair and watch any abnormal moment.
- Ask patient to do:
  - Extension.
  - Flexion.
  - Supination.
  - Pronation.

Palpation

Should include palpation of:

- Skin and soft tissue: muscles, ligaments, tendons, and epitrochlear lymph nodes. This lymph node is located just 1 cm above medical epicondyle in the antecubital fossa and then 1 cm distally on the shaft of the ulna. It is hard to feel in obese patients.
- Bony landmarks that should be palpated:
  - Medial epicondyle: any tenderness suggestive of medical epicondylitis.
  - Medial epicondylar ridge: any tenderness suggestive of elbow joint arthritis?

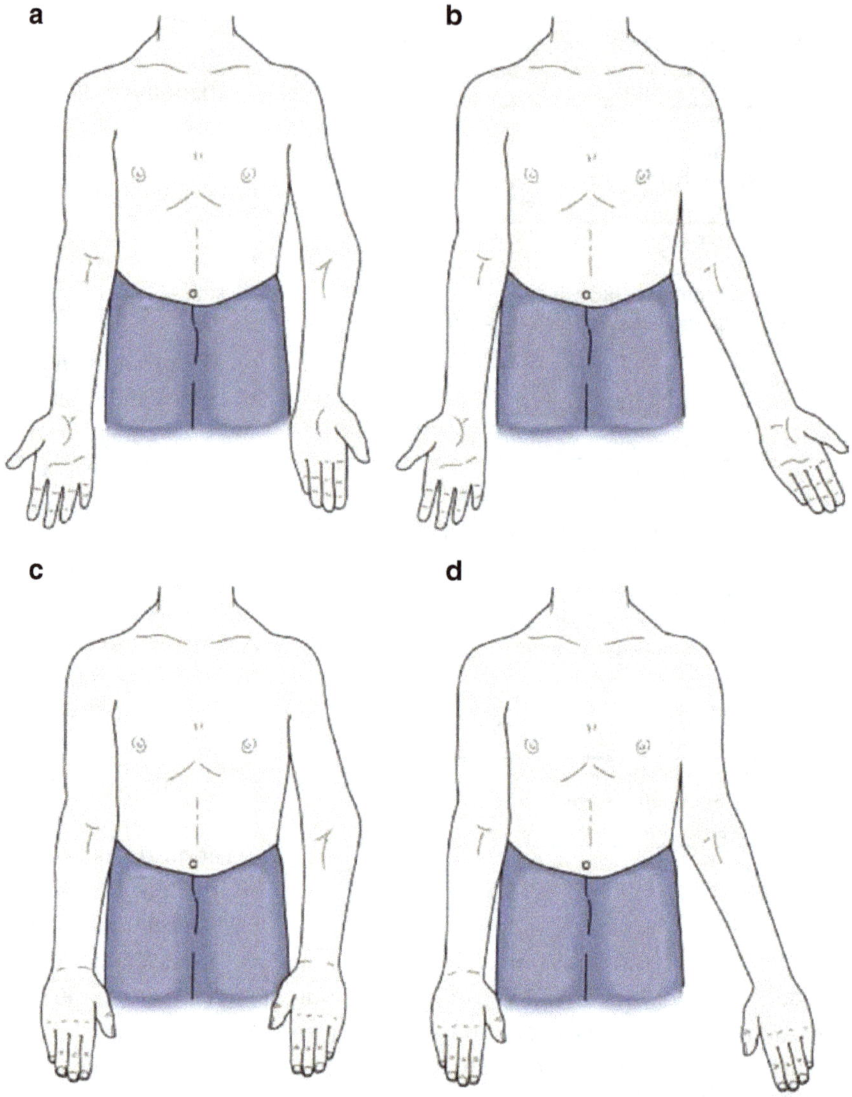

Fig. 2.9 Abnormality in carrying angle: (**b**, **d**) Cubitus valgus. (**a**, **c**) Cubitus varus (gunstock deformity). Effect of swelling: it holds the joint in partial flexion [4]

 - Lateral epicondyle: any tenderness suggestive of lateral epicondylitis?
 - Lateral epicondylar ridge: any tenderness.
 - Olecranon process: any tenderness suggestive of olecranon bursitis?
 - Superficial surface of the ulna (as far distal as the wrist).
 - Radial head.
- Elbow joint line: palpate for tenderness, effusion, and/or nodules.

> Ulnar nerve: runs in capital groove behind the medial epicondyle.

Start by palpating the posterior aspect: the three palpation landmarks (the medial epicondyle, the lateral epicondyle, and the apex of the olecranon) form an equilateral triangle when the elbow is flexed 90° and a straight line when the elbow is in extension. The points between the olecranon process while the elbow is in 90° of flexion and the medical or lateral epicondyle represent the joint line of the elbow joint (Fig. 2.11). If there is tenderness elicited while palpating these points, it indicates elbow joint arthritis. Otherwise, effusion may be elicited by palpation.

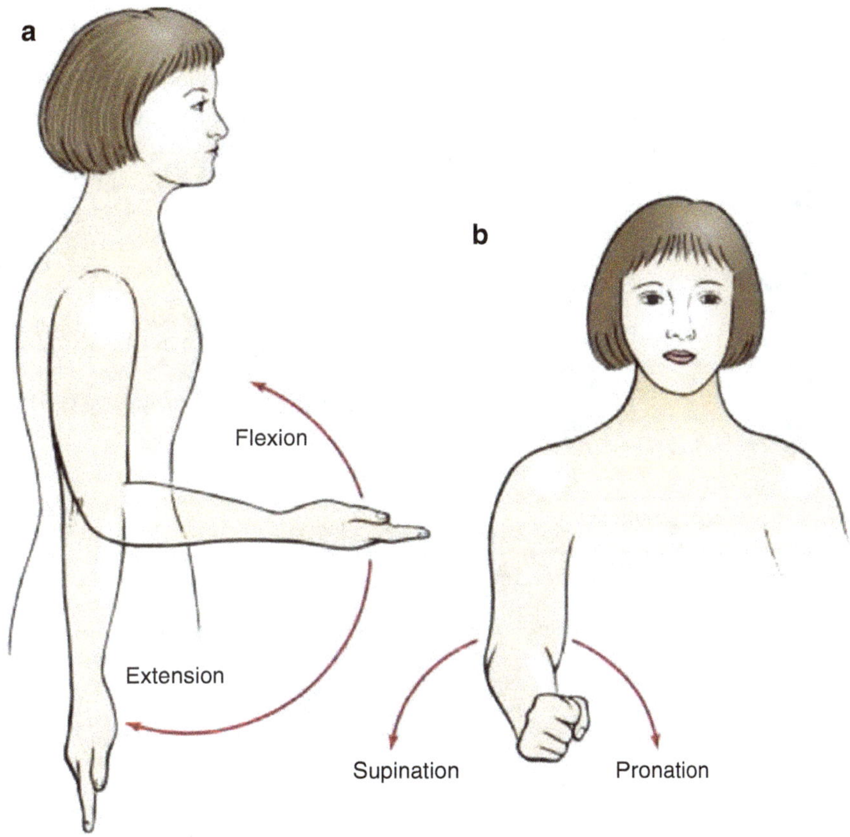

Fig. 2.10 Active range of motion of the elbow joint

Range of Motion

- You have done active ROM in your screening exam.
- Place one of your examining hands just above the elbow joint holding the distal end of the arm. The other hand should be holding the distal end of the forearm just few centimeters above the wrist joint. Examine passive range of motion for the following actions:
  - Flexion: bend the patient's elbow slowly by bringing both of your hands together.
  - Extension: move your hands away from each other to extend the patients elbow. Note that some patients particularly females may have hyperextensible joints that may cause few extra-degrees of elbow hyperextension.
  - Supination: with the hand holding the distal forearm, bring the palm of the patient to let it face upward.
  - Pronation: now let the palm face downward.

Presence of tenderness, limitation, stiffness, and/or end of range stiffness may indicate presence of arthritis.

Special Tests

Golfer's Elbow Test

This is to test for medial epicondylitis.

Ask the patient to have their elbow and fingers flexed. Palpate the medial epicondyle with one hand, and grasp the patient's wrist with the other hand, and then ask the patient to flex the elbow and wrist against resistance (Fig. 2.12). A positive test would be a complaint of pain or discomfort along the medial aspect of the elbow in the region of the medial epicondyle.

Tennis Elbow Test

This is to test for lateral epicondylitis.

Ask the patient to have their elbow and fingers extended. Palpate the lateral epicondyle with one hand, and grasp the patient's wrist with the other hand, and then ask the patient to

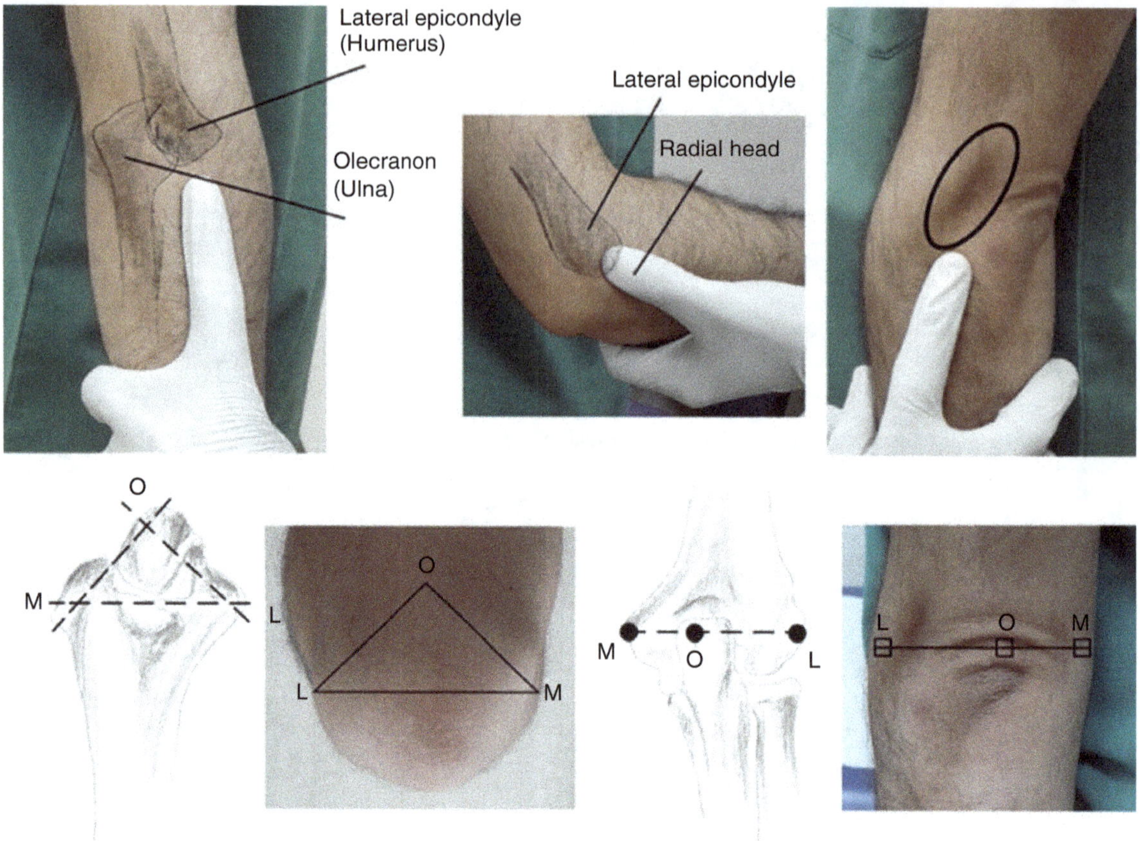

Fig. 2.11 Some anatomical landmarks in the elbow joint. O: olecranon process, M: medial epicondyle, L: lateral epicondyle

extend the elbow and wrist against resistance (Fig. 2.13). A positive test would be a complaint of pain or discomfort along the lateral aspect of the elbow in the region of the lateral epicondyle.

Elbow Flexion Test (Ulnar Nerve)

This test is to evaluate for cubital tunnel syndrome (Fig. 2.14).

Ask the patient to hold their elbows fully flexed for 3 min with their wrists in neutral position and their shoulders adducted at their sides. The test is considered to be positive if paresthesias were elicited within the ulnar nerve distribution of the hand.

2.5.3 The Shoulder Joint

2.5.3.1 First Step: The Anatomy (Fig. 2.15)

The shoulder consists of three bones, four articular surfaces, muscles, and ligaments. The bones include clavicle, proximal humerus, and scapula. The articular surfaces include sternoclavicular joint, acromioclavicular joint, gleno-

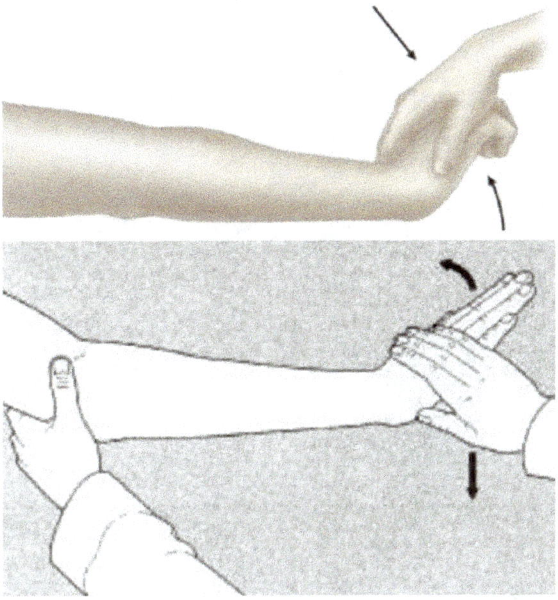

Fig. 2.12 A special test for medial epicondylitis

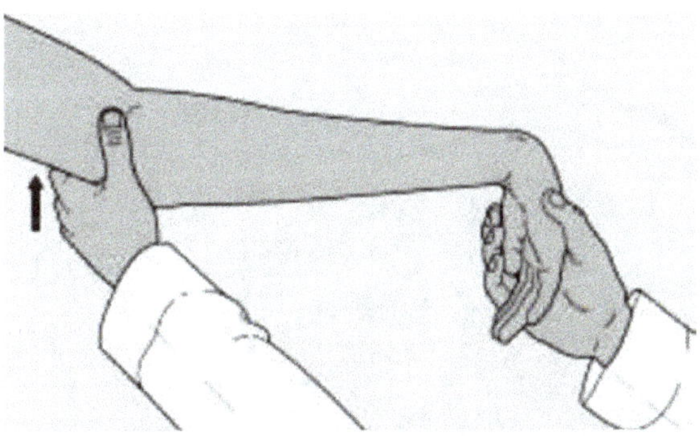

Fig. 2.13 A special test for lateral epicondylitis: see text

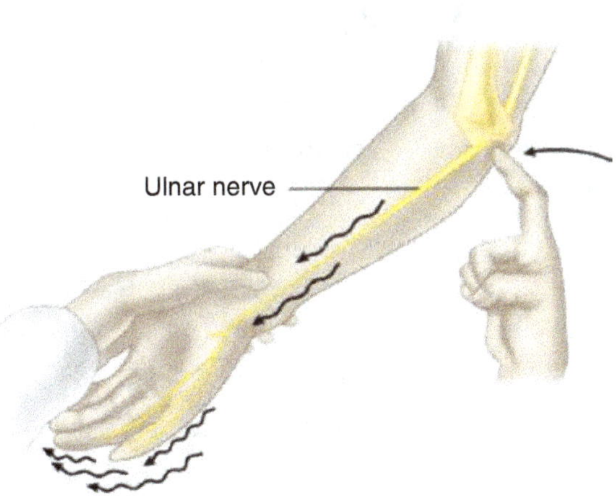

Fig. 2.14 Elbow flexion test

humeral joint, and scapulothoracic articulation. The muscles of shoulder are rotator cuff which includes supraspinatus, infraspinatus, subscapularis, and teres minor. The subscapularis muscle rotates the humerus internally, while the infraspinatus and teres minor rotate the humerus externally. Abduction of the humerus is accomplished by supraspinatus along with deltoid muscle.

For the ligaments of the shoulder, they are the glenohumeral ligaments which are superior, middle, and inferior glenohumeral ligaments.

Approach to Shoulder Pain

Shoulder pain represents either intrinsic or extrinsic pathologies. Intrinsic pathologies account for 85% of the cases and include traumatic, acute, and chronic causes. While extrinsic pathologies account only for 15% of the cases which represent referred pain that can be of cardiac, respiratory, gastric, or diaphragmatic in origin. The approach to patients present with shoulder pain should always start with:

- History.
- Physical examination.
- Differential diagnosis.

Start analysis of the shoulder pain by first determining the site of the pain. To assure accurate workup you may ask the patient to point one finger to the site of the pain by one finger. Shoulder pain can be classified into three categories according to the site: anterior, lateral, or posterior (Table 2.2).

Lateral shoulder pain is the most common, and it is classical for rotator cuff tendinitis. Anterior shoulder pain is classical for glenohumeral arthritis. Posterior shoulder pain, which is the least common, usually represents referred pain.

Following this step you need to cover other aspects of pain history to help you narrow the differential diagnosis according to the anatomical location and other important pieces of information you are going to collect from the patient. This should include the duration, nature, aggravating factors (with lifting, reaching or pushing) and

Fig. 2.15 Anatomy of the shoulder joint

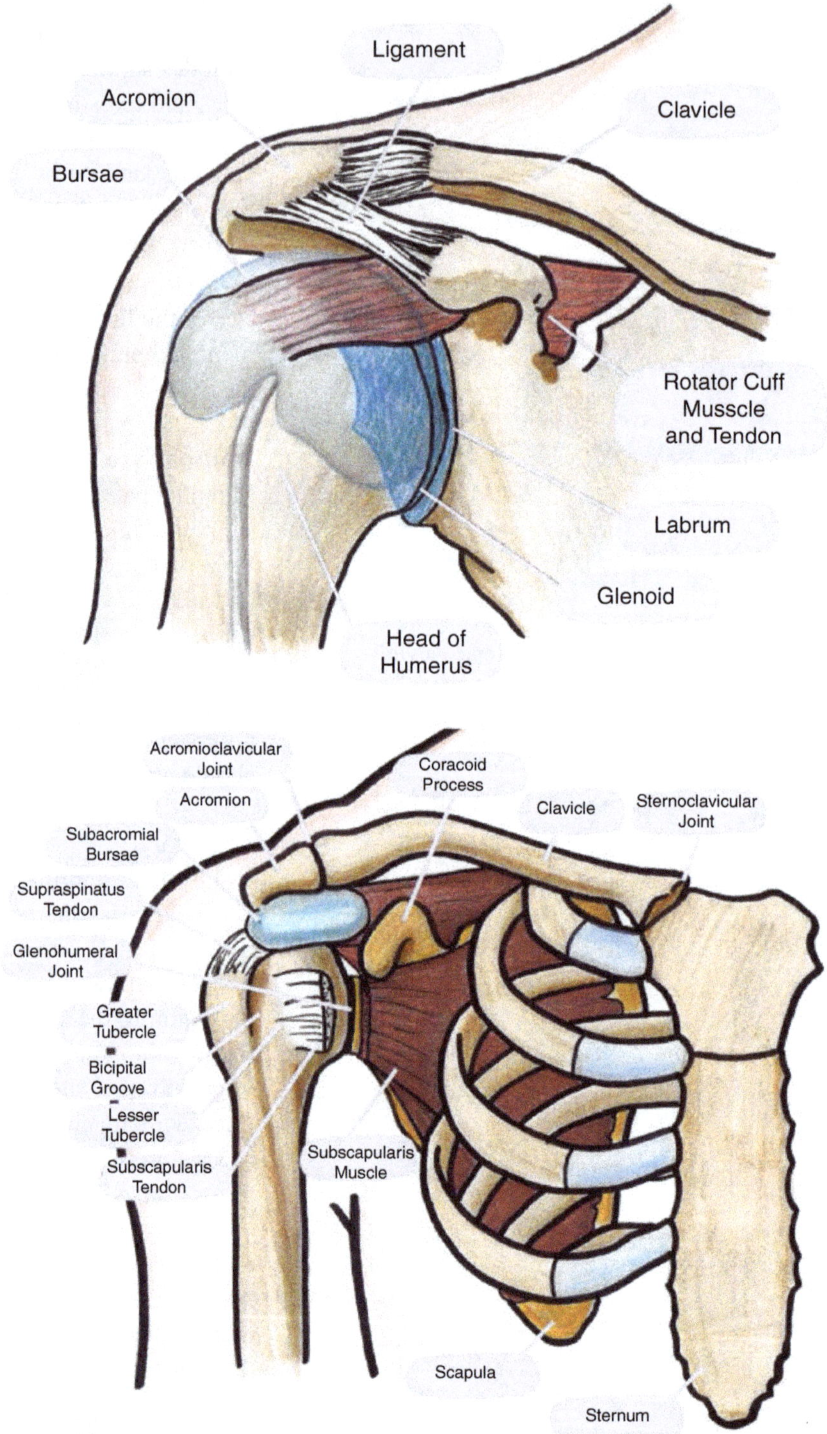

relieving factors, radiation (shoulder pain that radiates past elbow can be due to cervical pathology), history of trauma, and sports activities. Past medical history: diabetic and patients with thyroid diseases are at risk of developing adhesive capsulitis.

Table 2.2 Differential diagnosis of shoulder pain

Lateral shoulder pain	Anterior shoulder pain	Posterior shoulder pain
Rotator cuff tendinitis. Adhesive capsulitis	Adhesive capsulitis Acromioclavicular pathologies Glenohumeral joint arthritis Biceps tendinitis Sternoclavicular injuries	– Rotator cuff tendinitis involving the external rotators – Referred pain • Diaphragm • Gall bladder • Perforated duodenal ulcer • Heart • Spleen • Apex of lungs

2.5.3.2 Second Step: The Approach

It is always:
- Inspection
- Screening exam
- Palpation
- Range of motion
- Special tests

Remember:
- Always inspect anteriorly, laterally, and posteriorly

Inspection

- Skin: redness, scars, rashes.
- Muscles: wasting, atrophy of deltoid (squaring sign).
- Bones and joints: swelling particularly anteriorly obscuring the coracoid process area; this is in case of glenohumeral joint effusion, deformities (acromioclavicular (AC) joint, clavicle), scapula elevation (back), and asymmetry posteriorly (look at back exam for asymmetry).

Screening Exam

The aim is to screen for gross pathology.

- It is basically the active ROM testing (Fig. 2.16).
- Ask the patient to abduct (ABD) shoulders to 90°, then supinate forearms (externally rotating (ER) the shoulders), continue abduction to 180°, do painful arc by bringing both shoulders to zero position again (if the patient develops pain, it indicates positive painful arc test suggestive rotator cuff tendinitis (RCT)), then ask patient to bring his hands behind the neck (ER + ABD), and then move hands backward over the back internal rotation (IR) and adduction (ADD) (IR + ADD). Then try bringing your thumbs on your back as high as possible (Apley's scratch; Fig. 2.17), and finish with forward flexion and extension.
- Shoulder elevation, protraction, retraction, and circumduction.

Palpation

- Remember: shoulder (or glenohumeral joint) effusion is usually detected anteriorly (this is not a common finding).
- Palpate for bony and soft tissue structures: start with sternoclavicular joint (SC joint), then move to feel clavicle, AC joint, acromion, subacromial bursae (a lateral structure just below the acromion) (tenderness indicates RCT, greater trochanter (GT) (rotator cuff inserts here, you are feeling the capsular attachment of glenohumeral joint (GH joint) medially feel bicipital groove (long head of biceps), coracoid process where the short head of biceps inserts (it is painful!)
- Palpate for crepitus by simply feeling over the joints while moving the shoulder.

Range of Motion

- The aim is to differentiate between intra-articular and extra-articular pathology.
- In intra-articular pathology (arthritis), active and passive ROM are limited due to inflammation of the synovial membrane that moves during both active and passive ranges. There is usually effusion that might limit the ROM whether it was passive or active. Even if here was no effusion, the inflammation of the synovial membrane itself would limit the ROM passively and actively because of the pain.

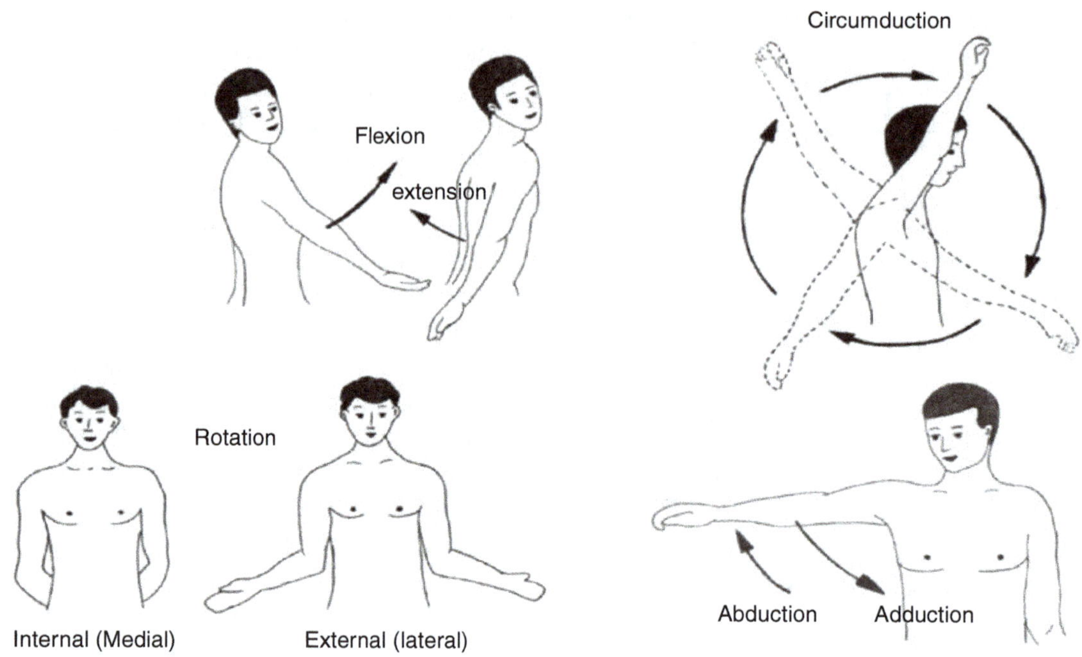

Fig. 2.16 Range of motion testing for shoulder joint

Fig. 2.17 Apley's scratch test

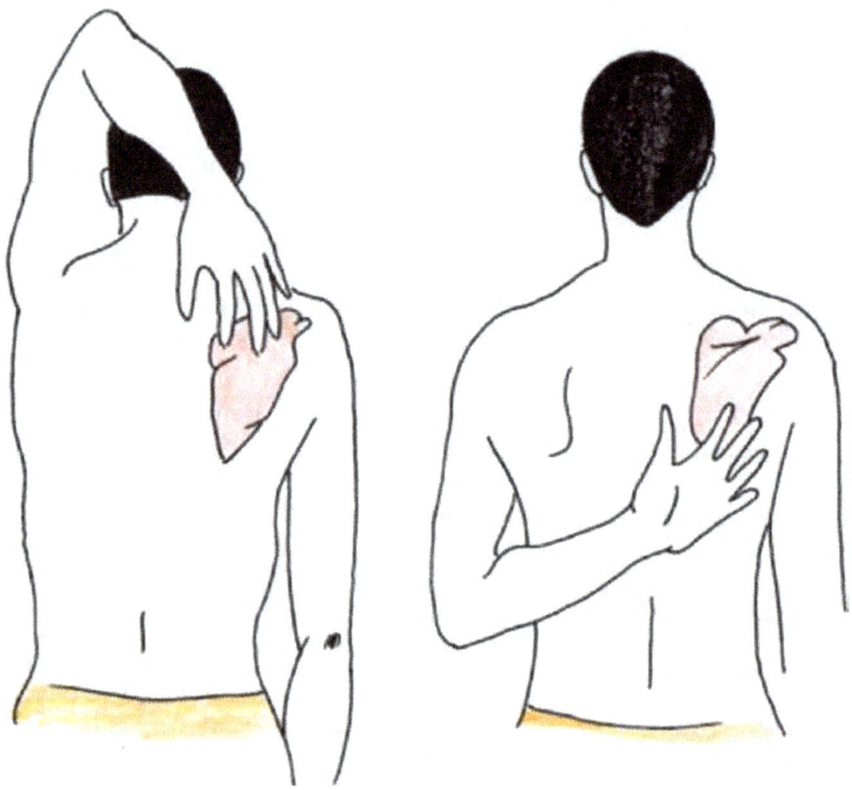

- In extra-articular pathology (periarthritis), the active range is limited only. Here, there is synovial membrane inflammation to limit any kind of movement in the joint. Instead, there is pathology in structures around the joint like in RCT or subacromial (subdeltoid) bursitis. Here the active ROM will be limited but the passive is not.
- You need to test two components to determine with accuracy the cause of the pain.
- Active ROM was assessed during the screening exam.
- For passive ROM: watch the location of your hands!
- Place your right hand on the right shoulder over AC joint firmly. This is to stabilize the scapula in order to do isolated GH joint movement without scapular elevation. The other hand should hold the proximal forearm.
- Do shoulder abduction up to 90°. This is a pure GH joint movement. Normally, there should be zero scapular elevation. Then do ER and IR, while the shoulder is abducted at 90°. Then adduct the shoulder back to zero position where the forearm and the elbow are just beside the body. Then do extension. Then remove your right hand on the right shoulder and do forward flexion.
- You can assess ER + IR while at zero abduction with arms on the sides.
- Repeat the same approach for the left shoulder with your left hand stabilizes the scapula over the left AC joint.

Principle
To assess tendons you need to stretch the tendon (impingement) and/or stress it!

Special Tests

Several MSK examination techniques will be described to assess for specific diseases affecting the shoulder joint. The emphasis should be as stated earlier on the combined evaluation for any patient with MSK complaints of the history and MSK examination findings in order to reach to a correct diagnosis. The diagnostic accuracy for majority of these tests is limited [5]. However, combining careful history taking skills with competent MSK examination findings should help improve the diagnostic accuracy at least to narrow your differential diagnosis rather than reaching an accurate diagnosis.

For RCT

- Painful arc (as described above): from 120° to 60°.
- Isometric resisted abduction while the arm is in zero degree. If there is pain developing, this could be due supraspinatus tendinitis.
- *Empty can sign:*
  (Shoulder abducted 90° + forward flexion 30° away from the body on horizontal line + thumb down (IR)—supraspinatus) (Fig. 2.18).

Infraspinatus and Teres Minor

- Isometric resisted ER (elbow flexed 90° with the arm at the side).
- In the same position, you can assess isometric resisted IR for subscapularis tendinitis (Fig. 2.19).

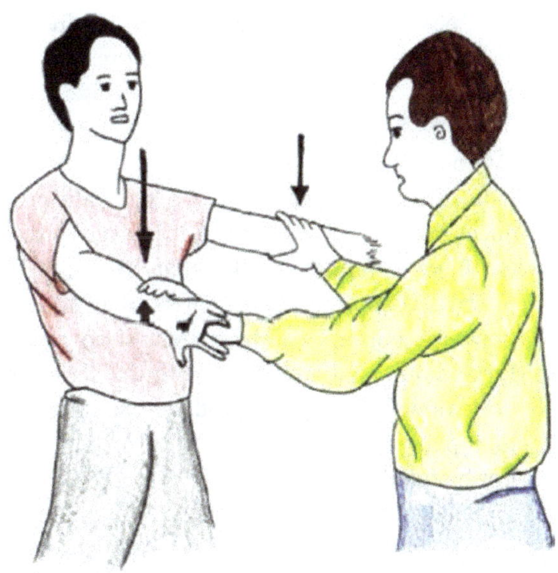

Fig. 2.18 Supraspinatus examination ("Empty can" test)

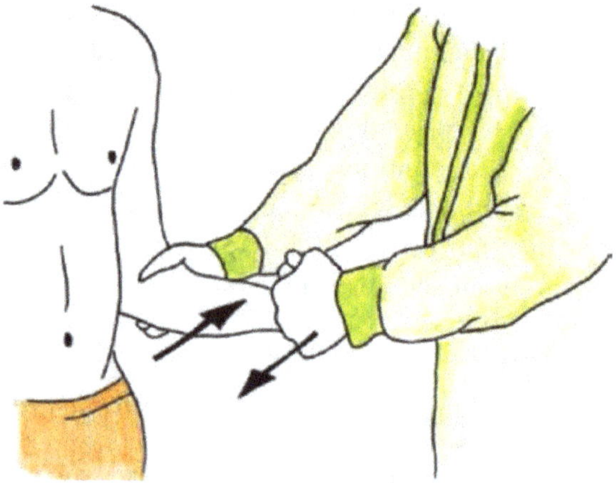

Fig. 2.19 Infraspinatus and teres minor examination

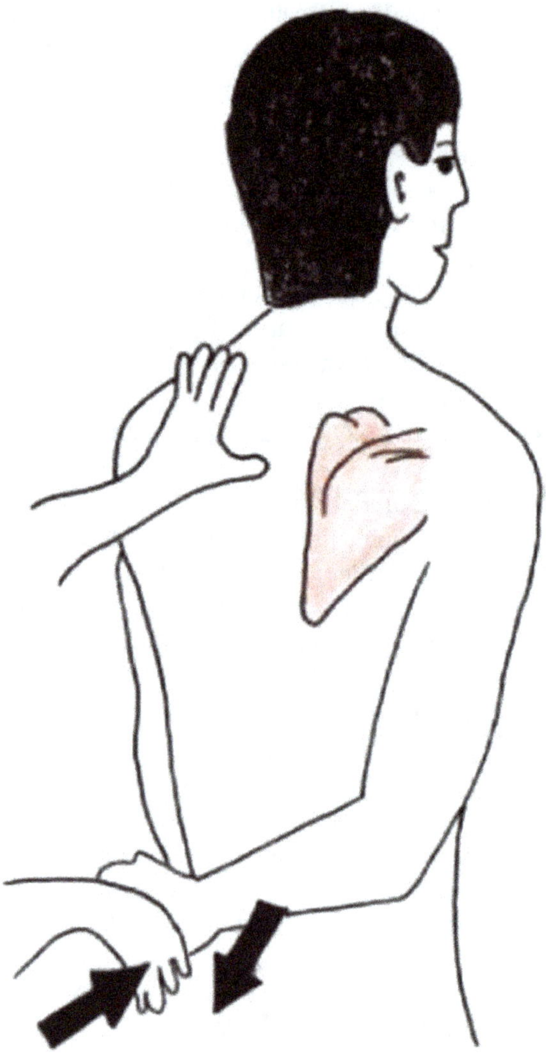

Fig. 2.20 Left off test

Left off Test

This test is performed with isometric resisted IR while the patient adducting his shoulder and internally rotating it. Presence of pain while resistance may indicate subscapularis tendinitis (Fig. 2.20).

Hawkins Impingement Sign

Shoulder horizontal adduction in 90° of flexion then adduct shoulder more with passive IR; this should reproduce symptoms (Fig. 2.21).

Drop Arm Test (Fig. 2.22)

This is to test for complete supraspinatus tear. Sudden push to an abducted shoulder may result in arm drop if there is complete supraspinatus tear.

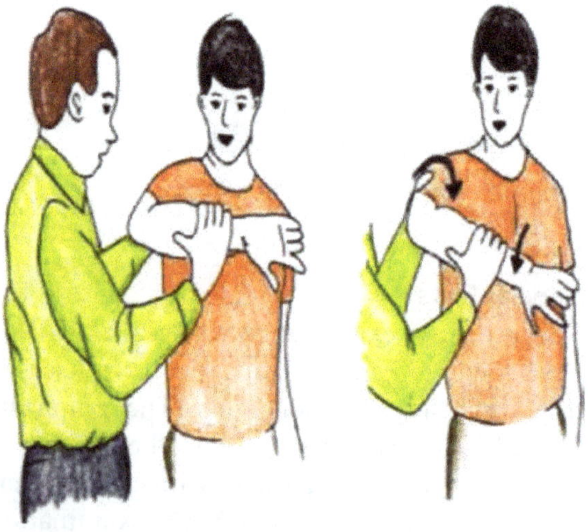

Fig. 2.21 Hawkins' test for subacromial impingement or rotator cuff tendinitis

For AC joint:

- Painful arc (as described above): when it produces pain from 180 to 120. It is usually due to AC joint pathology rather than RCT.
- There is another test called cross-body adduction test (Fig. 2.23). The patient simply performs horizontal adduction with the shoulder in flexion. This might reproduce pain due AC joint pathology.
- For bicipital tendinitis:
  - Speed's test: resisted shoulder flexion at 90° with elbow extended and forearm supinated.
  - Yergason's sign (Fig. 2.24): resisted supination of the forearm with elbow 90° flexion. It

has to be noted that rupture of the long head of biceps is rarely associated with significant weakness in elbow flexion. This is probably due to the fact that 85% of elbow flexion is from brachioradialis and short head of biceps rather than from long head of biceps.

- For glenohumeral joint instability:
- Anterior apprehension test (Fig. 2.25) (supine, 90 ABD and 90 ER, apply gentle forward pressure to posterior aspect of humeral head).

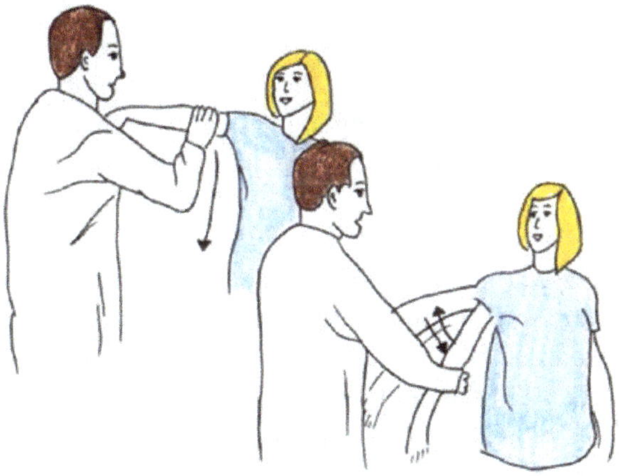

Fig. 2.22 Arm drop test

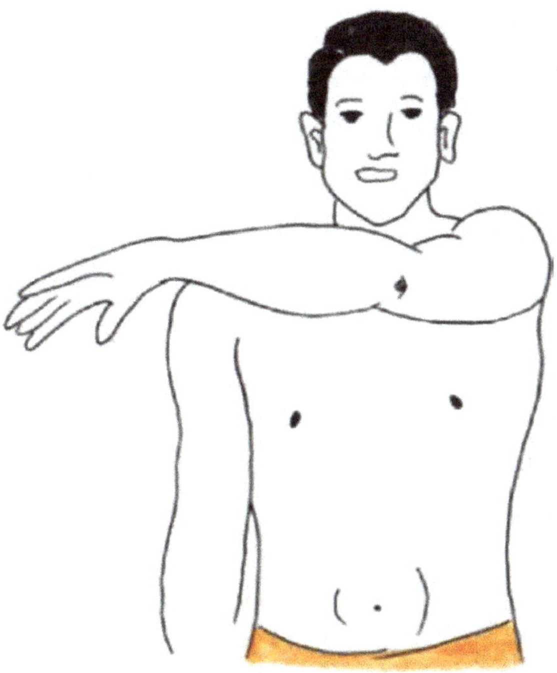

Fig. 2.23 Cross-arm test for acromioclavicular joint disorder

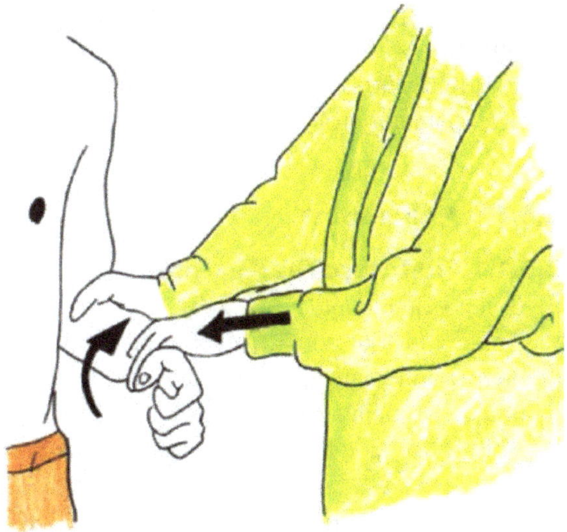

Fig. 2.24 Yergason test for biceps tendon instability or tendinitis

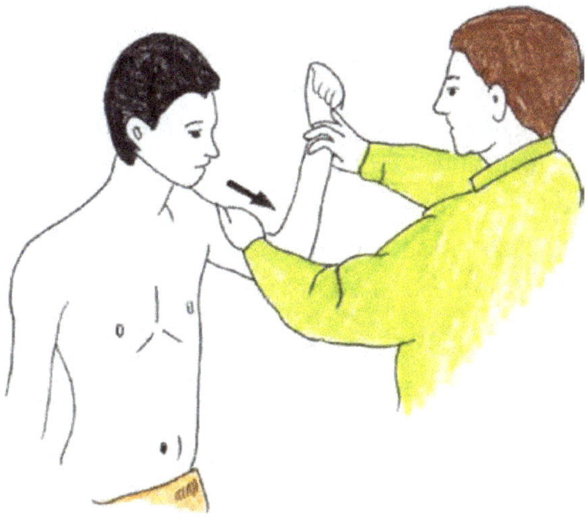

Fig. 2.25 Apprehension test for anterior instability

2.6 Musculoskeletal Examination of the Lower Limb Joints

The joints included in lower limb are ankle, knee, and hip. As in the upper limb section, there is a brief review of the important anatomical landmarks that should be mastered because it has clinical correlations. This will be referred to as the first step. Then an approach to pain originating from this joint will be discussed focusing on anatomical differential diagnosis. The second step will be to follow the stated approach in MSK examination with descriptions whenever it is necessary. Illustrations have been used sometimes as a self-explanatory toll.

2.6.1 Ankle Joint

2.6.1.1 First Step: The Anatomy

- Bones of the Foot (Fig. 2.26)
- Ankle and foot consist of 26 bones, 33 ligaments, and more than 100 muscles and tendons. The main structures are:
- **Bones:** tibia and fibula and tarsal bones, which are calcaneus, talus, navicular, and cuboid, and three cuneiforms bones, five metatarsals, 14 Phalanges (proximal, intermediate and distal), and two sesamoid bones.
- **Joints:** ankle joint, subtalar joint, metatarsophalangeal joints (MTP), and interphalangeal joints.
- **Ligaments**: anterior and posterior tibiofibular ligament, anterior and posterior, talofibular ligament (ATFL and PTFL) and deltoid ligament (Figs. 2.27 and 2.28).
- **Muscles and tendons:** anterior tibialis, peroneal, extensors, and flexors muscles and tendons (Fig. 2.29).

Approach to Ankle Pain

The approach of any patient presents with ankle pain should include:

- History.
- Physical examination.
- Differential diagnosis.

The first step in any history of a joint pain is determining the site of the pain. This simply can be achieved by asking the patient to point out by one finger the site of the pain. The following steps should focus on comprehensive approach to pain analysis including duration, progression, aggravating and relieving factors, and history of trauma. Here, it is important to ask about and examine the patient's shoes. RA classically affects MTPs and ankles. The first MTP joint can be affected classically by gouty arthritis. History of acute first MTP joint pain with swell-

Fig. 2.26 Bones of the foot

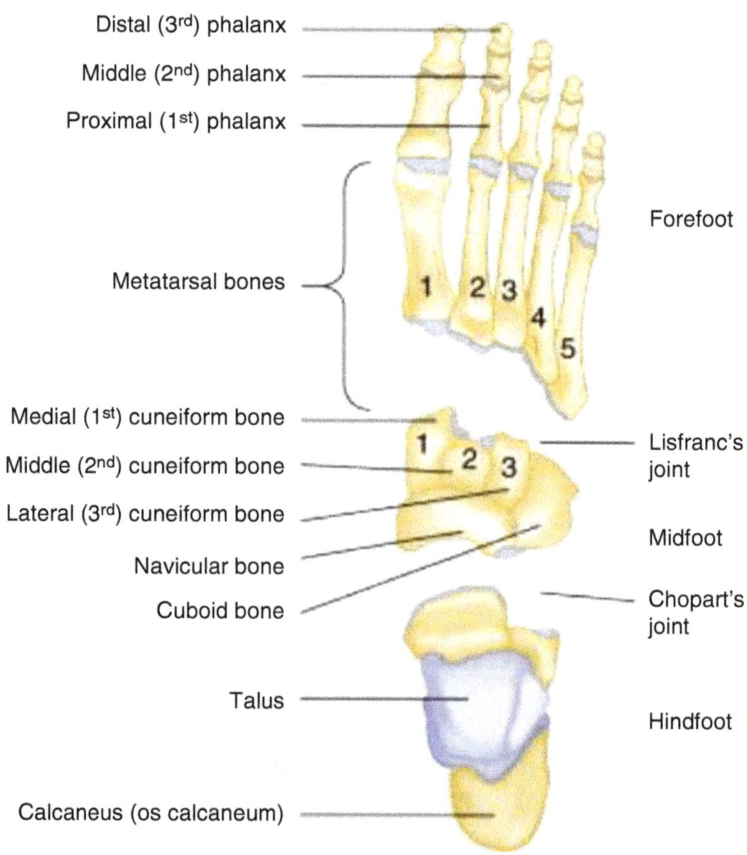

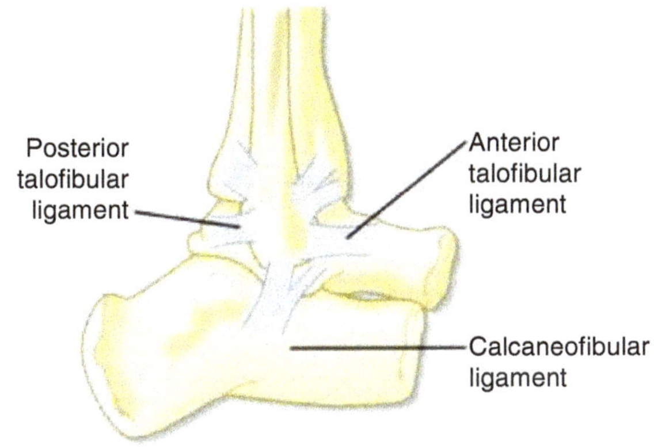

Fig. 2.27 Bones and ligaments of the ankle

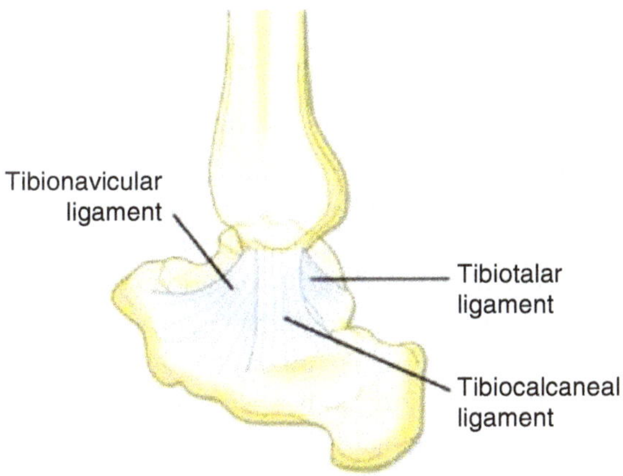

Fig. 2.28 Bones and ligaments of the ankle

ing and redness is diagnostic for gout. Acute gout might mimic cellulitis as it may cause soft tissue swelling and redness as well. The first MTP joint can be involved chronically in osteoarthritis. The interphalangeal joints can be involved in psoriatic arthritis (PsA) that might give identical presentation to RA. In addition, PsA might cause diffuse swellings in one or more than one toe called dactylitis. It may cause Achilles tendinitis and/or plantar fasciitis. Subtalar joint is classically affected in osteoarthritis. History of trauma-related pain should direct the attention immediately to soft tissue problems (periarthritis rather than arthritis). Table 2.3 lists the possible differential diagnosis according to the site of the ankle and foot joints pain.

2.6.1.2 Second Step: The Approach

It is always:
- Inspection
- Screening exam
- Palpation
- Range of motion
- Special tests

Inspection

Expose both ankles and feet and examine for asymmetry. Then follow the standard approach in inspection as it was explained at the introduction of this chapter.

Remember: Always examine anteriorly, medially, laterally, and posteriorly.

- Nail: evidence of psoriasis.
- Skin: scar, redness, rashes, wart, ulcers, blister, calluses, corn, erythema, ecchymosis, change in color.
- Muscle and tendons: wasting, atrophy, and swelling posteriorly for Achilles tendinitis.
- Bone and joint: swelling, deformity (hammer toe, clawing or crowding of the toes, hallux valgus of forefoot), arch of the foot.

Screening Exam

- The aim is to screen for gross pathology.
- It is basically the gait and active ROM testing. For any lower limb joint examined, gait examination is a mandatory step.
- Ask the patient to walk in a straight line and then on toes and on heels.
- Ask the patient to run a short distance (if it possible, this is of great value in assessing periarthritis).
- Ask the patient to hop five times on each foot (if it possible) and then squat and stand from squatting position.
- This quick screening tool actually has assessed the neuromuscular integrity for the lower limb. Walking on the toes, for example, assessed hyperextension of MTPs. If there is

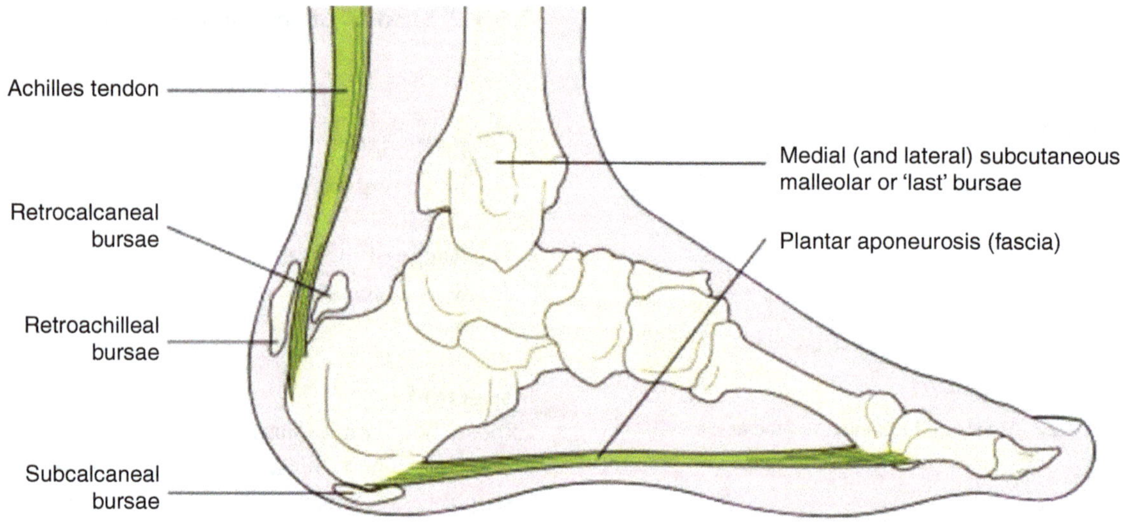

Fig. 2.29 Achilles tendon and plantar fascia

Table 2.3 Differential diagnosis according to the site of the ankle and foot joints pain

Anterior	– Rheumatoid arthritis – Gout arthritis – Osteoarthritis – Tendinitis
Lateral	– Peroneal tendinitis, rupture, or subluxation caused usually by rheumatoid arthritis
Medial	– Tarsal tunnel syndrome – Posterior tibial tendinitis
Posterior	– Achilles tendinitis/rupture – Retrocalcaneal bursitis
Planter	Plantar fasciitis

arthritis in these joints, the patient will not be able to perform this. In addition, walking on toes assessed plantar flexion in ankle joints and extension of knees and hips. Squatting and standing from squatting position have assessed, in addition of joints, the strength of proximal muscles. Walking on heels is an excellent screening for plantar fasciitis. The different steps applied in this screening exam assessed as well almost all the nerve roots for the lower limbs.

Palpation

The major aim is to look for evidence of arthritis in the form of warmth, effusion, and joint line tenderness. Tenderness might be felt laterally and/or medially if there is ligamentous pathology:

- Palpate skin and soft tissue (muscles, ligaments, and tendons).
- Determine joint lines and palpate for tenderness:
  - Ankle joint: (tibia, fibula, and talus joint) perform plantar flexion/dorsiflexion to locate joint line or just medial to the strong tendon of tibialis anterior as it passes over the ankle joint to be inserted at the base of first metatarsal bone.
  - Subtalar joint (talocalcaneal joint): perform inversion/eversion or adduction/abduction of the midfoot to locate this joint. Usually, it can be palpated below and anterior to lateral malleolus.
  - MTPs: Press firmly and intermittently with your thumb and index finger over these joints to illicit tenderness. It is much more reached from plantar aspect than the dorsal aspect of the feet.
  - Medially: Palpate the big toe at the site of the first MTP, and move along the first metatarsal to feel the metatarso-cuneiform joint. Palpate the navicular tubercle, the head of the talus, and the medial malleolus.
  - Laterally: Start palpating the fifth metatarsal bone to feel the styloid process, and then reach the cuboid bone to the calcaneus. Palpate for the peroneal tubercle to the lateral malleolus.

- Posteriorly: Feel the Achilles tendon and follow its insertion at the calcaneus for any tenderness. Just lateral and medial to the insertion of the Achilles tendon, feel for retrocalcaneal bursitis on both sides (lateral and medial) of the tendon.
- Inferiorly (plantar aspect): Feel for tenderness at the insertion of plantar fascia under the medial side of the heel.

In assessing dorsiflexion: the knee must be flexed for proper evaluation

Range of Motion (Fig. 2.30)

- You have done active ROM in your screening exam, but you may repeat active ROM now for detailed examination.
- Examination includes passive and active ROM for the following actions: plantarflexion, dorsiflexion, inversion, and eversion of the foot and flexion and extension of the toes, particularly the big toe.
- Hold the distal leg with one hand while the knee in a flexed position. Then hold the feet from central position just between the ankle and the MTP joints. Now, perform slowly full dorsiflexion (20° from neutral position) by bringing the ankle to the leg, and then push the ankle away from the leg for plantarflexion (50° from neutral position). Now, grasp the feet and perform inversion and eversion. In the same position, you may perform midfoot ad duction and abduction as well. Note any limitation of movement, tenderness, stiffness, and/or end range stiffness.

Special Tests

- Squeeze test (Fig. 2.31): This test aims to stress the MTPs looking for tenderness due to arthritis. Simply squeeze the sides of MTP joints at the level of the heads of phalanges.
- Peroneal subluxation test:
- This is to assess the peroneus longus tendon rupture or instability. Ask the patient to sit down and actively dorsiflexes and everts the foot against resistance; and simultaneously palpate the peroneal tendon posterior to the distal fibula. Pain, clicking, or sensation of instability may indicate subluxation of the peroneal tendon. This test is abnormal when 3–5 mm translocation is present compared with the opposite side.
- The anterior drawer test (Fig. 2.32):

  Evaluate stability of the anterior talofibular ligament (ATFL): stabilize the anterior portion of the distal tibia and fibula with your hand, and use your other hand to cup the heel of the patient foot and pull it toward yourself.
- The inversion stress test (Fig. 2.33):
- Evaluate the stability of the lateral ligament complex (the ATFL and the calcaneofibular ligament (CFL)).
  - Stabilize the anterior portion of the distal tibia and fibula with your hand, and use your other hand to cup the heel of the patient foot.
  - The ATFL is evaluated by maximally plantarflexing the ankle and then inverting the rear foot.
  - The CFL is evaluated by maximally dorsiflexing the foot and then inverting the rear foot.
  - The test is considered abnormal when 10°–15° more inversion is present, compared with the opposite side.
- Test for Morton's neuroma:
- Grasp consecutive metatarsal heads and compress them together. If a click, as well as reproduction of the patient's pain, occurs, a Morton's neuroma should be suspected.
- Thompson test (Fig. 2.34):

  Ask the patient to lie in prone position with the foot hanging off the table, and then squeeze the gastrocnemius muscle. If the foot does not plantarflex, rupture of the Achilles tendon must be considered.

2.6.2 Musculoskeletal Examination of the Knee Joint

2.6.2.1 First Step: The Anatomy (Fig. 2.35)

The bones and articulation of knee joints consists of four bones, which are femur, tibia, fibula, and patella. There are three articulations: medial tib-

Fig. 2.30 Range of motion of the ankle joint

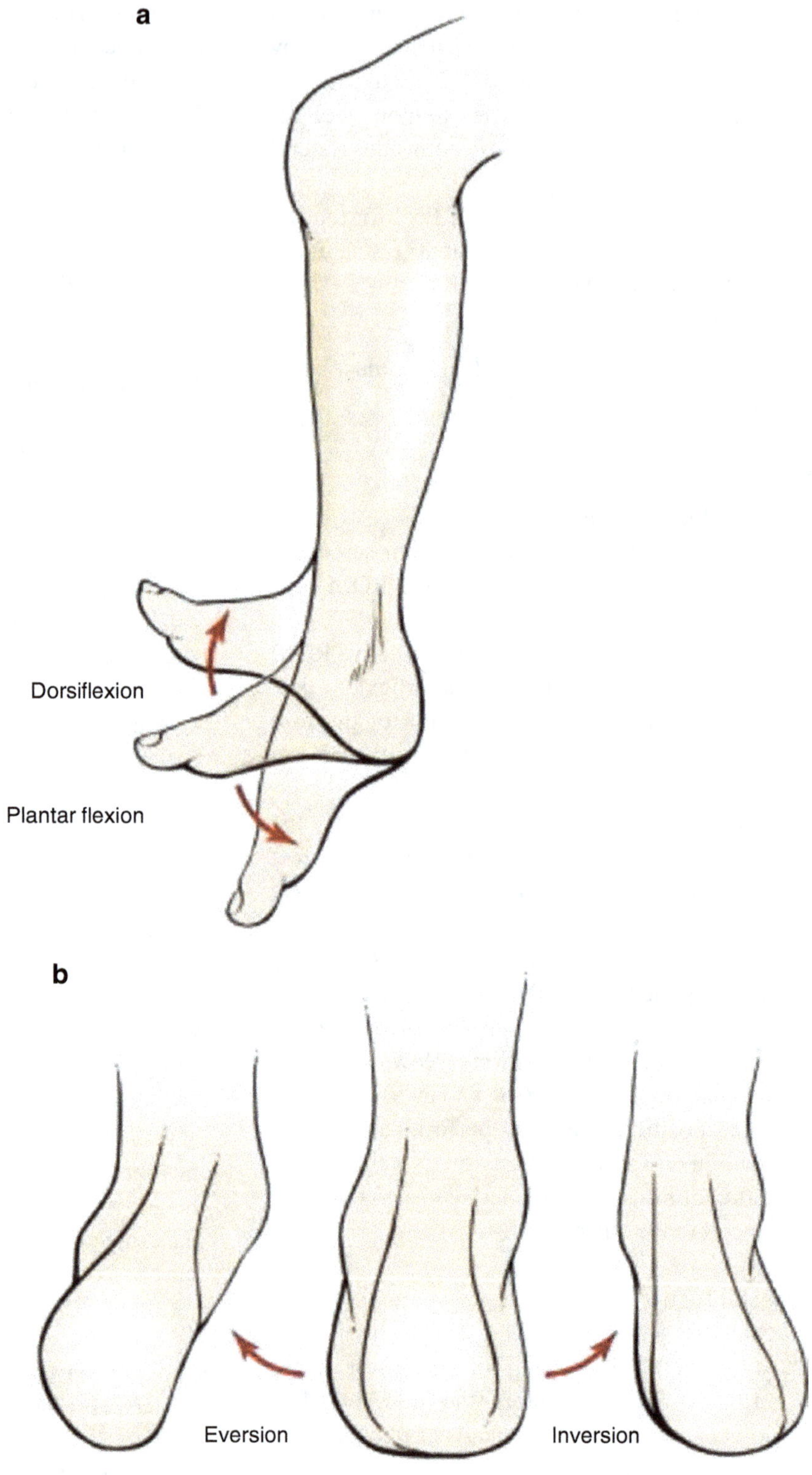

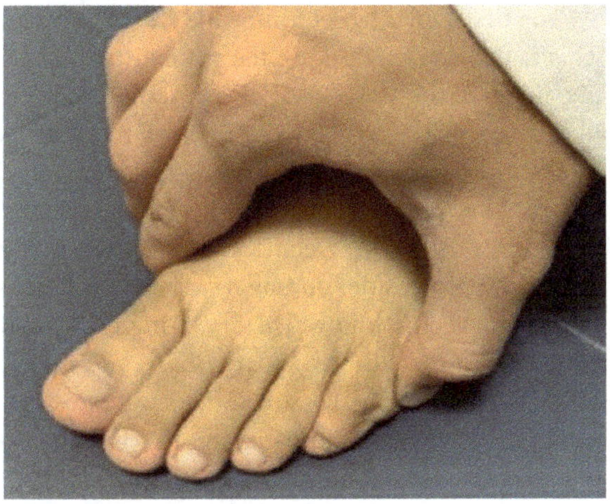

Fig. 2.31 Squeeze test

iofemoral, lateral tibiofemoral, and patellofemoral articulation. The knee joint has many bursae: in the anterior aspect suprapatellar bursae, prepatellar bursae, and superficial and deep patellar bursae and in the medial aspect pes anserine. Cartilage and ligaments of the knee are anterior and posterior cruciate ligaments, medial and lateral collateral and medial and lateral menisci.

Approach to Knee Pain

The approach of any patient presents with knee pain should include:

- History.
- Physical examination.
- Differential diagnosis.

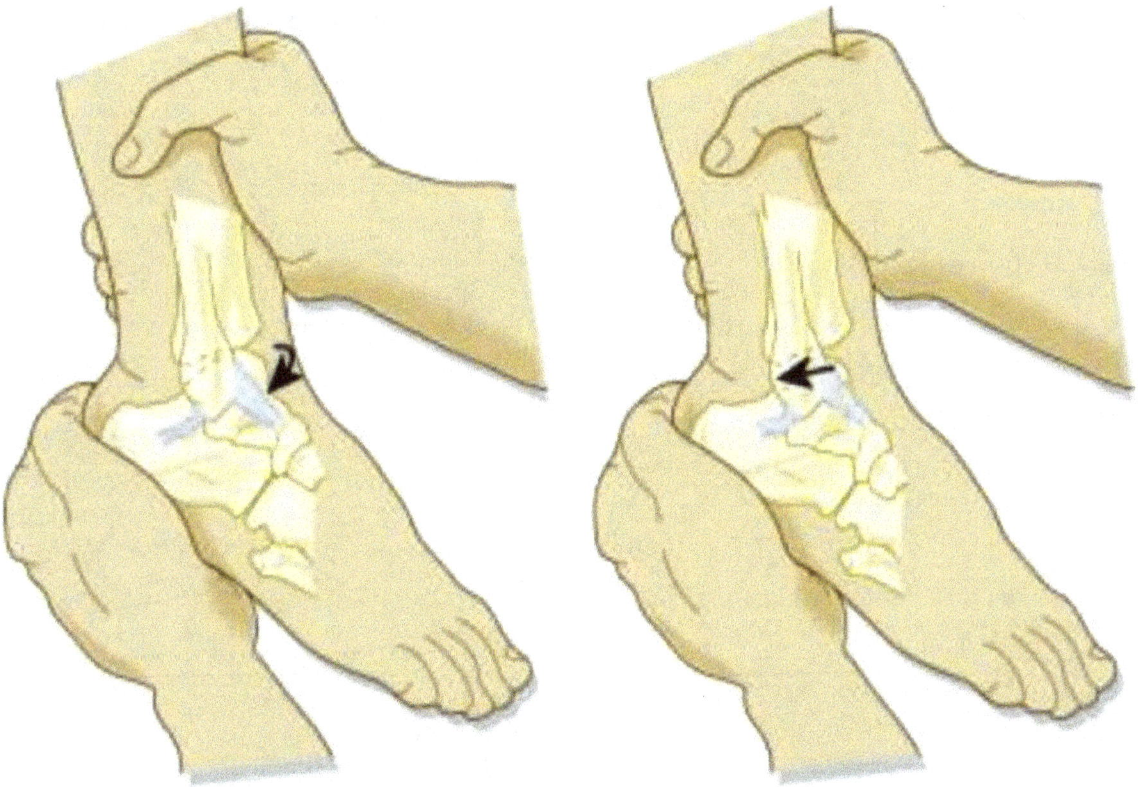

Fig. 2.32 Anterior drawer test

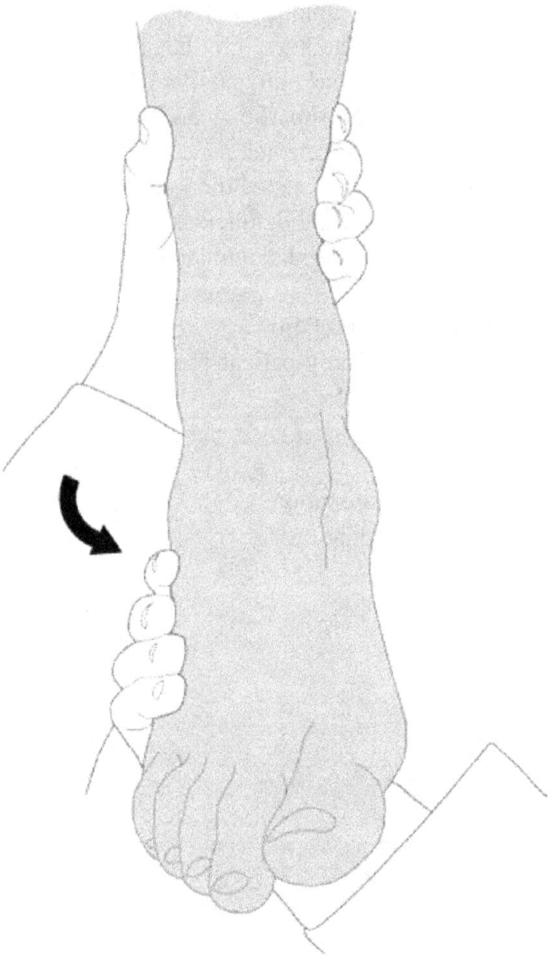

Fig. 2.33 The inversion stress test

The first step is to determine the site of the pain. This is achieved by asking the patient to point by one finger to the site of the pain. In some condition like anserine bursitis, the location of the pain is totally away from joint line. Determining the site of the pain is extremely an important step for reaching accurate diagnosis. Detailed history including duration, progression, and aggravating and relieving factors should follow. History of trauma should be clearly outlined particularly if it was sports related. There are many soft tissue structures that can be affected with traumatic injuries. The knee is the most common joint involved in septic arthritis. Symptoms suggestive of an infectious process like fever should be obtained as well. The knee as well is a common joint in osteoarthritis and crystal deposition diseases (like pseudogout).

Table 2.4 provides a classification of the knee pain according to the site of the pain and its differential diagnosis.

2.6.2.2 Second Step: The Approach

> It is always:
> - Inspection
> - Screening exam
> - Palpation
> - Range of motion
> - Special tests

Fig. 2.34 Calf squeeze test

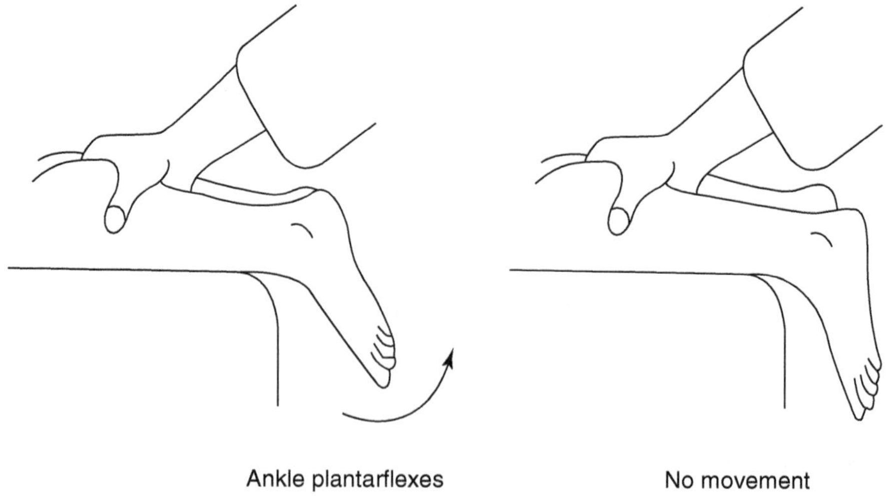

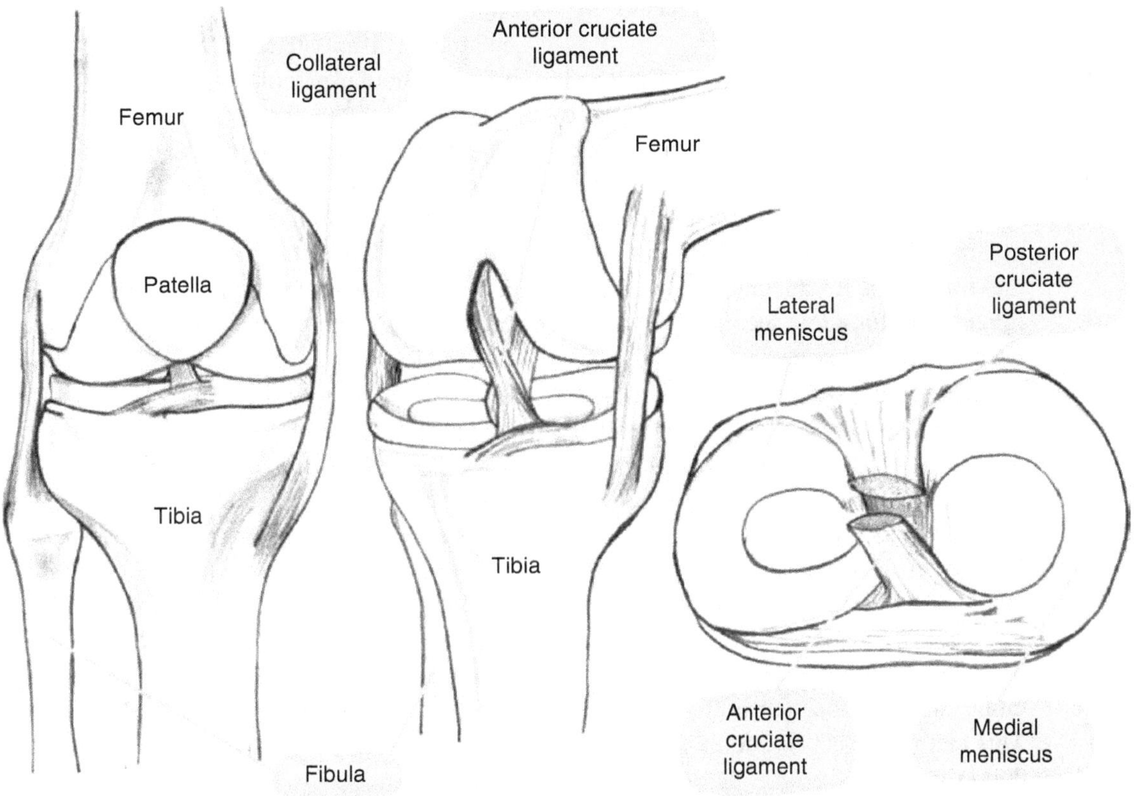

Fig. 2.35 Anatomy of the knee

Table 2.4 A classification of the knee pain according to the site of the pain and its differential diagnosis

	Common	Not to be missed
Anterior	– Arthritis – Osteoarthritis – Prepatellar bursitis – Jumper's knee (patellar tendinitis)	– Ligamentous injury – Tibial apophysitis (Osgood-Schlatter lesion) – Patellofemoral pain syndrome (chondromalacia patellae)
Lateral	– Iliotibial band tendinitis	– Lateral collateral ligament sprain – Lateral meniscal tear
Posterior	– Popliteal cyst (baker's cyst)	– Posterior cruciate ligament injury
Medial	– Pes anserine bursitis	– Medial collateral ligament sprain – Medial meniscal tear

Inspection

- Skin: redness, scars, rashes.
- Muscles: wasting (note medial fibers of quadriceps), atrophy.
- Bones and joints: swelling, deformities – genu varus (common in osteoarthritis of the knee joint) and genu valgus deformities.

Screening Exam

- The aim is to screen for gross pathology.
- It is basically the gait and active ROM testing.
- Ask the patient to walk and comment if the gait is normal or abnormal.
- Ask the patient to walk on toes, heels, and squat and stand up from the squatting position (see details in ankle joint exam above).

Palpation

- The major aim is to look for evidence of arthritis in the form of warmth, effusion, and joint line tenderness.
- Palpate for tenderness over the patella, patellar tendon, suprapatellar bursae, prepatellar bursae (housemaid knees), anserine bursae (medially below joint line, just 2 cm from tibial tuberosity), and tibial tuberosity (where the

patellar tendon inserts, it can be tender in patellar tendinitis).

- Palpate for crepitus, osteophytes, and popliteal cyst.
- The maneuvers used to detect effusion:
  1. Bulge sign:
     - Milk the knee with the palmar or dorsal aspect of your fingers 1–3 times from the tibial side to medial side of the femur. Wait for a few seconds.
     - Now with your fingers, milk the fluid down from the femur side to the tibia laterally. Note the bulge of fluid on the medial side. This method detects mild effusion.
  2. Patellar tap test:
     - Compress the suprapatellar pouch with one hand. With the tips of the fingers of the other hand, give a sharp downward push on the patella. Feel the patella's clunk against the femoral condyles. This method detects moderate effusion.
  3. Balloon sign:
     - Compress the suprapatellar pouch with one hand. Place the thumb and index (or long) finger of the other hand on either side of the patella at the level of the joint line. Now if you press with these fingers, you should feel the fluid pushing away the other hand. This test is positive for large effusion.

Range of Motion

The aim is to differentiate between intra-articular and extra-articular pathology.

- In intra-articular pathology (arthritis), active and passive ranges of motion are limited (see explanation in shoulder joint exam).
- In extra-articular pathology (periarthritis), the active range is limited only.
- You need to test two components: active and passive ROM.
- Ask the patient to bring both heels toward the pelvis as much as possible (flexion), and then ask the patient to put his knees flat on the bed (extension).
- For passive ROM testing, ask the patient to relax. With one hand covering the entire knee anteriorly and the other holding the heel, flex the knee and then extend it. You should comment on tenderness, stiffness, end of range stiffness, and/or limitation of movement.

Special Tests

- The aim is to look for the integrity of menisci and ligaments around the knee.
- For menisci integrity, you can use the McMurray test (Fig. 2.36): hold the knee with one hand, while the patient is in supine position. Bring the knee to full flexion. Now, extend the knee slowly with applying valgus stress from the lateral aspect of the knee you

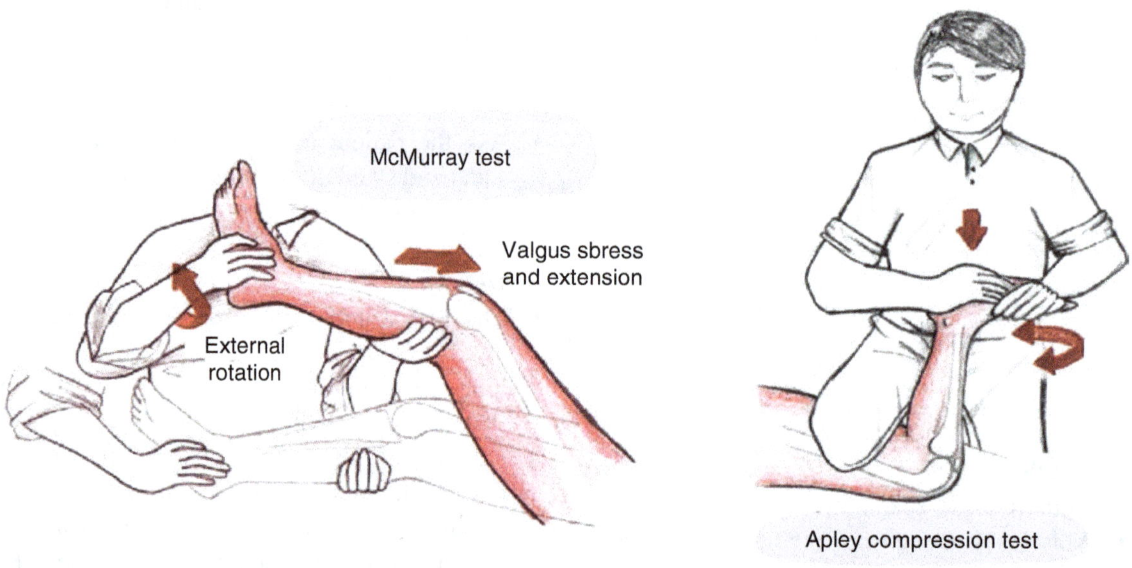

Fig. 2.36 McMurray test and Apley compression test

are holding with your hand, while the other hand is externally rotating the knee from the ankle. The test is considered positive if there is pain and/or popping sound.

- Apley's compression test: here the patient lies in prone position with the knee being examined flexed at 90°. You should stabilize the knee by placing your leg pressing over posterior aspect of the patient's thigh. Apply now compressing pressure over the knee from the ankle with external rotation force. The test is considered positive if it produces pain.
- For cruciate ligaments (CL), you can use the anterior drawer test (Fig. 2.37): you should sit on the patient's feet for stabilization the flexed knees to around 90°. Place your hands on the tibial plateau from medical and lateral aspects, and then try to push tibia anteriorly over the femur toward your side (anterior drawer test) or posteriorly (posterior drawer test). Any displacement particularly when compared with the other knee is considered positive for cruciate ligament instability. The Lachman test: the patient here is in supine position. You should place one of your hands above the knee joint line with a good grasp, while the other is just below the knee joint line. In around 20–30° of passive knee flexion, try to apply contradicting forces by two hands; one pushes anteriorly while the other pushes posteriorly. Any excessive displacement is considered positive (Fig. 2.38). The validity of these tests has been questioned [5]. In general, this test is more sensitive than the anterior drawer test [4].
- For collateral ligaments, you can apply valgus and varus stresses, while the knee is held in 40–70° of flexion to assess for medial and lateral collateral ligaments, respectively. With positive result, there will be laxity and wide openings of the joint.

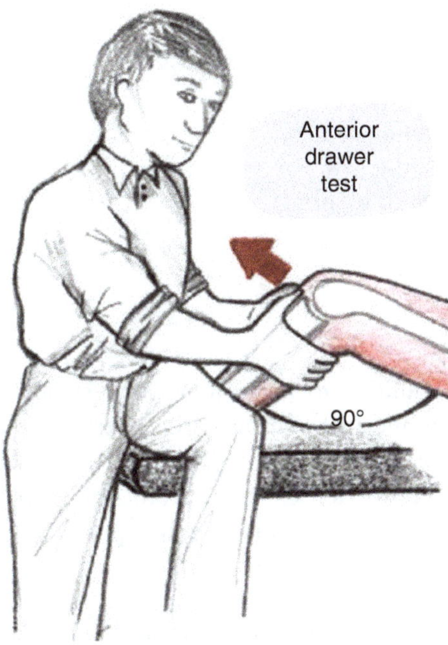

Fig. 2.37 Anterior drawer test

2.6.3 Musculoskeletal Examination of the Hip Joint

2.6.3.1 First Step: The Anatomy (Fig. 2.39)

The hip joint is formed by the articulation between the round head of the femur and the acetabulum. It is a ball and socket joint with one part, the acetabulum, which is fixed in the body. Three bones compose the acetabulum: Ilium, ischium, and pubis. Femoral neck, Greater Trochanter (GT), and lesser trochanter are bony structures of anatomical significance. Femoral neck is vulnerable site for osteoporotic fractures. This site is used to measure bone mineral density to diagnose osteoporosis. The insertion of hip abductors and extensors are at the GT. While the hip flexor (iliopsoas) inserts at the lesser trochanter. An important bursae covers the GT which can be inflamed and cause symptoms. Symphysis pubis is a fibrocartilage that can cause symptoms.

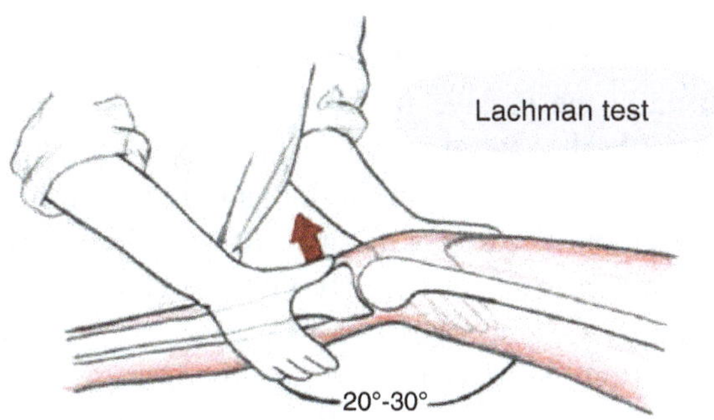

Fig. 2.38 Lachman test

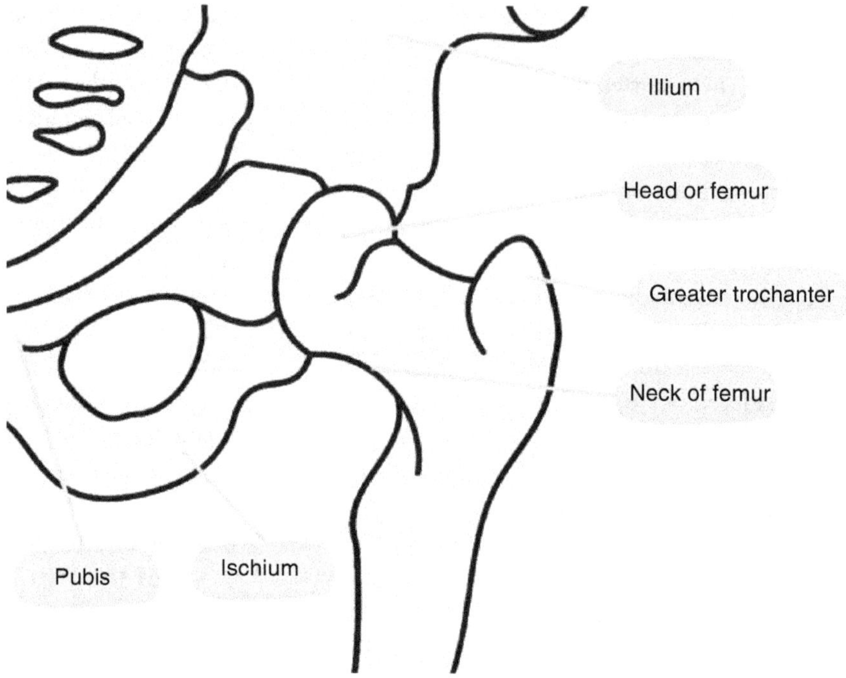

Fig. 2.39 Anatomy of the hip joint

Approach to Hip Pain

It is important to determine the site of pain. This is an essential step in the history of any joint pain. True hip joint pain (due to arthritis of head of femur articulating with the acetabulum) can be felt only anteriorly in the groin region. In the case of hip arthritis, you can expect to find, in addition to groin pain, severe limitation in the ROM actively and passively. Hip joint is a deeply seated joint; for this reason aspiration is always performed under fluoroscopic or US guidance. Pains that felt elsewhere in the hip region could be due other structures around the hip joint and still called by patients as "hip pain." Trochanteric bursitis is a classical example of a lateral hip pain in moderately obese female. Here there is tenderness by palpation in the lateral hip, and the active adduction and/or abduction may be painful, but usually the passive ROM is intact. In meralgia paresthesia (lateral cutaneous nerve entrapment), there is usually pain in the anterolateral hip region with entirely normal ROM. There are many structures posteriorly that can cause pain. Sacroiliac joint gives rise to posterior hip pain and usually referred to by some patients as buttock pain. Lumbar radiculopathy is another differential diagnosis. The patient should be asked then to point to the site of hip pain by one finger to exactly determine it. Table 2.5 summarizes the most important differential diagnosis of hip pain according to its site.

2.6.3.2 Second Step: The Approach

> It is always:
> - Inspection
> - Screening exam
> - Palpation
> - Range of motion
> - Special tests

Inspection

- You should start inspection from standing position and inspect anteriorly, laterally, and posteriorly. Then you can continue your examination after screening exam and palpation, while the patient is in supine position.
- Standing:
  - Back:

    Skin: redness, scars, rashes.

    Muscles: wasting, atrophy.

Table 2.5 Classification of the hip pain according to the site of the pain and its differential diagnosis

Site of the pain	Common	Less likely	Not to be missed
Anterior	Arthritis Synovitis Osteoarthritis Chondropathy Osteitis pubis	Stress fracture Hip joint instability	Synovial chondromatosis Avascular necrosis (AVN) of the head femur Slipped capital femoral epiphysis (SCFE) Tumor Legg-Calve-Perthes disease
Lateral	Trochanteric bursitis Greater trochanter pain syndrome	Referred pain from lumbar spine	Fracture of neck of femur Nerve root compression Tumor
Posterior	Sacroiliac joint disease, Lumbar radiculopathy Inferior hip joint osteophytes associated with hip arthritis		

Bones and joints: assess symmetry and pelvic obliquity – inspect posterior superior iliac spine (PSIS) (dimples of Venous) as they should be align to one level. Asymmetry may give clues to cases with chronic low back pain without apparent etiology. Inspecting gluteal folds, tip of scapula can assess symmetry.

- Lateral: inspect for lumbar lordosis and possible swelling or redness over greater trochanter.
- Anterior: symmetry can be assessed by inspecting anterior superior iliac spine (ASIS). Rarely, fullness in the groin region may indicate hip arthritis. However, significant hip joint pathology can occur without apparent swelling. Inspect also for rashes, redness, and scars.

Screening Exam

- Apparent leg length: from xiphoid cartilage or umbilicus to medial malleolus
- True leg length: from ASIS to medial malleolus

- The aim is to screen for gross pathology.
- It is basically the gait and active ROM testing.
- Note position: external rotation (ER) indicates hip joint pathology as internal rotation (IR) is lost first in arthritis.
- See ankle joint exam above for details of gait assessment. Simply you should ask the patient to walk/turn/walk on toes/on heels/squat (if possible) and stand from squatting position. This is a comprehensive evaluation of the neuromuscular integrity of the lower limb. Walking by itself is a good screening for hip flexion and extension. Squatting position is a good screening again for hip flexion and extension.
- Assess Trendelenburg sign: ask the patient to stand on the affected side that has classically hip joint arthritis (diseases like osteoarthritis) with week hip abductors and extensors. Then ask the patient to raise the normal side. Normally, the pelvis in the unsupported side will be raise due to the tone of strong muscles from the other supported side. In this sign and because of weakness of hip muscles from arthritis, the muscle tone here cannot support the pelvis in the other unsupported side, and this will result in pelvis drop in the unsupported side with positive sign. Trendelenburg gait is basically the same explanation, but when the patient needs to walk, bending laterally toward the supported side will raise the dropping unsupported pelvis producing the classical waddling gait with bilateral involvement of both hips.
- Note the type of gait (Fig. 2.40).

Palpation

- You can start palpation, while patient is still in standing position.
- Back: palpate paraspinal muscles, sacroiliac joint (SI joint) (1 inch medical + inferior to PSIS), iliac crest, and ischial tuberosity (IT)

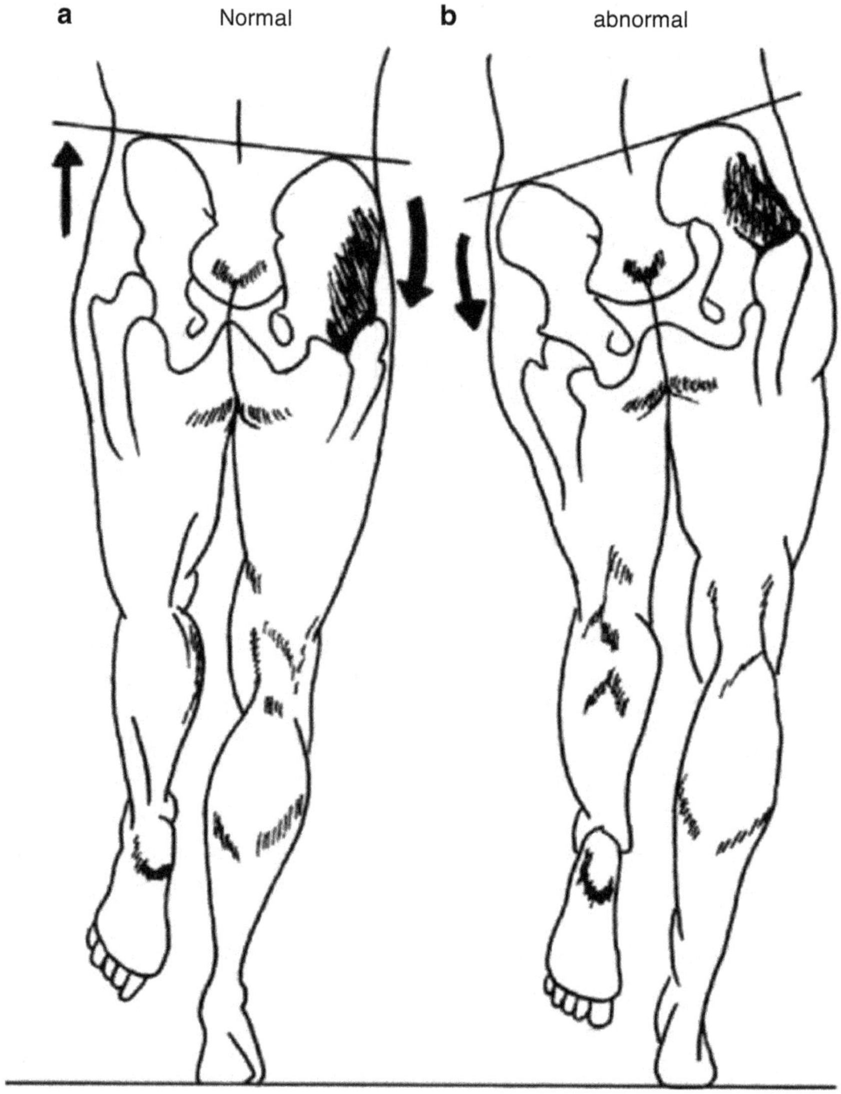

Fig. 2.40 Types of gait: normal (**a**) and abnormal (**b**)

(you may ask the patient to step on a stool using the limb under examination), feel GT, and feel sciatic nerve between the IT and GT.

- Lateral: palpate trochanteric bursae (Fig. 2.41).
- Anterior: palpate groin region – lymph nodes, pulses, hernia, ASIS, hernial orifice, pubic tubercle (where adductor longus originates), symphysis pupis – note any discrepancies in leg length.
- You may continue your palpation now, while the patient is in supine position.
- Quick screening: "frog" leg position—external rotation (ER) + abduction (ABD) + knee flexion—then compare both sides. In this position you may feel adductor longus tendon by asking the patient to adduct the hip against resistance and then just follow the adductor longus tendon until its origin from the pubic tubercle. Eliciting pain here may give you the diagnosis of adductor longus tendinitis.
- Flex hips and knees then extend them and look for leg length discrepancy.

Range of Motion

- You have done active ROM in your screening exam for two important hip movement flexion and extension. Now, you need to do comprehensive assessment of ROM (Fig. 2.42).
- In supine position: ask the patient to flex hip as much as possible; you may combined hip

Fig. 2.41 Trochanteric and iliopsoas bursae

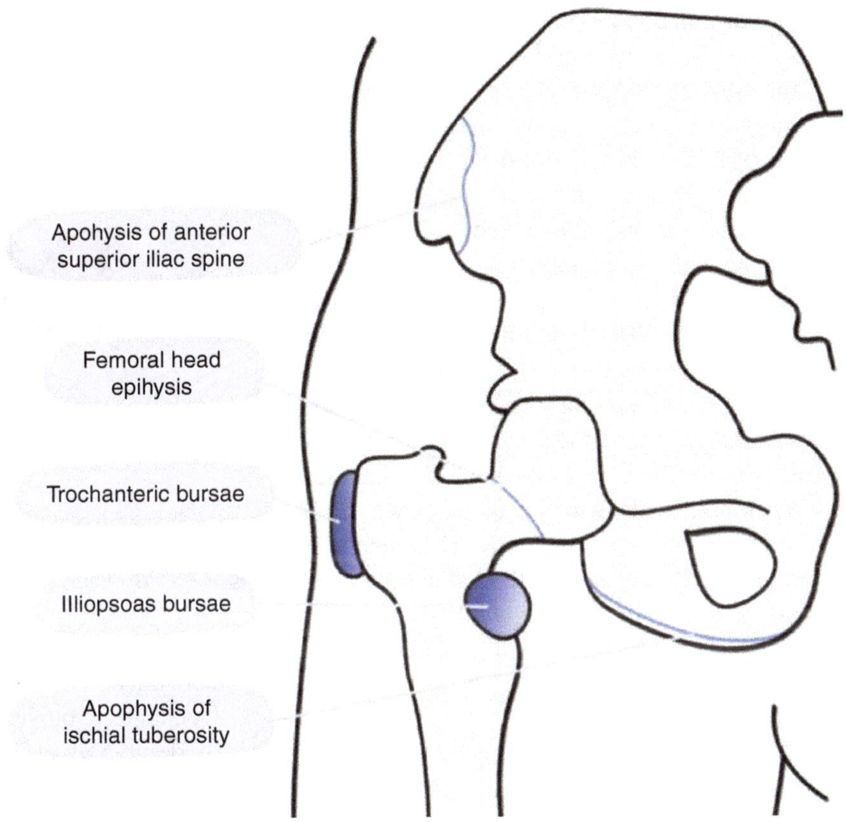

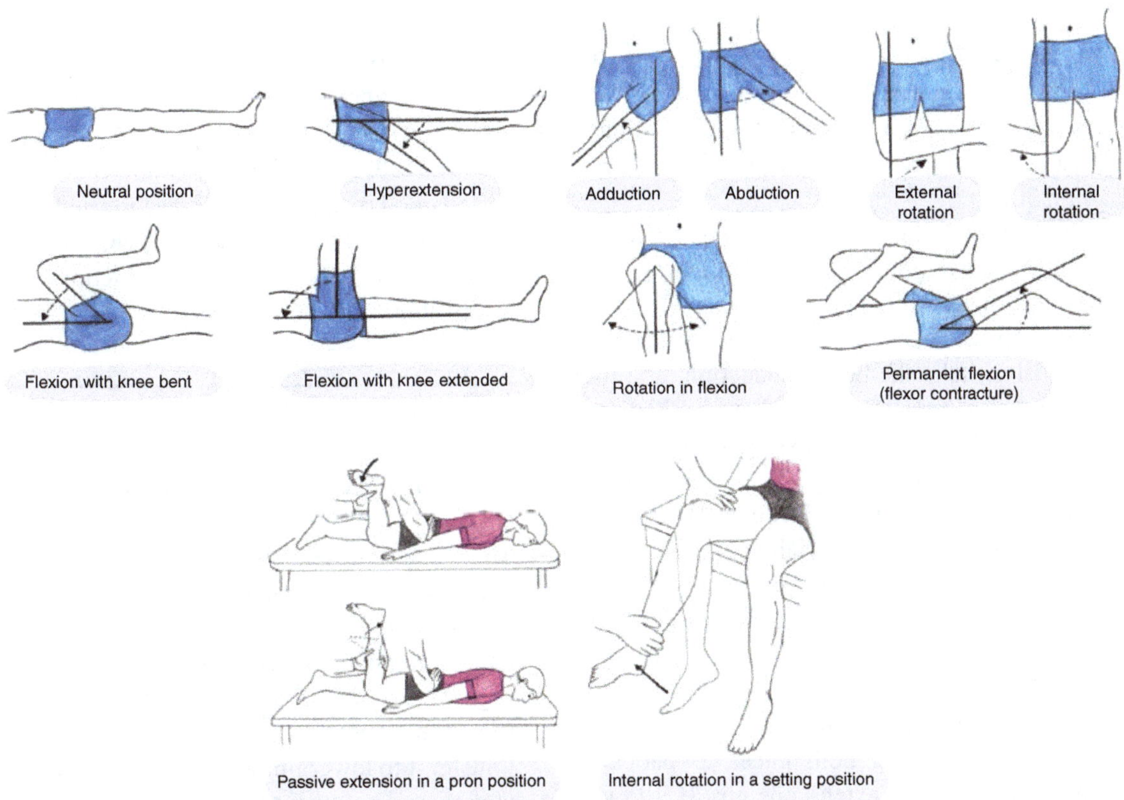

Fig. 2.42 Range of motion testing for hip joint

and knee active flexion by asking the patient to bring the knee to abdomen. Back to supine position and ask patient to abduct the hip laterally to as much possible and return to each hip one at time and ask the patient to cross midline. This is adduction. Back to supine position, and ask the patient to bring both plantar surfaces of both feet together facing each other with both knee flexed. This is external rotation (ER), and it is called "frog" leg position. The opposite of this position is the assessment of internal rotation (IR). The other position for active ER and IR is while patient is sitting at the edge of the bed with the knees and hips flexed. Bringing the leg away is IR and toward the midline is ER. The same technique can be done while the patient is supine. Extension can be assessed while the patient is in lateral decubitus position with the hip moved posteriorly.

- Active: Flexion 120°
  - Abduction 50°
  - Adduction 30°
  - Frog leg (for ER) 45°
  - Opposite of frog leg (for IR) 35°
  - Or in prone position: do active ER + IR
  - Assess ER + IR through leg rolling while hips are extended.
- In lateral decubitus position: you may palpate trochanteric bursae and perform active extension 30°.
- The passive ROM can be assessed, while the patient is in supine position. Flex the hip and try to bring it to patient's abdomen. Back to neutral position, and while putting one hand on the pelvis, take the hip to abduction, and use the same technique for the other hip. Perform passive adduction by crossing midline. For ER, flex hip and knee to 90°, then hold knee with one hand and the heel with the other hand, and then bring heel medially. For IR: bring heel laterally. Assess passive extension in lateral decubitus position or in prone position.

Special Tests

- Hip fixed flexion deformity:
- Thomas test: bring both knees to patient's abdomen and then extend one hip. If it failed to extend fully, there is fixed flexion hip deformity.

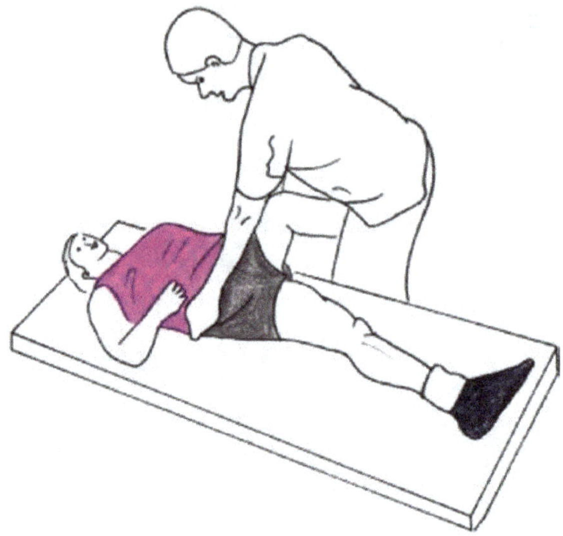

Fig. 2.43 Testing for piriformis syndrome

- Trochanteric bursitis:
- Tenderness over GT with pain elicited by resisted abduction.
- Radiculopathy:
- Straight leg raising test and slump test (see back exam).
- Piriformis syndrome:
- Resisted abduction while hip is flexed at 90° and adducted (Fig. 2.43).
- Tightness in iliotibial band (Ober's test):

In lateral decubitus, neutralize hip and knee at 90°, and then abduct hip: a tight iliotibial band prevents the hip from adducting passively (Fig. 2.44).

2.7 Back Examination

2.7.1 First Step: The Anatomy

- The spine represents the axial skeleton of the back, and it is composed of 32–33 small bones, called vertebrae (7 cervical, 12 thoracic, 5 lumbar, 5 fused sacral, and 3 or 4 coccygeal) (Figs. 2.45 and 2.46). The vertebrae bear the majority of the body weight and transfer it to lower limbs and also provide protection and support to spinal cord. A typical

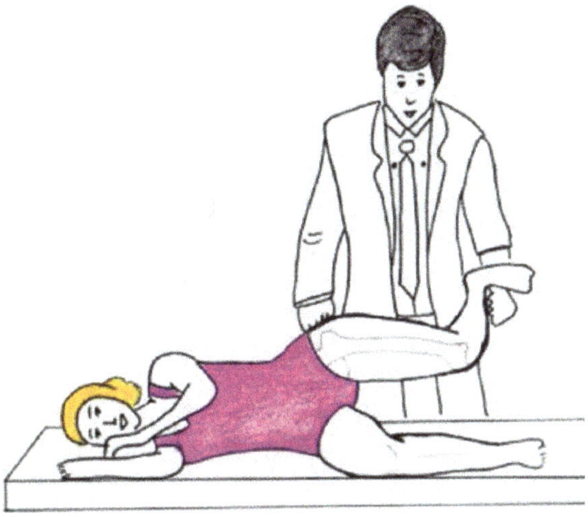

Fig. 2.44 Ober's test

vertebra is consisted of anterior body and posterior arch enclosing the vertebral canal where the spinal cord extends from the brain to the area between the end of first lumbar vertebra and top of second lumbar vertebra (L1 or L2 vertebral levels). Between each vertebra is a cartilaginous joint, called intervertebral disc. The discs limit the movements between the individual vertebrae and also act as a shock absorber (Fig. 2.47). The vertebral bodies are strictly attached to the intervertebral discs by two main ligaments: anterior and posterior longitudinal ligaments. Each pair of vertebrae is also connected by a synovial joint called facet joints. This is formed by the inferior articular process of one vertebra joining the superior articular process for the vertebra just below it. The facet joints give the spine its flexibility as there are two facet joints between each pair of vertebrae, one on each side. While the joints allow flexibility, the mobility of the spine is provided by the surrounded paraspinal muscles extended laterally along the spine.

- In the vertebral foramen posteriorly, the spinal cord extends down to the end of the second lumbar vertebra. Below this level, the spinal canal forms a group of nerve fibers, called the cauda equina. This group of nerves goes to the pelvis and lower limbs. Attached to each segments of the spinal cord, there is a pair of 31 spinal nerves exiting the vertebral foramina through vertebral notches of the adjacent pedicles. The spinal nerves exit the intervertebral foramina in relation to vertebral levels as the following: nerves of C1-C7 exit superior to the pedicles of the same-numbered level, C8 nerve inferior to C7 pedicles, and then T1 and below exit inferior to the pedicles of the same-numbered level.
- Different injuries and diseases may affect the components of spine and its surrounded paraspinal muscles resulting in back pain (Figs. 2.48 and 2.49) (See Chap. 6).

2.7.2 Second Step: The Approach

It is always:
- Inspection.
- Screening exam.
- Palpation.
- Range of motion.
- Special tests.

2.7.2.1 Inspection

You may start your examination by explaining to your patient the steps of your exam. After proper exposure, start your inspection, while the patient is standing. You may ask one of the family members to be around.

Always inspect the patient posteriorly, laterally, and anteriorly.

- **Alignment:** you should be familiar with the normal alignment of the spine. This is to help inspect for abnormal alignment that may give rise to chronic back pains: kyphosis, scoliosis, and exaggerated or lost lumbar lordosis. In patients with ankylosing spondylitis (AS), lumbar lordosis is usually lost from spondylitis. This also can be lost due to severe muscle spasm over the lower back.
- **Skin:** Inspect for erythema, hair patch, café au lait spots, nodules, and/or scars.
- **Muscles:** wasting, atrophy.

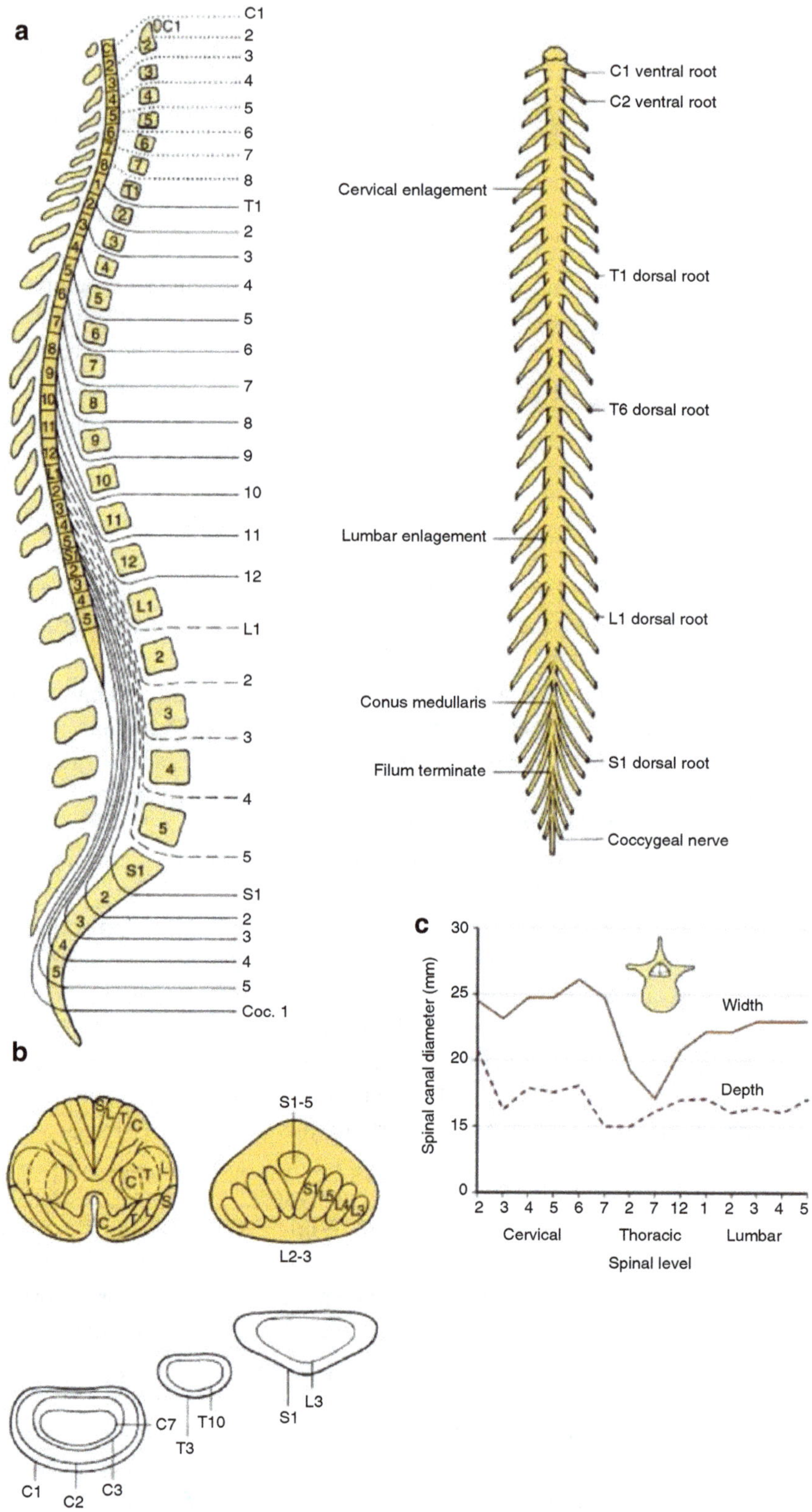

Fig. 2.45 Bones of the spine [6]

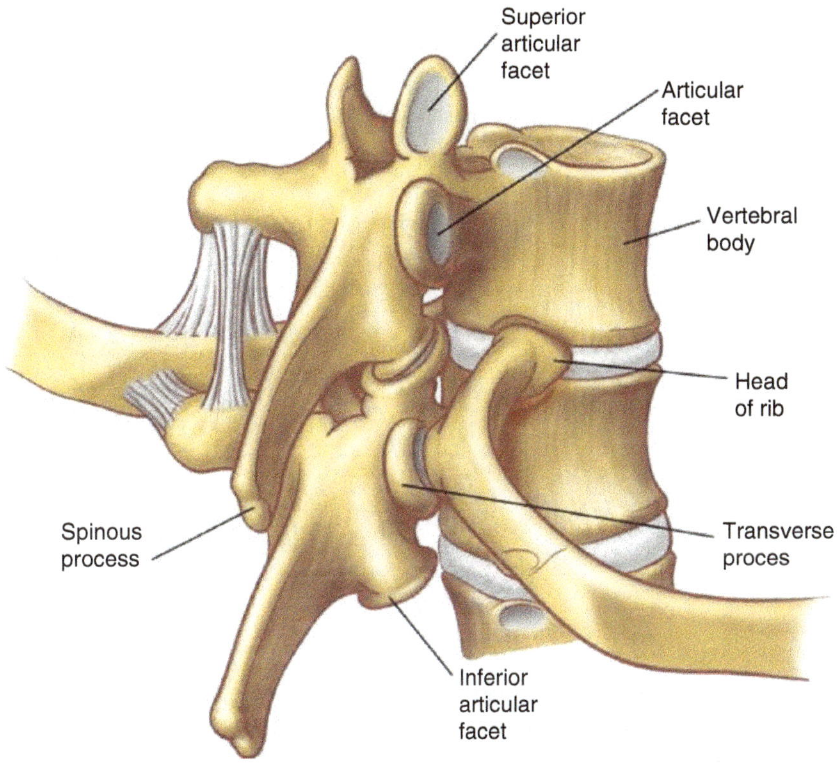

Fig. 2.46 Structures of lateral spine

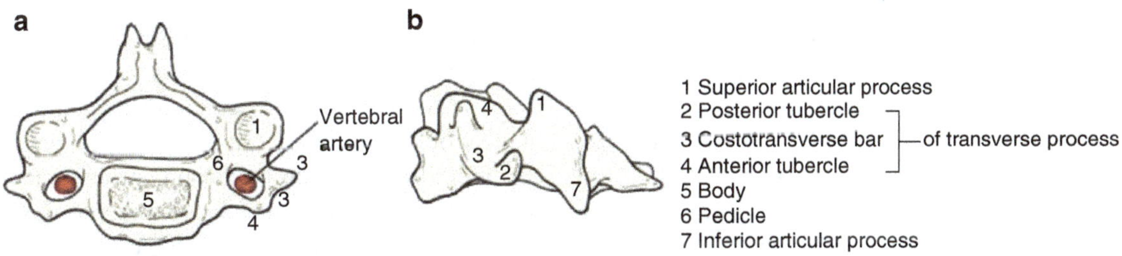

Fig. 2.47 Structure of a vertebra

- **Symmetry**: check symmetry of the back by assessing whether tips of scapulae are at one level or not. Also for the iliac crests and gluteal folds. Inspect PSIS (dimples of Venous) as they should be align to one level. You may ask the patient to flex the hip and observe while you are standing behind the patient the symmetry and whether the asymmetry is corrected or not.

2.7.2.2 Screening/Gait Assessment

- **Gait:** straight walking while watching for abnormal flexion (suggestive of spinal stenosis or facet joint pathology), abnormal extension (suggestive of disc pathology), or Trendelenburg gait (Fig. 2.50).
- **Screening for neurological integrity:** walking on toes (L5, S1) and then on heels (L4, L5), knee extension (L3, L4); then ask patient

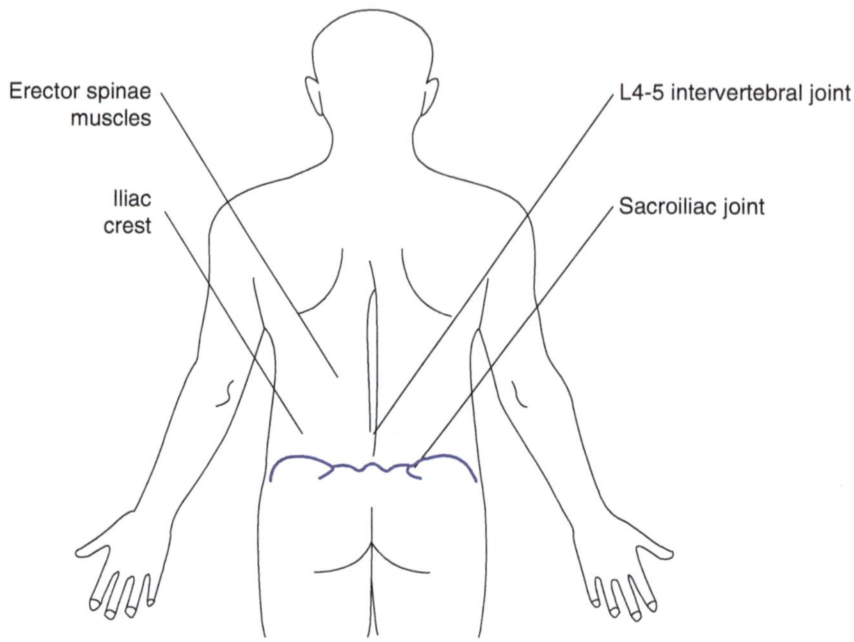

Fig. 2.48 Some surface anatomy landmarks

to squat and stand from squatting position, hip flexion (L2, L3), and hip extension (L5, S1).

- **Position:** watch as patient changing position.
- **Asses Trendelenburg sign (see hip joint exam):** the patient stands on affected side and then raises the normal side, and in a positive test, the unsupported side will drop.
- **Note the type of gait:** normal gait passes through two phases stance and swing phases. The stance phase consists of heel strike, mid-stance, and toe off. The swing phase has an acceleration and deceleration components. A common gait abnormality in rheumatology is antalgic gait which is simply short stance phase gait due to pain in one of the lower limb joints.

2.7.2.3 Palpation

Start palpation while patient is in prone position. Palpate spinous processes over the midline from cervical down to sacral regions (Fig. 2.51). You may percuss to illicit severe tenderness that might indicate discitis. You may palpate now the para-median spinal structures including muscles (for tenderness and/or spasms as majority of low back pain is caused by muscle strain and/or spasm), interspinous or supraspinous ligaments, and facet joints. Keep in mind the low specificity of these techniques. You may palpate now iliac crests for tenderness suggestive of enthesitis a hall mark feature of spondyloarthritis, while palpation observe any skin and/or soft tissue fluid collection suggestive of an abscess. Palpate the dimples of Venus at the level of S2 as the sacroiliac joints lie beneath them. It can be severely tender in sacroiliitis. You may ask the patient to stand and put his feet on a chair or a stool and you can posteriorly identify by palpation two bony prominences: the ischial tuberosity medially and the GT laterally. The sciatic nerve can be palpated in the area between these two. Severe tenderness can be illicit in patients with sciatica and/or piriformis syndrome.

2.7.2.4 Range of Motion

This can be assessed by asking the patient to perform the following:

- **Flexion:** ask patient to bend forward with extended knees and bring fingers to floor. The distance between the long finger and the floor can be documented and used to follow up response of treatment in cases of spondylitis.
- **Extension:** stabilize the pelvis and ask the patient to extend the back as much as possible. Figure 2.52 demonstrates ROM of cervical spine.

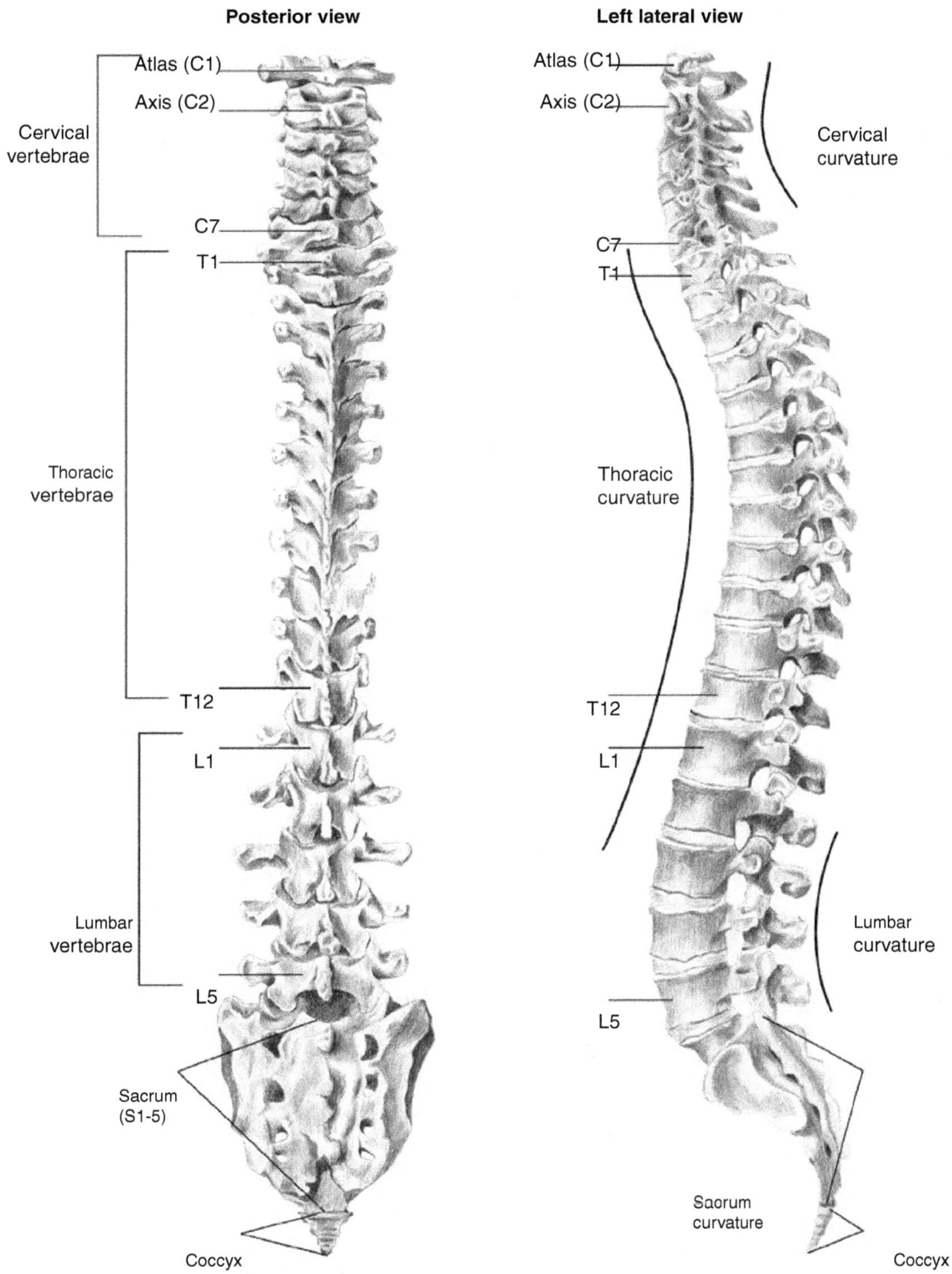

Fig. 2.49 Vertebral column [7]

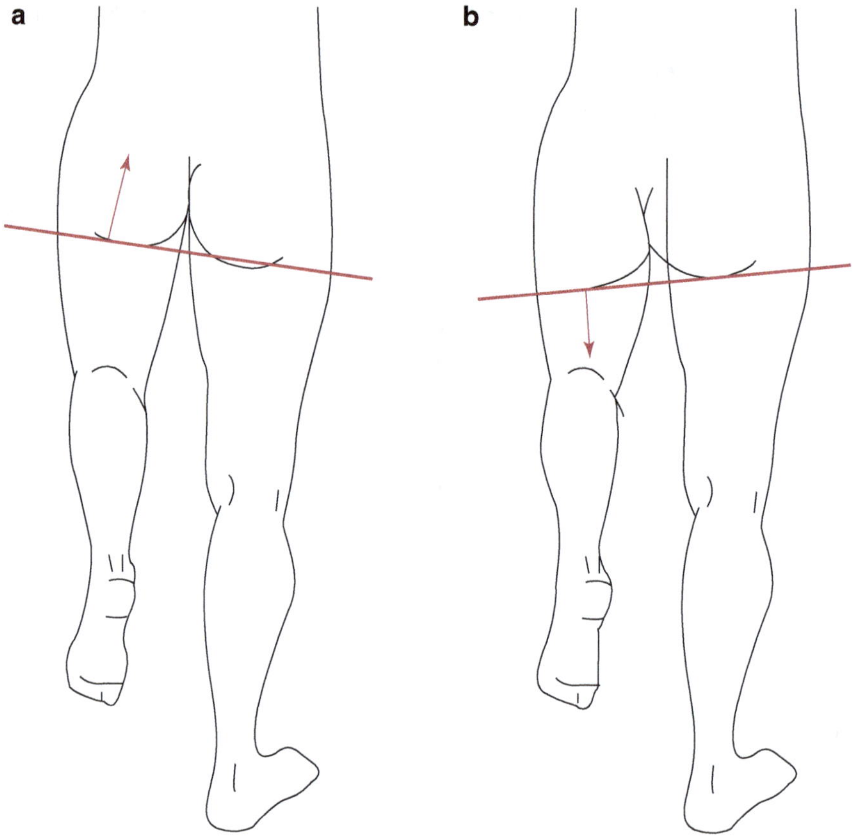

Fig. 2.50 Trendelenburg sign: (**a**) normal response. (**b**) Abnormal response with drop of the pelvis in the unsupported leg due to weakness in the opposite (supported leg) muscles. This will result in Trendelenburg gate

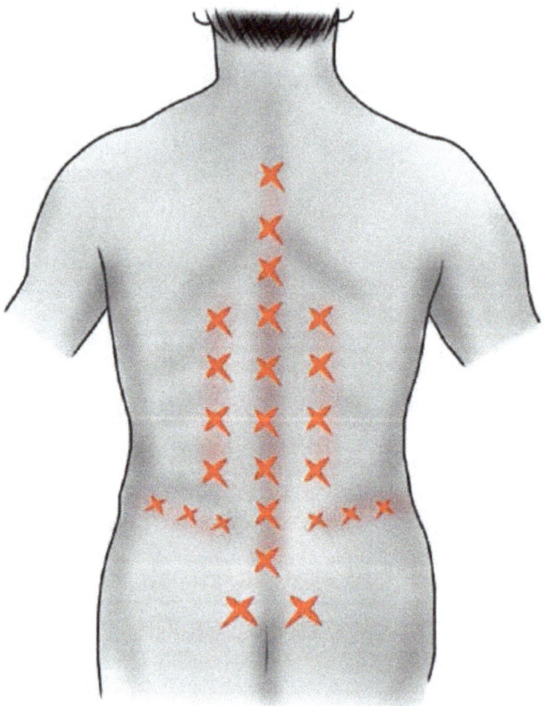

Fig. 2.51 Areas for palpation

- **Lateral flexion:** The patient may stand against the wall and bend laterally and trying to slide the fingers to fibula. The distance between the long finger and the fibula or the floor can be documented and used in monitoring response to therapy in spondylitis (Fig. 2.53).
- **Thoraco-lumbar rotation:** This is best examined while the patient is sitting at the edge of the bed. Ask the patient to turn to the side without moving the pelvis as much as possible; up to 70° can be achieved normally. This movement can be checked passively to examine for any tenderness, stiffness, limitation, and/or end of range stiffness (Fig. 2.53).

2.7.2.5 Special Tests

Straight Leg Raising Test (SLRT) (Fig. 2.54)

This is to test for radiculopathy of L5-S1. Keep the patient in supine position with extended hip and knee. Then flex the hip slowly until a complaint of shooting radicular pain or tightness is

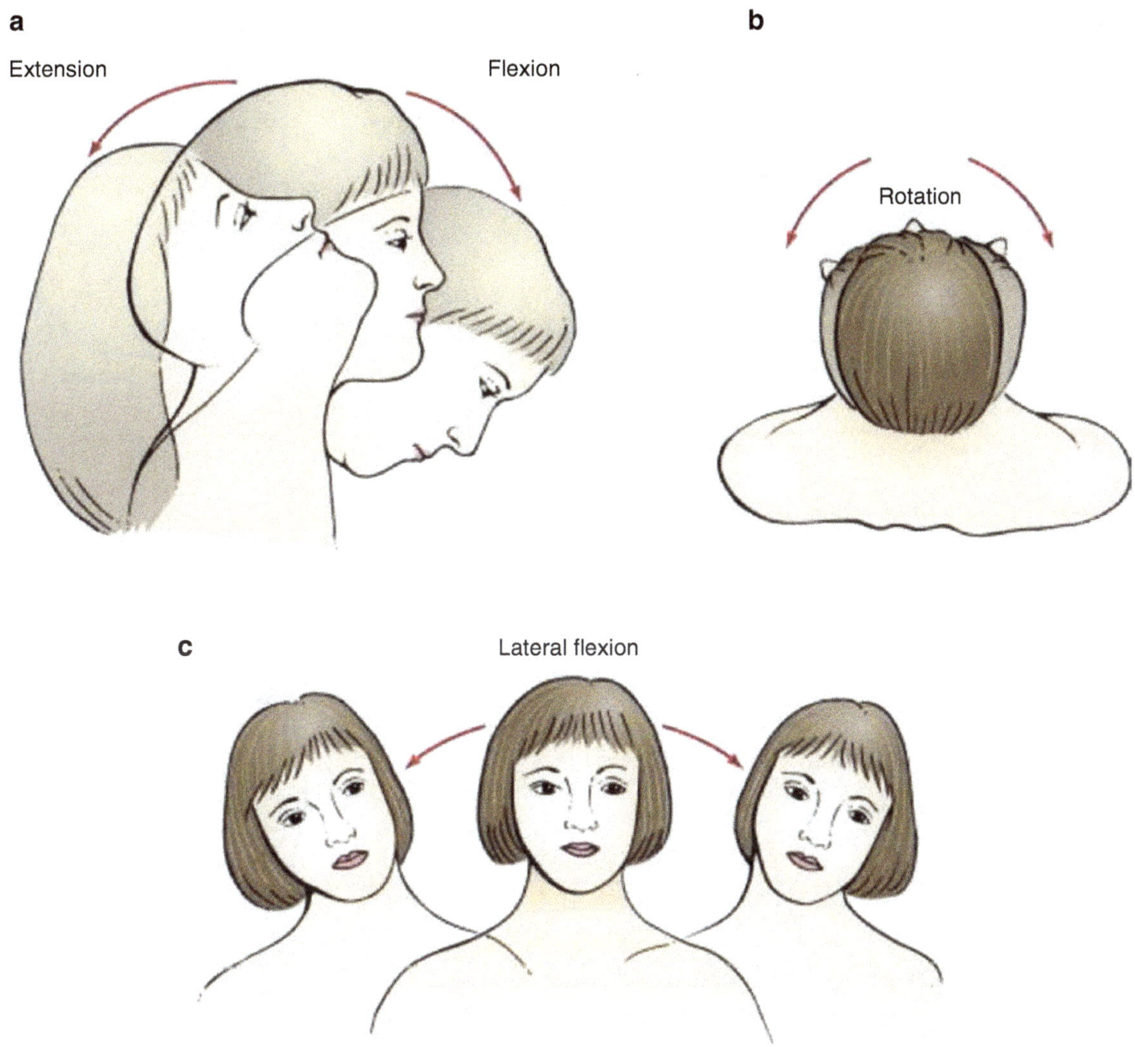

Fig. 2.52 Range of motion of cervical spine

reached. The test can be considered positive with classical radiation of the pain at 30–70° of leg elevation. Just lowering the examined leg few degrees before the pain appeared and then passive dorsiflexion of the ankle is performed as a confirmatory technique. Symptoms should recur in strongly positive test (Fig. 2.55).

Slump Test (Fig. 2.56)

This test is performed again to look for radiculopathy at L5-S1. The patient should be sitting at the edge of the bed with both arms stabilized over the back. You should flex the outstretched extended leg to be examined by holding the toes or the ankle, and at the same time, ask the patient to flex the neck and bring the chin to the chest wall. A shooting radicular pain might result from this stretch indicating a positive test.

Sacroilliac Joints Exam

Patrick test and compression test: perform (FABER test (flexion abduction external rotation test)) Fig. 2.57. Flex the hip, abduct, and externally rotate it while the other leg in extended. Then compress over the iliac crest of the extended leg and over the knee of the flexed leg. A positive test produces pain in the sacroiliac joint of the leg being tested.

Modified Schober's Test

This test is to assess for limited lumbar spinal flexion. Mark the PSIS (dimple of venous) by

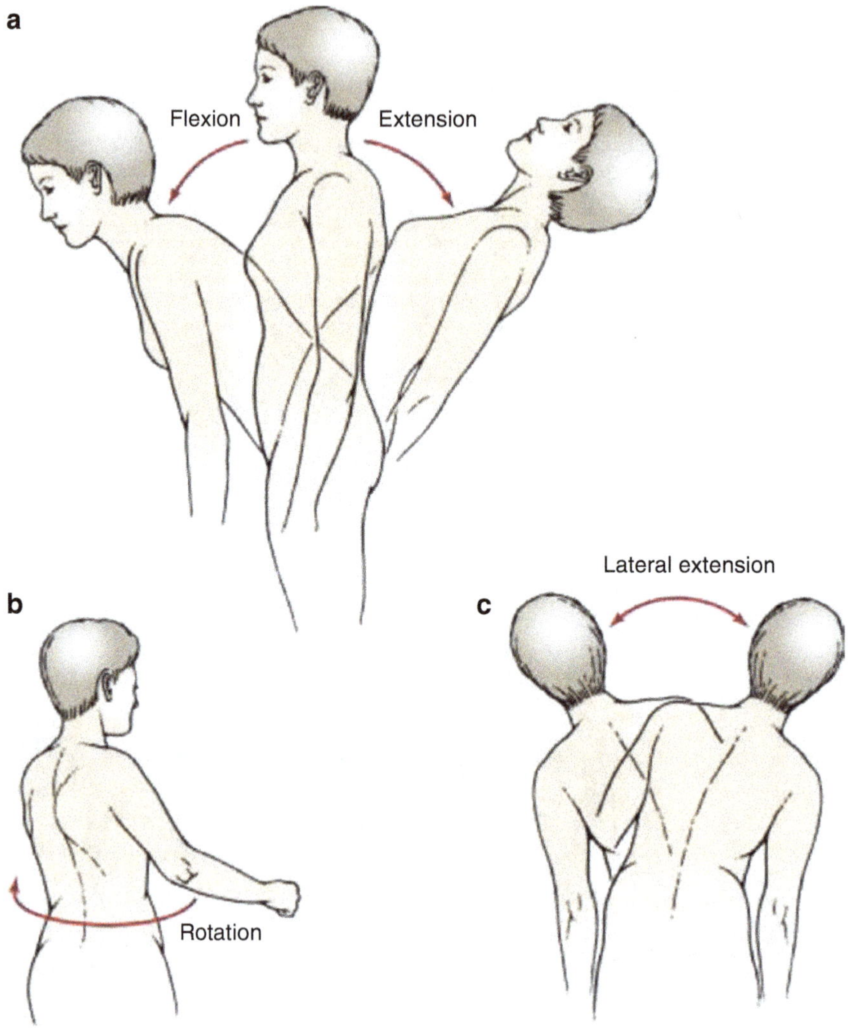

Fig. 2.53 Range of motion of thoraco-lumbar spine. (**a**) Flexion and extension. (**b**) Rotation. (**c**) Lateral extension

drawing a line connecting both points. At the center of this line, mark a point. Using a tape measure placed at the center point, mark 5 CM below this line and 10 CM above this line. Then ask the patient to bend forward without bending the knees. Now, measure the distance between the points. The distance between the two points should be more than 15 by 5 additional CM (≥ 20 CM). Any movement that results in less than this is considered abnormal.

Neurological Exam

Detailed neurological exam should be conducted. The motor findings are reliable and should direct further intervention with the patient. One of the simple tests to perform is muscle bulk by a tape measure from a fixed bony prominence. More than 1 CM difference is considered abnormal for patients presenting with radicular symptoms. Rectal tone (S3,4,5) should be also performed in the right clinical settings. Fig. 2.58 represents a quick tool to examine in brief the roots of the lower limb. This quick approach includes examining the power of the following movement (note that it goes for simplicity from 2 to 5): hip flexion (L2), knee extension (L3), ankle dorsiflexion (L4), big toe extension (L5), and ankle plantar flexion (S1). This is in addition to sensory exam as shown in Fig. 2.59. Sensory level is an important clinical finding to be determined in the right clinical setting in order to decide on further intervention and follow-up. Figure 2.60 summarizes the steps of back examination.

Acknowledgments The authors are grateful for the help provided by Mohamed Cheikh, Mawaddah Al hadeedi, Abdulrahman Kabli, Rehab Simsim, and Waleed Hafiz in composing this chapter.

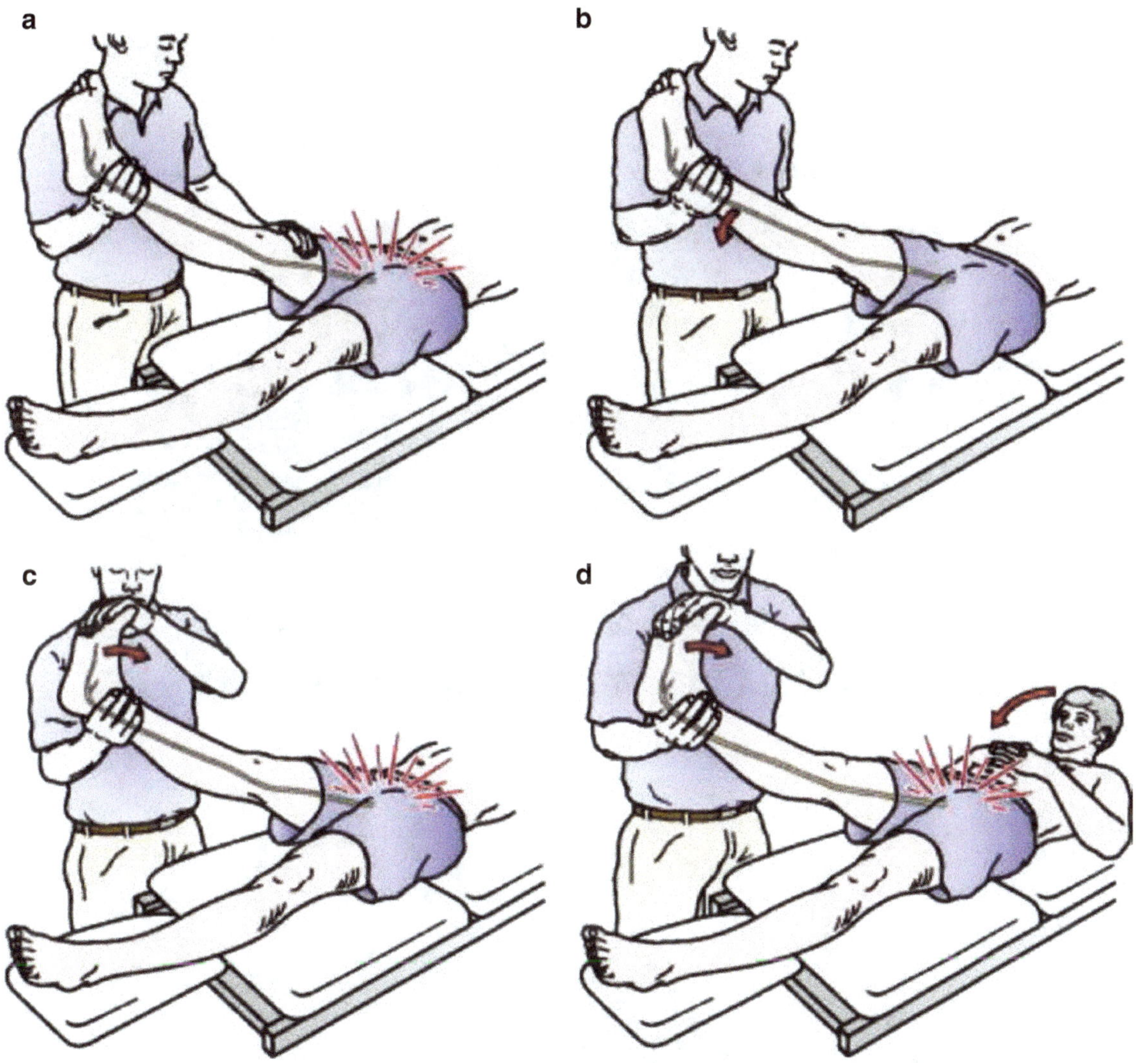

Fig. 2.54 Straight leg raising test

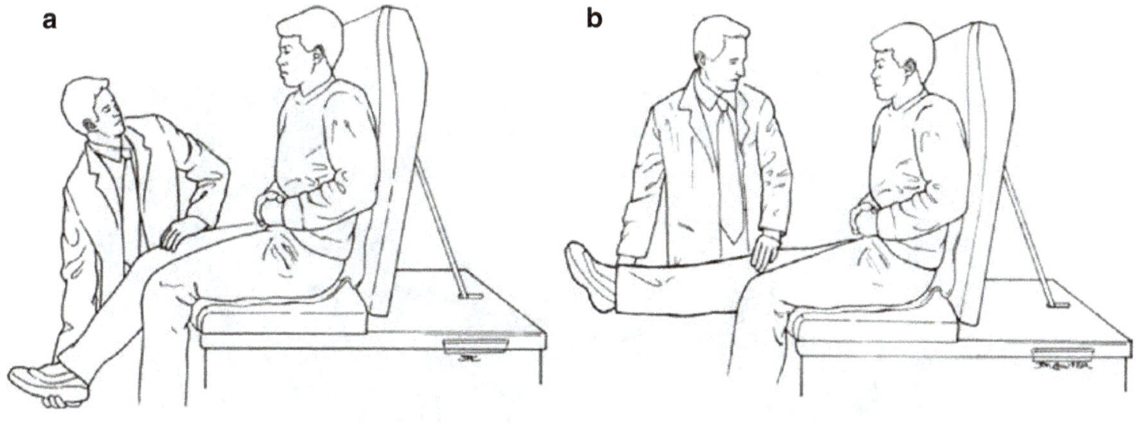

Fig. 2.55 Another approach to test for radiculopathy at L5-S1

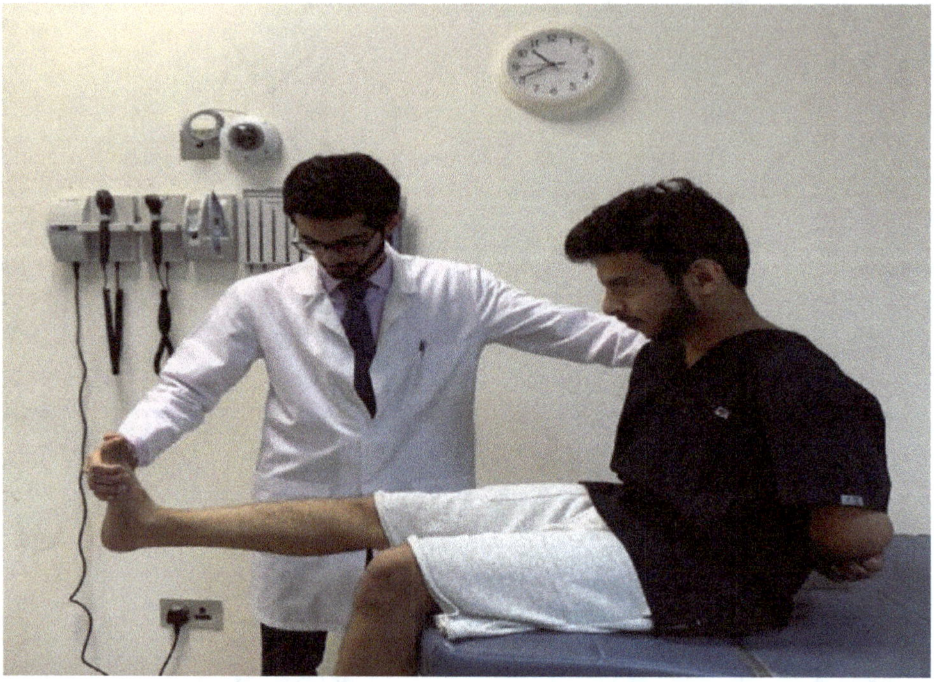

Fig. 2.56 Slump test

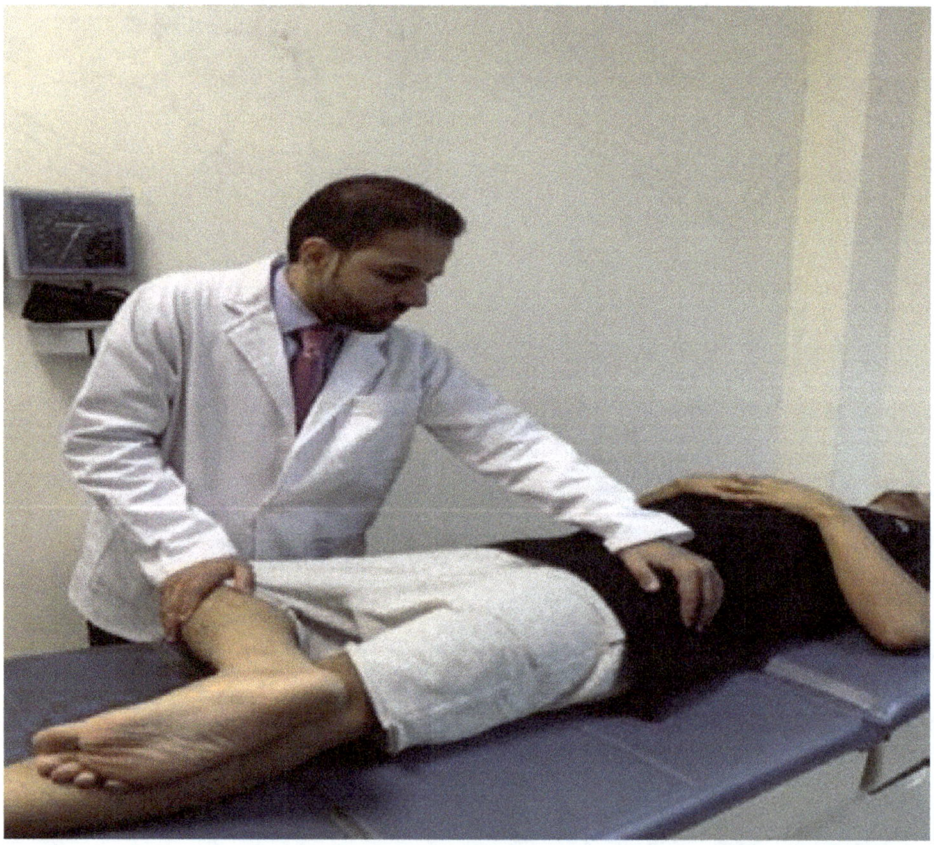

Fig. 2.57 FABER test (flexion abduction external rotation test)

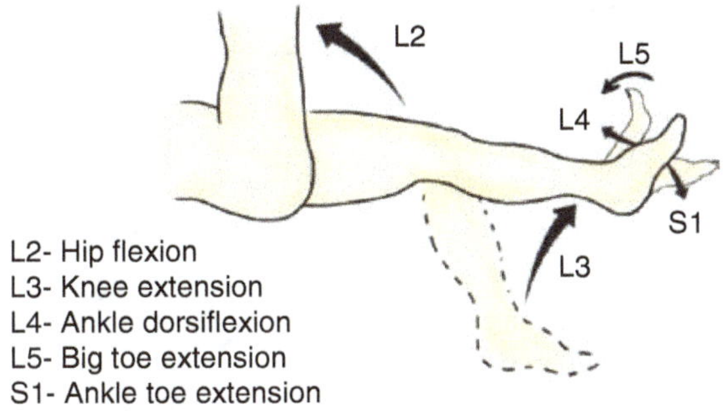

Fig. 2.58 Quick tool to examine in brief the roots of the lower limb

Fig. 2.59 Levels of principle dermatomes of the lower limb

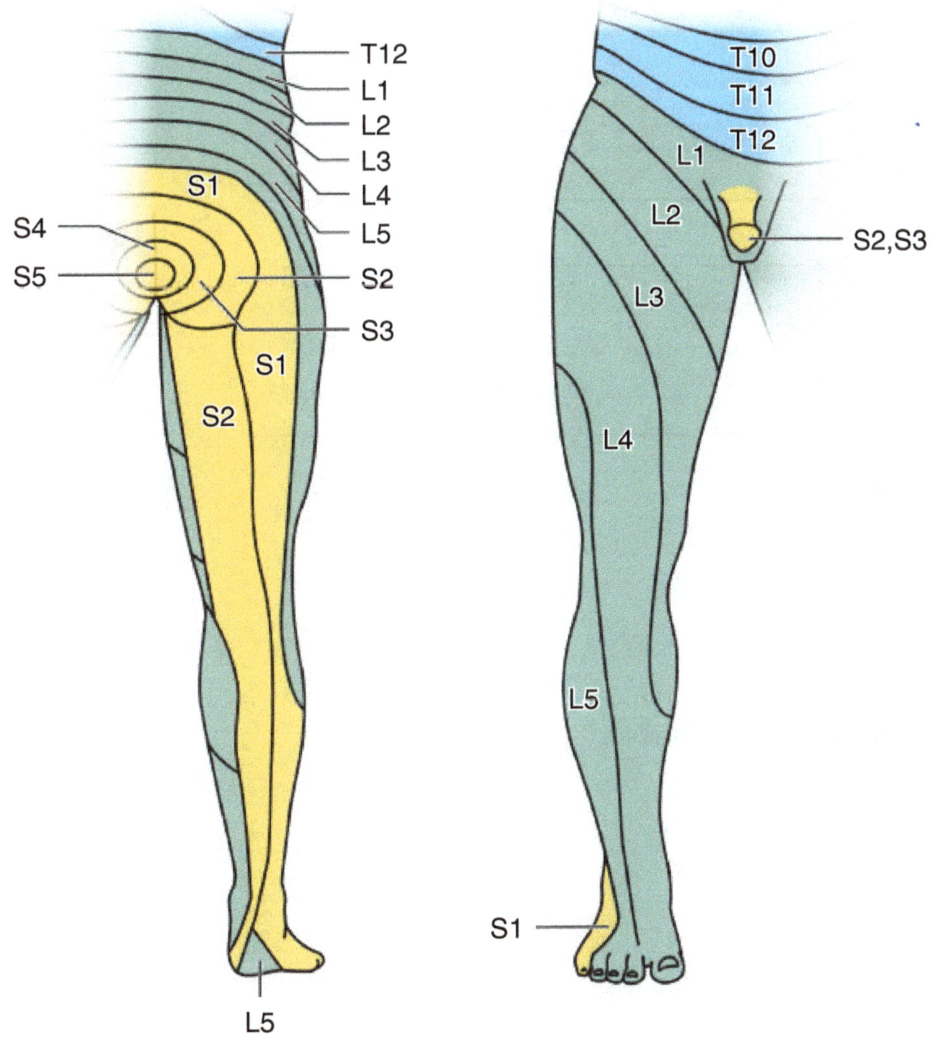

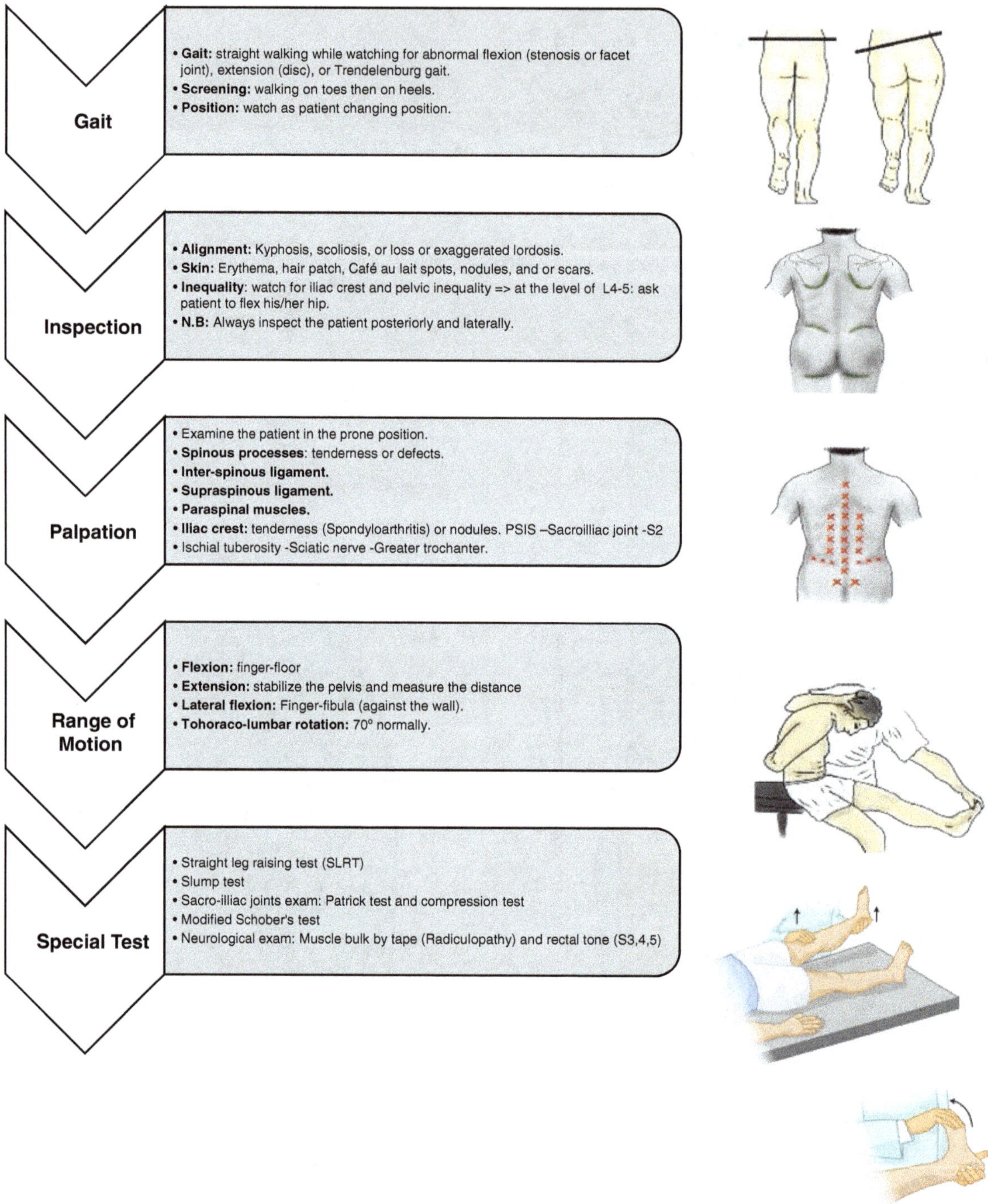

Fig. 2.60 Summary of back examination

References

1. Woolf AD, Walsh NE, Akesson K. Global core recommendations for a musculoskeletal undergraduate curriculum. Ann Rheum Dis. 2004;63(5):517–24.
2. Woolf AD, Pfleger B. Burden of major musculoskeletal conditions. Bull World Health Organ. 2003;81(9):646–56.
3. Almoallim H, et al. Sensitivity of standardised musculoskeletal examination of the hand and wrist joints in detecting arthritis in comparison to ultrasound findings in patients attending rheumatology clinics. Clin Rheumatol. 2012;31(9):1309–17.
4. Solomon DH, et al. The rational clinical examination. Does this patient have a torn meniscus or ligament of the knee? Value of the physical examination. JAMA. 2001;286(13):1610–20.
5. Hegedus EJ, et al. Physical examination tests of the shoulder: a systematic review with meta-analysis of individual tests. Br J Sports Med. 2008;42(2):80–92; discussion 92
6. Yoganandan N, Dickman CA, Benzel EC. Spine surgery. Copyright © 2012, Copyright © 2012, 2005, 1999 by Saunders, an imprint of Elsevier Inc.
7. Hansen JT. Netter's Clinical Anatomy. Copyright © 2014, Copyright © 2014 by Saunders, an imprint of Elsevier Inc.

3

Rheumatic Diseases: Lab Testing, Interpretation and Classification

Altaf Abdulkhaliq and Manal Alotaibi

3.1 Introduction

Generally the diagnosis of rheumatic diseases is based on a set of clinical, serological, and radiological measures. The discovery of a novel test that appears to be considerably more disease-specific and preferably sensitive would be of value for the early diagnosis and immediate, effective therapy to prevent joint deterioration, functional disability, and unfavorable disease outcome [1].

However, components of acute phase reaction proteins such as erythrocyte sedimentation rate (ESR) and C-reactive protein (CRP) or rheumatoid factor (RF) lack specificity and sensitivity and could not reach the expectation of earlier diagnosis of specific rheumatic diseases. Therefore, the discovery of immunologic laboratory tests has occupied a valued position in the practice of rheumatology and has helped define the pathophysiology of various rheumatic conditions such as the immunologic basis of rheumatoid arthritis (RA) [2, 3] and explain the contribution of genetic basis to autoimmune disease via the association of ankylosing spondylitis (AS) with HLA-B27 and RA with certain HLA-DR alleles [4, 5].

Hence the salient existence of such immunologic laboratory tests has assisted the more precise diagnosis of diverse rheumatologic conditions that may share some clinical characteristics. In addition, these tests can provide valuable evidence concerning disease manifestation, activity and prognosis, and therapeutic monitoring.

Essential terms concerning the laboratory tests are needed to be defined such as sensitivity, specificity, and positive and negative predictive values. *Sensitivity* refers to the ability of the test to detect the proportion of patients with a disease which usually have a positive test result. However, *specificity* refers to the ability of the test to detect the proportion of patients without the disease which usually have a negative test result. *Predictive value* refers to the likelihood of disease or non-disease based on a positive or negative test result. A high positive predictive value test indicates that the patient with a positive test result most probably has the disease in question. Similarly, a high negative predictive value test indicates that the patient with a negative test result most likely does not have the disease in question.

Unlike with sensitivity and specificity of the test, the predictive value is markedly affected by disease prevalence. For instance, the predictive value of a positive rheumatologic test in patients with polyarthralgia is likely to be higher in a rheumatology clinic than in a family physician's clinic [6].

A. Abdulkhaliq (✉)
College of Medicine, Umm Al-Qura University, Makkah, Saudi Arabia
e-mail: aaabdulkhaliq@uqu.edu.sa

M. Alotaibi
Northwestern University Feinberg School of Medicine, Chicago, IL, USA

Internal Medicine Department, College of Medicine, Umm Al-Qura University, Makkah, Saudi Arabia

The subsequent sections will discuss the step-wise approach to the diagnostic workup of rheumatic diseases and are presented as follows:

- Inflammatory markers (ESR and CRP)
- Rheumatoid factor (RF)
- Antinuclear antibody (ANA) profile, for instance, anti-double-stranded DNA antibodies (anti-dsDNA) and anti-ribonucleic protein (RNP) antibodies
- Other disease-specific antinuclear antibodies and cytoplasmic antibodies
- Complement deficiencies and decreased complement activity in certain medical conditions
- Components and classification of synovial fluid analysis
- Other biochemical tests: renal function tests and urine analysis (this section is not in the scope of the current chapter but it will be discussed in details in the chapter of "Renal System and Rheumatology")

3.1.1 Objectives

By the end of the current chapter, the candidates should be able to:

- Identify the rule of acute phase reaction proteins in rheumatic diseases.
- Interpret the auto-antibodies' results based on clinical findings.
- Classify various types of joint effusions based on clinical and laboratory analysis of synovial fluid.

3.2 Acute Phase Reactants

Acute phase reactants (APRs) or proteins are defined as those proteins whose serum concentrations increase or decrease by at least 25% during inflammatory states. Changes in levels of APR largely result from the effects of cytokines, including interleukin (IL)-6, IL-1 beta, tumor necrosis factor-alpha (TNF-alpha), and interferon gamma.

Serum APR level measurements are useful because they frequently reflect the presence and intensity of an inflammatory process. The assessment of APR may be most helpful in patients with RA, polymyalgia rheumatica, and giant cell arteritis.

However, APR measurements in clinical use are not specific to any particular disease.

The most widely used indicators of the acute phase response are the ESR and CRP [7].

ESR and CRP definitions, measurements, uses, and other important aspects are addressed in Table 3.1.

3.3 Rheumatoid Factor (RF) and Anti-citrullinated Protein Antibody (ACPA)

3.3.1 Definition

RF is an antibody directed against the Fc fragment of immunoglobulin G (IgG). It may be of any isotype: IgG, IgA, IgE, and IgM. RF-IgM is the only one measured in clinical practice. The origin of RF is incompletely understood [7]. ACPAs are antibodies that are targeted against citrulline which is situated on proteins. Important clinical features of RF including measurement and common issues while dealing with it in clinical practice are all addressed in Table 3.2.

3.4 Antinuclear Antibodies (ANAs)

3.4.1 Definition

ANAs are serologic hallmarks of patients with systemic autoimmune disease. These antibodies should be ordered when the clinical assessment of the patient suggests the presence of an autoimmune or connective tissue diseases [7]. Clinical aspects of ANAs are discussed in Table 3.3.

Table 3.1 ESR versus CRP

<table>
<tr><td rowspan="2">Definition</td><td colspan="2">ESR</td><td>CRP</td></tr>
<tr><td colspan="2">ESR is an indirect measurement of serum acute phase protein concentrations, defined as the rate (mm/hour) at which erythrocytes suspended in plasma settle when placed in a vertical tube, reflects a variety of factors, most notably the plasma concentration of fibrinogen [7]</td><td>CRP is defined as a pentameric protein comprised of five identical, non-covalently linked 23-KD subunits arranged in cyclic symmetry in a single plane. It is a component of the innate immune response and has both pro-inflammatory and anti-inflammatory actions. CRP can activate the complement system and enhance the apoptotic cell clearance [7]</td></tr>
<tr><td rowspan="3">Methods of measurement</td><td colspan="2">Cont. ESR</td><td>Cont. CRP</td></tr>
<tr><td>The Westergren method</td><td>The Wintrobe method</td><td rowspan="2">It is measured by immunoassay technique or nephelometry [7]</td></tr>
<tr><td>Uses a 200-mm tube and has a dilution step that correct for the effect of anemia.
It is the preferred method and can detect an ESR more than 50–60 mm/h [7, 8]</td><td>Uses a 100-mm tube and has no dilution step [7, 8]</td></tr>
<tr><td rowspan="2">Sensitivity and specificity</td><td colspan="2">An advanced rate does not diagnose a specific disease, but it does indicate that an underlying disease may exist [7, 8]</td><td>Although CRP is a sensitive reflector of inflammation, it is not specific for inflammation [9]</td></tr>
<tr><td colspan="3">An elevated ESR observed together with a normal CRP is often a false-positive value for the ESR; this may reflect the effects of blood constituents, such as monoclonal immunoglobulins, that are not related to inflammation but that can influence the ESR. However, this conclusion is not always valid. As an example, the ESR may be markedly elevated in patients with active systemic lupus erythematosus (SLE), while the CRP response is muted. These variations may be explained by differences in the production of specific cytokines or their modulators in different diseases [10]</td></tr>
<tr><td>Normal result</td><td>– Normal values for the Westergren method are:
Men = 0–15 mm/h
Women = 0–20 mm/h
Children = 0–10 mm/h
– A normal value does not rule out the disease
– Non-inflammatory conditions that can elevate ESR include aging, female sex, obesity, pregnancy, and race [7, 8]
– The age-adjusted upper limit of normal for ESR is:
Male = age/2
Female = (age+10)/2</td><td colspan="2">– Normal value is less than 0.08 mg/dl
– CRP levels vary with age, sex, and race [7]
– The age-adjusted upper limit of normal for CRP is:
Male = age in years/50
Female = (age in years/50) + 0.6 [9]</td></tr>
</table>

(continued)

Table 3.1 (continued)

Abnormal results	**1-Causes of marked ESR elevation (more than 100 mm/hr):** 1. Infection (bacterial 33%) 2. Connective tissue diseases (gain cell arteritis, polymyalgia rheumatica, SLE, vasculitides 25%) 3. Malignant neoplasms and renal disease 17% 4. Inflammatory disorders 14% [7, 11] **Causes of marked decreased in ESR (0 mm/h):** 1. Afibrinogenemia/ dysfibrinogenemia 2. Agammaglobulinemia 3. Increased plasma viscosity 4. Extreme polycythemia [7, 11]	**Values between 0.3 and 1 mg/dL may indicate:** 1. Minor degrees of inflammation, e.g., periodontitis 2. Minor degrees of metabolic malfunction (non-inflammatory states), e.g., obesity and insulin resistance [7, 9] **Values greater than 1 mg/dL can indicate:** Clinically significant inflammation [9] **Values greater than 8–10 mg/dL may indicate:** 1. Bacterial infection 2. Systemic vasculitis 3. Metastatic cancer 4. Trauma, burns, and surgery [7, 9]
Advantages and disadvantages	1. Inexpensive, familiar, and easy to perform 2. As a patient's condition worsens or improves, the ESR changes are relatively slow [12] 3. A literature review was conducted for all clinical trials and observational studies of disease-modifying medications and corticosteroids in RA to elaborate on the laboratory results of both ESR and CRP before treatment and 4 weeks to 24 weeks after treatment in the same patients, and it has been concluded that the ESR was more sensitive to change than the CRP at 12 weeks and 24 weeks of treatment [13]	1. It rises more quickly and falls more quickly than ESR [11] 2. Measurements of CRP concentrations are of prognostic value in rheumatoid arthritis and can help guide management [11, 13–15] 3. CRP alone may have been in favor as a simple, validated, reproducible, non-age-dependent test for disease activity assessment [12] 4. CRP had been found to be more sensitive and specific marker for diagnosing bacterial infections in SLE compared to procalcitonin (PCT) [14, 15]. However, further meta-analysis report of studies describing the role of PCT or CRP as a biomarker of infection in autoimmune diseases has determined that PCT test is more specific than sensitive [16]. In addition, a later study has confirmed that PCT test is superior to CRP test in detecting superimposed bacterial infections in active SLE patients, where the PCT levels are correlated with the progression of bacterial infection and used to monitor the response to antibiotic treatment [17]
	The serum protein electrophoresis is the most sensitive test for detecting inflammatory changes. It is the most expensive, directly quantifies the acute phase response [7]. However, there is no single best laboratory test to reflect inflammation The optimal use of acute phase protein measurements may be to obtain several measurements, most commonly ESR and CRP, rather than a single test [9, 14, 18] **Additional tests** suggest systemic inflammation: Low albumin and mild elevation of hepatic alkaline phosphatase [7]	

3.4.2 Methods of Measurement

- Indirect immunofluorescence method using "fluorescence microscope" is the gold standard method to detect ANAs. Currently most laboratories use human epithelial cell tumor line (HEp2 cells) as a substrate to detect antibodies that bind to various nuclear antigens (ANAs) instead of frozen section of rodent organ cells.
- Other methods that can be used for detection of specific ANA include ELISA, immuno-blotting, and Western-blotting methods.

Table 3.2 Characteristics of RF

<table>
<tr><td>Measurement</td><td colspan="3">It is measured by nephelometry, radioimmunoassay, enzyme-linked immunosorbent assay (ELISA), and latex agglutination techniques, although there is no single technique that has clear advantage over others. Automated methods, such as nephelometry and ELISA, tend to be more reproducible than manual methods [7]. The most commonly used technique to measure ACPA is the ELISA for antibodies against cyclic citrullinated peptides (CCP).</td></tr>
<tr><td>Sensitivity and specificity</td><td colspan="3">• The sensitivity of RF in RA has ranged from 26% to 90%
• The reported sensitivity of the RF test in RA has been as high as 90%. However, population-based studies, which include patients with mild disease, have found much lower rates of RF-positive RA (26 to 60%) [19]
• The sensitivity of ACPA testing is similar to RF at around 75%. However it provides much higher specificity rates at around 95%.
• The specificity is 85% [19]
• The specificity to a young healthy population is about 96% [19, 23]</td></tr>
<tr><td rowspan="3">Positive results
Cont. Positive results</td><td colspan="3">The common denominator for the production of RF (positive result) is chronic immune stimulation</td></tr>
<tr><td>Healthy individuals</td><td>Non-rheumatic disorders</td><td>Rheumatic disorders</td></tr>
<tr><td>• RF is present in some healthy individuals, especially the elderly (3–25%), male and female are affected equally, and only 20% of cases is the RF level significantly positive
• RF has been found in 2–4% of young, healthy individuals [7, 20]</td><td>1. Chronic infection, e.g., AIDS, mononucleosis, parasitic infections, chronic viral infection (hepatitis B or hepatitis C (HCV) 54–76%), chronic bacterial infections (tuberculosis, subacute bacterial endocarditis (SBE))
2. Cryoglobulinemia 40–100% especially with HCV
3. Pulmonary disorders, such as sarcoidosis
4. Malignancy, especially after radiation or chemotherapy and B-cell neoplasms
5. Primary biliary cirrhosis [7, 21]

Positive ACPA can be found in the following non rheumatological diseases:
1. Active tuberculosis (varying rates)
2. Chronic obstructive pulmonary disease (5%)
3. It is important to note that unlike RF, ACPAs are rarely found in patient with hepatitis C virus</td><td>1. Rheumatoid arthritis 26–90%
2. Sjögren's syndrome 75–95%
3. Mixed connective tissue disease 50–60%
4. Mixed cryoglobulinemia (types II and III) 40–100%
5. Systemic lupus erythematosus 15–35%
6. Polymyositis or dermatomyositis 5–10%
7. Sarcoidosis 15% [7, 21]

ACPAs were found to be positive in the following autoimmune diseases:
1. SLE and primary Sjogrens Syndrome (17%)
2. Psoriatic arthritis (8-16%)</td></tr>
<tr><td>Can RF be used as a screening test?</td><td colspan="3">• Measurement of RF is a poor screening test to diagnose or exclude rheumatic disease in either healthy populations or in those with arthralgias but have no other symptoms or signs of rheumatic disease [20]
• In a population study, it has been found that the presence of both RF and anti-citrullinated protein antibody (ACPA) in apparently healthy people substantially increases the probability of having RA. So the presence of the two autoantibodies (RF and ACPA) is associated with a relative risk of approximately 70% [20]
• The RF has a higher positive predictive value (PPV) if ordered more selectively in patients with a modest or higher chance of having an RF-associated rheumatic disease such as RA, Sjögren's syndrome, or the mixed cryoglobulinemia syndrome. Included in this group are patients with prominent morning stiffness, with sicca symptoms, or with arthralgia or arthritis in a rheumatoid distribution (i.e., symmetric polyarthritis involving small joints) [19]
• Higher titers of RF have a higher positive predictive value for RA [19].</td></tr>
</table>

(continued)

Table 3.2 (continued)

Significance of measuring RF and ACPA in known RA cases	• RF-positive patients with RA may experience more aggressive and erosive joint disease and extra-articular manifestations than those who are RF-negative. Similar findings have been observed in juvenile idiopathic arthritis [19] • RF status may be useful in combination with other indicators, including HLA-DRB1, CRP, the ESR, and severity of synovitis on physical exam, to predict progression of radiographic changes in RA patients and to guide treatment [19] • ACPA positivity was found to be associated with more erosive joint disease, especially apparent on radiographs. It was also found to be better at predicting these changes than RF
RF and monitoring of rheumatic diseases	• The change in RF level does not reflect changes in RA disease activity • RF should not be used routinely to monitor RA disease activity in clinical practice • RF titer may fall with effective treatment of RA in patients who are originally RF-positive [19, 22] • In Sjögren's syndrome, the disappearance of a previously positive RF may herald the onset of lymphoma. That is why some clinicians check RF repeatedly in patients with Sjögren's syndrome. The clinical utility of this practice, however, has not been critically assessed [19, 22]
Antibody status (ACPA/RF)	• RF and ACPA have the potential to revert and convert during the early course of disease. Fluctuations in RF and ACPA were not associated with clinical outcomes [23] • Repeated measurement of ACPA or RF during the first year after onset of arthritis does not offer major additional information [24]
RF and the mortality	Patients with RA with positive RF, especially IgA and IgM isotypes, carry a risk of dying earlier than patients without these serological findings [25]

Table 3.3 ANA characteristics

Positive result	• It is defined as the level of ANA that exceeds the level seen in 95% of the normal population • In most laboratories, this level is a titer of 1:40 to 1:80 that are reported positive • Clinically significant titers in laboratories that use HEp-2 cells as substrate are usually more than or equal to 1:160 [7, 26]			
	Systemic autoimmune diseases	**Organ-specific autoimmune diseases**	**Infections**	**Others**
	1. SLE 93% 2. Scleroderma 85% 3. Mixed connective tissue disease 93% 4. Polymyositis/ dermatomyositis 61% 5. Rheumatoid arthritis 41% 6. Rheumatoid vasculitis 33% 7. Sjögren's syndrome 48% 8. Drug-induced lupus 95–100%; (e.g., procainamide, hydralazine, isoniazid, and quinidine) 9. Discoid lupus 15% 10. Pauci-articular juvenile chronic arthritis 71% [7, 26]	1. Hashimoto's thyroiditis 46% 2. Graves' disease 50% 3. Autoimmune hepatitis 63–91% 4. Primary biliary cirrhosis 10–40% 5. Primary autoimmune cholangitis 100% 6. Idiopathic pulmonary arterial hypertension 40% 7. Multiple sclerosis 25% [7, 26]	– Chronic infectious diseases (mononucleosis, hepatitis C infection, SBE, tuberculosis, and HIV) and some lympho-proliferative diseases – Malignancy (rare) with the exception of dermatomyositis [7, 26]	1. Highly relatives of patient 15–25% 2. Normal elderly 20% 3. Patients with silicone breast implant 15–25% [7]
Is ANA used as a screening test?	– No, it cannot be used as a screening test for autoimmune disorders in the general healthy population in the absence of clinical findings as it may be present in very low specificity titer in normal population 5% – It should be used primarily as a confirmatory test when the clinicians strongly suspect SLE or autoimmune disorders – A patient with a negative ANA and strong clinical evidence of SLE or another SS-A-associated disease, antibodies to SS-A should be ordered [7]			

(continued)

Table 3.2 (continued)

Is ANA used for monitoring diseases?	– No, there is no evidence about use of ANA titer as a monitor to follow disease activity in patients with SLE and autoimmune diseases [7]				
ANA patterns	The pattern type has been found to have relatively low sensitivity and specificity for different autoimmune disorders, and thus tests for specific antibodies have largely replaced the use of patterns				
	The homogeneous or diffuse pattern Represents antibodies to the DNA-histone complex (anti-DNP (LE cell) and anti-histone)	**The peripheral or rim pattern** It is produced by antibodies to DNA (anti-dsDNA) and antibodies to nuclear envelope antigens (anti-laminin)	**The speckled pattern** It is produced by antibodies to SM, RNP, Ro/SSA, La/SSB, Scl-70, centromere, proliferating cell nuclear antigen (PCNA), and other antigens	**The nucleolar pattern** It is produced by antibodies to RNA polymerase I, proteins of the small nucleolar RNP complex (fibrillarin, Mpp10, and hU3–55 K), Th/to, B23, PM-Scl, and NOR-90, and other antigens	**The centromeric pattern** It is produced by antibodies to proteins that are associated with the site of chromosomal constriction. Proteins designated, CENP-A, CENP-B, CENP-C, etc., are only present on active centromeres (i.e., during meiosis and mitosis) [7, 26]
ANA titer	– The presence of very high concentrations of antibody (titer >1:640) should arouse suspicion of an autoimmune disorder. However, its presence alone is not diagnostic of disease – If no initial diagnosis can be made, it is our practice to watch the patient carefully over time and to exclude ANA-associated diseases – An accurate ANA with titer, in combination with a full history and physical examination, can be extremely useful in the diagnosis and exclusion of connective tissue disease [26]				
	– 1–2% of patients who have active and untreated SLE will have a negative ANA, and this is because the substrate used in ANA test did not contain a sufficient antigen to detect SS-A antibodies – 10–15% of SLE patients will become ANA-negative with treatment or inactive disease – 40–50% of SLE patients with end-stage renal disease on dialysis will become an ANA-negative [7]				

3.5 ANA Profile

3.5.1 Definition

An ANA profile consists of many antibodies to measure specific ANAs for certain nuclear antigens. It should be performed when the screening test for ANA is positive and when further information is needed regarding the type of autoimmune disorder [7].

ANA profile antibodies and their specific uses are elaborated on Table 3.4.

3.6 Other Disease-Specific Antinuclear Antibodies and Cytoplasmic Antibodies

These antibodies have to be ordered individually according to the set-up diagnosis based on patient's symptoms and clinical presentations, and they include:

1. **Anti-histone antibodies**: sensitive (70%) for drug-induced lupus but nonspecific and have limited diagnostic utility because they may also be present in patients with SLE. The best test to conduct in patient with suspected drug-induced lupus is antichromatin antibody test, not anti-histone antibody test [7]. However, anti-histone antibody test might be of value in patients having a positive ANA test with history of exposure to medications-induced lupus, such as procainamide (Pronestyl) and isoniazid (INH) [27].
2. **Anti-Th/To antibodies**: crest syndrome 20% [7].
3. **Anti-SCL-70 antibodies** (topoisomerase1): diffuse **systemic** sclerosis (scleroderma) 22–40% [7]. They are highly specific but not sensitive for scleroderma [29].
4. **Anti-tRNA synthetase antibodies (anti-Jo-1, other)**: polymyositis 20–30% [7].
5. **Anti-neutrophil cytoplasmic antibodies (ANCAs)**:

Table 3.4 The standard ANA profile

Measured antibodies	Associated diseases	Characteristics
Anti-dsDNA antibodies (directed against double-stranded DNA)	SLE 60%	– It is very specific for SLE – It is the one that used to follow SLE disease activity; high titers are associated with lupus nephritis or a flare of lupus activity [27]
Anti-U1 RNP antibodies (ribonuclear protein)	SLE 30%, progressive systemic sclerosis (low titer), and mixed connective tissue disease (MCTD)	– A very high level of this antibody is highly suggestive of MCTD [28]
Anti-SM (smith) antibodies	SLE 30%	– It is very specific for SLE – The sensitivity of anti-dsDNA and anti-Sm for the diagnosis of SLE is relatively low – Anti-Sm antibodies generally remain positive, even when a patient has entered remission; therefore it may be especially useful diagnostically when a SLE patient's disease is relatively inactive [28]
Anti-SS-A (RO) antibodies	SLE 30%, primary Sjögren's syndrome 70%, neonatal lupus, sub-acute cutaneous lupus (SCLE), secondary Sjögren's syndrome (rare) [28]	
Anti-SS-B (LA) antibodies	SLE 15%, Sjögren's syndrome 60% [28]	
Anti-centromere antibodies	Crest syndrome 98%, diffuse scleroderma 22–36% [28]	

- **Cytoplasmic anti-neutrophil cytoplasmic antibodies (C-ANCA)**, the most common c-ANCA target is serine proteinase-3: granulomatous polyangiitis (GPA) (Wegener granulomatosis) 90%, microscopic polyangiitis (MPA), eosinophilic granulomatosis with polyangiitis (EGPA) (rare). Its titer can correlate with GPA disease activity [30].
- **Perinuclear anti-neutrophil cytoplasmic antibodies (P-ANCA)**, the most common p-ANCA target is myeloperoxidase: MPA 70%, pauci-immune glomerulonephritis, and EGPA, or myeloperoxidase (−)—ulcerative colitis, chronic infection, and neoplasm (rare) [30].

6. **Anti-mitochondrial antibodies (AMAs)**: primary biliary cirrhosis 80% [7].
7. **Antibodies to the gp210 and p62 proteins of the nuclear pore complex**: primary biliary cirrhosis 10–40% [7].

3.7 Circulatory Complement Components

Complement is an important effector pathway of innate immunity and has a role in the pathogenesis of some of rheumatic conditions, namely, SLE.

Causes of Decreased Circulatory Complement Components

- Hereditary complement deficiencies (decreased production)
- Secondary complement deficiencies (acquired) [31]

3.7.1 Mechanism of Acquired Complement Deficiencies

1. Increased level of circulatory immune complexes (increased consumption of complements) due to:
   - Infectious causes
   - Glomerulonephritis
   - Rheumatic diseases:
     (a) **SLE**: Low C4 and C3 levels occur in about 50% of patients with SLE. Levels of C3 and C4 are decreased with increased severity of SLE, especially renal disease. A return to normal levels with treatment is a good prognostic sign. Serial observations reveal decreased levels preceding clinical exacerbation.
     (b) **Cryoglobulinemia**: The complement profile shows decreased levels of C4 and C2 with normal or slightly lowered C3.
     (c) **Systemic vasculitis** especially polyarteritis nodosa, urticarial vasculitis: 50% of patients with polyarteritis may have decreased serum complement levels. Its values can be helpful in assessing the clinical course, especially the response to therapy.
     (d) **RA** with extra-articular manifestation (rare) [7, 32].
2. Reduced hepatic synthesis (uncommon)
3. Loss of complement components in the urine (rare) [30]

3.8 Synovial Fluid Analysis

The presentation of one or more hot, swollen joints is a common medical emergency, and synovial fluid aspiration, the so-called arthrocentesis, is the single most important test helping in the diagnosis of different types of arthropathies [33].

Therefore, specialized laboratories analyze synovial fluid to either confirm the diagnosis of crystal-associated arthropathies, support the diagnosis of septic arthritis, or establish other rheumatologic diagnoses such as mono-arthritis or joint effusion [34].

The complete analysis of synovial fluid includes macroscopic (gross appearance), microscopic, and specific stain tests to provide detailed information about the joint's condition and helps in establishing the diagnosis and treatment [35]. Description of macroscopic analysis of synovial fluid includes color, clearance, volume, and viscosity. However, the microscopic analysis can differentiate between inflammatory and infectious processes by measuring a complete leukocyte count. In addition, a differential of the synovial WBC count should be ordered, so that if the results came positive for infectious process, the performance of Gram-stain and culture tests will provide guidance to diagnosis and/or antibiotic therapy [36].

Microscopic examination specifically can also allow the detection and identification of various types of crystal by using polarized light microscope. Refer to Table 3.5 for an overview on important issues as regards arthrocentesis and synovial fluid analysis. However, Table 3.6 shows the classification of joint effusions into normal, inflammatory, non-inflammatory, and septic effusion based on clinical and laboratory analysis of synovial fluid with the causes of each type [37, 38]. Indications, contraindications, complications, and specimen analysis of synovial fluid are presented in Table 3.5. Classification and causes of joint effusions based on laboratory analysis of synovial fluid are presented in Table 3.6. Fig. 3.1 is the clinical diagnostic approach for painful peripheral joint.

3.9 Key Notes

- The likelihood diagnosis of septic arthritis is markedly increased with higher synovial WBC counts. It has been illustrated that for synovial WBC count the likelihood ratio (LR) of having septic arthritis is as follows [34]:
  - WBC count <25,000/μL, the LR is 0.32 at 95% CI.
  - WBC count ≥25,000/μL the LR is 2.9 at 95% CI.
  - WBC count >50,000/μL, the LR is 7.7 at 95% CI.

Table 3.5 Overview on arthrocentesis and synovial fluid analysis

Indications	Contraindications	Complications	Specimen handling	Synovial fluid analysis
1. According to the American College of Rheumatology (ACR), synovial fluid analysis should be performed in the febrile patient with an acute flare of established arthritis to rule out superimposed septic arthritis 2. Unexplained joint, bursa, or tendon sheath swelling 3. Suspected crystal-induced arthritis 4. Repeated aspiration and analysis may be indicated to follow up the response of septic arthritis to treatment and may also be valuable for diagnosis of some cases of gout in which the initial aspirate does not have detectable crystals [34]	1. There is no absolute contraindication 2. Bleeding diatheses and cellulites are considered as relative contraindication; it could make the approach to the joint space difficult due to the overlying swelling [37]	1. Infection 2. Hemarthrosis 3. Pain 4. Cartilage injury 5. Vasovagal syncope [37]	1. Aspiration is performed under aseptic technique with quick transfer of specimen for culture to the sterile tubes and plated as soon as possible 2. If the transfer is delayed more than 6 hours, many changes would occur, for example, decrease in leukocyte count or decrease in crystal numbers [36]	The WBC count and the percentage of PMN cells can help to differentiate between non-inflammatory, inflammatory, and septic joint conditions. These tests are the best diagnostic tool available for detecting bacterial arthritis [36] 1. Gram stain and cultures should be ordered even with relatively low suspicion of infection 2. Crystal search using polarized light microscopy 3. Chemistry analysis should not be routinely ordered [37]

Table 3.6 Classification and causes of joint effusions based on laboratory analysis of synovial fluid

Fluid features	Normal	Non-inflammatory	Inflammatory	Pyarthrosis or septic arthrosis
Appearance	Clear, highly viscous, colorless	Clear to slightly turbid	Slightly turbid, yellow or yellow-green	Turbid to very turbid, yellow or yellow-green
Total WBC count/ MM3	0–200	200–2000	2000–50,000	50,000–150,000
Polymorphonuclear cell (PMN)%	<10%	<20%	20–70%	≥75%
Causes		– Osteoarthritis – Joint trauma – Hypertrophic osteoarthropathy – Neuropathic arthropathy – Avascular necrosis [37, 38]	– RA – Gout – Pseudogout – Psoriatic arthritis – AS – SLE – Reiter syndrome – Sarcoidosis – Rheumatic fever – Wegener granulomatosis – Infectious arthritis – SBE [37, 38]	1. It is a septic arthritis until proven otherwise by the fluid culture 2. Pseudosepsis include reactions to intra-articular injections, gout, Reiter's syndrome, leukemic infiltration, and RA [37, 38]

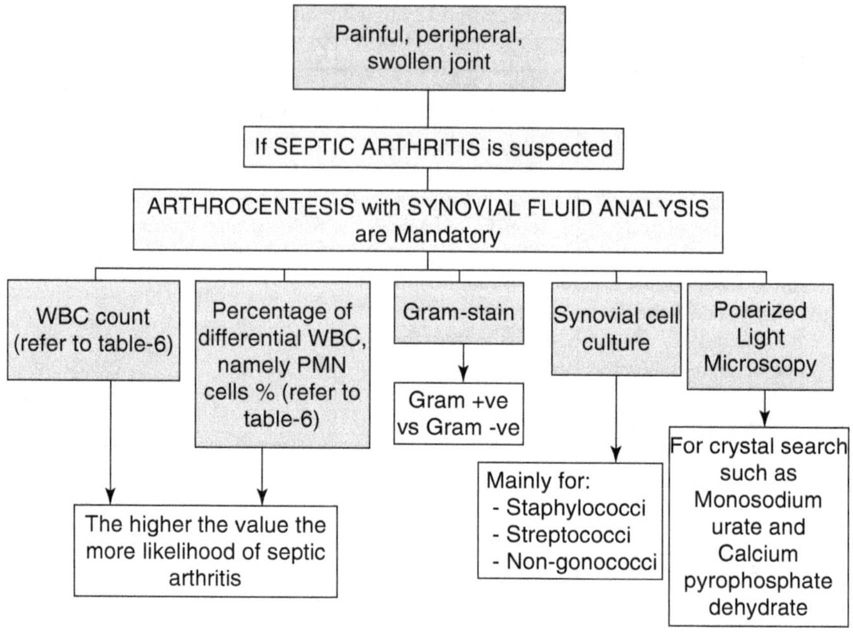

Fig. 3.1 Clinical approach for painful peripheral joint

  - WBC count >100,000/μL, the LR is 28.0 at 95% CI.
- Polymorphonuclear (PMN) cells of 90% are associated with increasing likelihood of septic arthritis of 3.4, while if the percentage of PMN cells is less than 90%, the likelihood decreases down to 0.34 (95% CI) that supports the clinician's suspicion of bacterial arthritis [38, 39].
- Eosinophilic cells in the synovial fluid suggest parasitic infection, allergy, Lyme disease, or neoplasm [40].
- If there is a suspicion of joint involvement by a neoplasm or hematologic malignancy, formal cytological examination should be ordered [38].
- Hemorrhagic effusions may be caused by hemophilia, anticoagulation or other bleeding diathesis, scurvy, trauma, neuropathic arthropathy, and tumors [38].

3.9.1 Gram Stain

- It is used to identify common bacterial organisms (Gram-positive versus Gram-negative coverage) for the diagnosis and treatment of septic arthritis.
- It may be the only evidence of infection with fastidious organisms that are not able to grow in culture [41].
- The *sensitivity* is not known precisely.
  - In non-gonococcal bacterial arthritis, it is in range from 50% to 70%.
  - In gonococcal arthritis, it is <10% [41].
- The *specificity* is high when performed and interpreted by an experienced clinician or technician [41].

3.9.2 Synovial Fluid Culture

- The synovial fluid samples should be routinely sent for culture for staphylococci followed by streptococci and Gram-negative bacteria (non-gonococcal causes).
- Antibiotics should generally not be given prior to joint aspiration [42, 43].
- **The specificity**: Positive synovial culture should be indicative of septic arthritis in 100% of cases with exclusive of contamination and laboratory error [42, 43].
- **The sensitivity**: It is not known precisely because of the lack of an alternative gold standard. The joint aspirate should be cultured for

Table 3.7 Gout versus pseudo-gout

	Crystal	Shape	Birefringence	Color of crystals parallel to axis of red-plate compensator
Gout	Monosodium urate (MSU)	Needle	Negative	Yellow
Pseudogout	Calcium pyrophosphate dehydrate (CPPD)	Rhomboid or rectangular	Positive	Blue [48]

N. gonorrhoeae or unusual organisms (TB, Lyme disease, or fungal infections) when the history is suggestive [42, 43].

3.9.3 Diagnostic Approach

- It should be noted that the absence of organisms on Gram stain or a negative subsequent synovial fluid culture does not rule out the diagnosis of septic arthritis especially if clinical suspicion is high. In such condition, an empirical treatment of the case as septic arthritis should be implemented [44–46].
- Moreover, it has been suggested that the "gold standard" for the diagnosis of septic arthritis is the level of clinical suspicion by an expert physician in the management of patients with musculoskeletal disease [35, 45].
- Similarly, another study had concluded that combining Gram stain and culture of synovial fluid with clinical follow-up is the best approach used to detect patients missed by Gram stain and culture alone [36].

3.9.4 Crystal Search Using Polarized Light Microscopy

Polarized light microscope (PLM) is a fundamental tool for detection and identification of various types of crystals present in synovial fluid depending on their shape (needle, rhomboid, cigar-shaped, etc.) birefringence, location (intracellular or extracellular), and quantity (scarce or plentiful). The obtained results of PLM help the clinicians in diagnosing and managing a case of monoarthritis. However, the presence of artifacts in microscopic analysis can confuse the inexperienced observer; therefore, a suitable interpretation of the synovial fluid analysis using PLM requires at least two experienced observers [47]. The microscopic features of common types of crystals that can differentiate between clinical cases of gout and pseudogout are illustrated in Table 3.7.

3.10 Summary

Due to the fact that musculoskeletal symptoms are exceedingly common compared with the prevalence of systemic rheumatic disease, the pretest probability of systemic rheumatic disease in the population is rather low compared with musculoskeletal symptoms that are nearly ubiquitous. Therefore, establishing the diagnosis of a rheumatic disease may require exclusion of other differential diagnoses that present in a similar fashion. Even the disease established-guidelines, which are often used by clinicians, perform poorly during the assessment of a patient presenting with new polyarthritis [49]. As a consequence, widely used laboratory tests can be very specific and permit rapid diagnosis and appropriate management. However, clinicians should be aware of the false-positive tests that may result in inappropriate management and unnecessary concern.

Generally, serum rheumatologic tests are most helpful for confirming a clinically suspected diagnosis. For instance, testing for RF is appropriate when suspecting RA, Sjögren's syndrome, or cryoglobulinemia, whereas ANA testing is highly sensitive for SLE and drug-induced lupus. Although an elevated ESR is a sensitive test for polymyalgia rheumatica and temporal arteritis, its specificity is quite low. In addition, ESR levels are frequently linked to the disease activity in rheumatoid arthritis and may found to be of value for monitoring therapeutic response. However, anti-double-stranded

DNA antibodies are usually associated with lupus nephritis, and their titer often correlates with disease activity in SLE. On the other hand, cytoplasmic anti-neutrophil cytoplasmic antibody test is highly sensitive and specific for GPA.

In order to increase the utility and decrease the cost-effectiveness of the laboratory testing of rheumatic disease, these tests should be used more selectively and avoid absolute overreliance on lab results. However, a logic combination of the clinical background and the testing results would provide the appropriate diagnosis of the rheumatic conditions. Finally, as Shmerling RH has stated, "the passage of time is one of most useful diagnostic tests as many patients with musculoskeletal symptoms improve over time without a clear diagnosis" [50].

Acknowledgments The authors would like to thank Dr. Waleed Hafiz for his assistance in the development of this chapter.

Abbreviations

(IL)-6	Interleukin-6
AMAs	Anti-mitochondrial antibodies
ANA	Antinuclear antibody profile
ANCAs	Anti-neutrophil cytoplasmic antibodies
anti-dsDNA	Anti-double-stranded DNA antibodies
anti-gp210	Anti-glycoprotein-210 antibodies
anti-p62	Anti-protien-62 antibodies
anti-SCL-70	Anti-topoisomerase1 antibodies
anti-Th/To	Antibodies to Th/To ribonucleoprotein
APRs	Acute phase reactants or proteins
AS	Ankylosing spondylitis
C4 and C3	Complements
C-ANCA	Cytoplasmic anti-neutrophil cytoplasmic antibodies
CI	Confidence interval
CRP	C-reactive protein
EGPA	Eosinophilic granulomatosis with polyangiitis
ELISA	Enzyme-linked immunosorbent assay
ESR	Erythrocyte sedimentation rate
GPA	Granulomatous polyangiitis
HEp2 cells	Human epithelial cell tumor line
HLA-B27	Human leukocyte antigen B27
HLA-DR	Human leukocyte antigen MHC class II
IgG	Immunoglobulin G
IL-1	Interleukin-1
INH	Isoniazid
LR	Likelihood ratio
MPA	Microscopic polyangiitis
MPA	Myeloperoxidase
P-ANCA	Perinuclear anti-neutrophil cytoplasmic antibodies
PLM	Polarized light microscope
PMN	Polymorphonuclear cells
Pronestyl	Procainamide
RF	Rheumatoid factor
RNP	Anti-ribonucleic protein antibodies
SLE	Systemic lupus erythematosus
TNF-alpha	Tumor necrosis factor-alpha
WBC	White blood cell count

References

1. Szodoray P, Szabo Z, Kapitany A, Gyetvai A, Lakos G, Szanto S, et al. Anti-citrullinated protein/peptide autoantibodies in association with genetic and environmental factors as indicators of disease outcome in rheumatoid arthritis. Autoimmun Rev. 2010;9(3):140–3.
2. Rose HM, Ragan C, et al. Differential agglutination of normal and sensitized sheep erythrocytes by sera of patients with rheumatoid arthritis. Proc Soc Exp Biol Med. 1948;68(1):1–6.
3. Ragan C. The history of the rheumatoid factor. Arthritis Rheum. 1961;4:571–3.
4. Schlosstein L, Terasaki PI, Bluestone R, Pearson CM. High association of an HL-A antigen, W27, with ankylosing spondylitis. N Engl J Med. 1973;288(14):704–6.
5. Stastny P. Mixed lymphocyte cultures in rheumatoid arthritis. J Clin Invest. 1976;57(5):1148–57.
6. Lane SK, Gravel JW Jr. Clinical utility of common serum rheumatologic tests. Am Fam Physician. 2002;65(6):1073–80.
7. Sterling G. Rheumatology secrets. 3rd Edition. Philadelphia, PA; 2002. ISBN: 9780323641869.
8. Simple rule for calculating normal erythrocyte sedimentation rate. Br Med J. 1983;286(6364): 557–8.

9. Kushner I, Rzewnicki D, Samols D. What does minor elevation of C-reactive protein signify? Am J Med. 2006;119(2):166. e17-28
10. Gaitonde S, Samols D, Kushner I. C-reactive protein and systemic lupus erythematosus. Arthritis Rheum. 2008;59(12):1814–20.
11. Fincher RM, Page MI. Clinical significance of extreme elevation of the erythrocyte sedimentation rate. Arch Intern Med. 1986;146(8):1581–3.
12. Crowson CS, Rahman MU, Matteson EL. Which measure of inflammation to use? A comparison of erythrocyte sedimentation rate and C-reactive protein measurements from randomized clinical trials of golimumab in rheumatoid arthritis. J Rheumatol. 2009;36(8):1606–10.
13. Ward MM. Relative sensitivity to change of the erythrocyte sedimentation rate and serum C-reactive protein concentration in rheumatoid arthritis. J Rheumatol. 2004;31(5):884–95.
14. van Leeuwen MA, van der Heijde DM, van Rijswijk MH, Houtman PM, van Riel PL, van de Putte LB, et al. Interrelationship of outcome measures and process variables in early rheumatoid arthritis. A comparison of radiologic damage, physical disability, joint counts, and acute phase reactants. J Rheumatol. 1994;21(3):425–9.
15. Kim HA, Jeon JY, An JM, Koh BR, Suh CH. C-reactive protein is a more sensitive and specific marker for diagnosing bacterial infections in systemic lupus erythematosus compared to S100A8/A9 and procalcitonin. J Rheumatol. 2012;39(4):728–34.
16. Wu JY, Lee SH, Shen CJ, Hsieh YC, Yo PH, Cheng HY, et al. Use of serum procalcitonin to detect bacterial infection in patients with autoimmune diseases: a systematic review and meta-analysis. Arthritis Rheum. 2012;64(9):3034–42.
17. Yu J, Xu B, Huang Y, Zhao J, Wang S, Wang H, et al. Serum procalcitonin and C-reactive protein for differentiating bacterial infection from disease activity in patients with systemic lupus erythematosus. Mod Rheumatol. 2014;24(3):457–63. https://doi.org/10.3109/14397595.2013.844391. Epub 2013 Oct 21. PMID: 24252006.
18. Gabay C, Kushner I. Acute-phase proteins and other systemic responses to inflammation. N Engl J Med. 1999;340(6):448–54.
19. Shmerling RH, Delbanco TL. How useful is the rheumatoid factor? An analysis of sensitivity, specificity, and predictive value. Arch Intern Med. 1992;152(12):2417–20.
20. Lawrence RC, Felson DT, Helmick CG, Arnold LM, Choi H, Deyo RA, et al. Estimates of the prevalence of arthritis and other rheumatic conditions in the United States. Part II. Arthritis Rheum. 2008;58(1):26–35.
21. Shmerling RH, Delbanco TL. The rheumatoid factor: an analysis of clinical utility. Am J Med. 1991;91(5):528–34.
22. van der Heijde DM, van Riel PL, van Rijswijk MH, van de Putte LB. Influence of prognostic features on the final outcome in rheumatoid arthritis: a review of the literature. Semin Arthritis Rheum. 1988;17(4):284–92.
23. Nishimura K, Sugiyama D, Kogata Y, Tsuji G, Nakazawa T, Kawano S, et al. Meta-analysis: diagnostic accuracy of anti-cyclic citrullinated peptide antibody and rheumatoid factor for rheumatoid arthritis. Ann Intern Med. 2007;146(11):797–808. https://doi.org/10.7326/0003-4819-146-11-200706050-00008. PMID: 17548411.
24. Mjaavatten MD, van der Heijde DM, Uhlig T, Haugen AJ, Nygaard H, Bjorneboe O, et al. Should anti-citrullinated protein antibody and rheumatoid factor status be reassessed during the first year of followup in recent-onset arthritis? A longitudinal study. J Rheumatol. 2011;38(11):2336–41.
25. Sihvonen S, Korpela M, Mustila A, Mustonen J. The predictive value of rheumatoid factor isotypes, anti-cyclic citrullinated peptide antibodies, and anti-neutrophil cytoplasmic antibodies for mortality in patients with rheumatoid arthritis. J Rheumatol. 2005;32(11):2089–94.
26. Solomon DH, Kavanaugh AJ, Schur PH, American College of Rheumatology Ad Hoc Committee on Immunologic Testing G. Evidence-based guidelines for the use of immunologic tests: antinuclear antibody testing. Arthritis Rheum. 2002;47(4):434–44.
27. Smeenk R, Brinkman K, van den Brink H, Termaat RM, Berden J, Nossent H, et al. Antibodies to DNA in patients with systemic lupus erythematosus. Their role in the diagnosis, the follow-up and the pathogenesis of the disease. Clin Rheumatol. 1990;9(1 Suppl 1):100–10.
28. Tokano Y, Yasuma M, Harada S, Takasaki Y, Hashimoto H, Okumura K, et al. Clinical significance of IgG subclasses of Anti-Sm and U1 ribonucleoprotein antibodies in patients with systemic lupus erythematosus and mixed connective tissue disease. J Clin Immunol. 1991;11(6):317–25.
29. Moder KG. Use and interpretation of rheumatologic tests: a guide for clinicians. Mayo Clin Proc. 1996;71:391–6.
30. Seo P, Stone JH. The antineutrophil cytoplasmic antibody-associated vasculitides. Am J Med. 2004;117(1):39–50.
31. Saeki T, Ito T, Yamazaki H, Imai N, Nishi S. Hypocomplementemia of unknown etiology: an opportunity to find cases of IgG4-positive multi-organ lymphoproliferative syndrome. Rheumatol Int. 2009;30(1):99–103.
32. Guidelines for the initial evaluation of the adult patient with acute musculoskeletal symptoms. American College of Rheumatology Ad Hoc Committee on Clinical Guidelines. Arthritis Rheum. 1996;39(1):1–8.

33. Al-Shakarchi ICG. The treatment and care of hot, swollen joints. Rheumatol Pract. 2009;7(7):9.
34. Swan A, Amer H, Dieppe P. The value of synovial fluid assays in the diagnosis of joint disease: a literature survey. Ann Rheum Dis. 2002;61(6): 493–8.
35. Dieppe PAH, Swan A. Synovial fluid analysis. Annu Meet Int Soc Technol Assess Health Care Meet 2000; 16 (112).
36. Mathews CJ, Kingsley G, Field M, Jones A, Weston VC, Phillips M, et al. Management of septic arthritis: a systematic review. Ann Rheum Dis. 2007;66(4):440–5.
37. Margaretten ME, Kohlwes J, Moore D, Bent S. Does this adult patient have septic arthritis? JAMA. 2007;297(13):1478–88.
38. Kerolus G, Clayburne G, Schumacher HR Jr. Is it mandatory to examine synovial fluids promptly after arthrocentesis? Arthritis Rheum. 1989;32(3):271–8.
39. Krey PR, Bailen DA. Synovial fluid leukocytosis. A study of extremes. Am J Med. 1979;67(3):436–42.
40. Kortekangas P, Aro HT, Tuominen J, Toivanen A. Synovial fluid leukocytosis in bacterial arthritis vs. reactive arthritis and rheumatoid arthritis in the adult knee. Scand J Rheumatol. 1992;21(6):283–8.
41. Kay J, Eichenfield AH, Athreya BH, Doughty RA, Schumacher HR Jr. Synovial fluid eosinophilia in Lyme disease. Arthritis Rheum. 1988;31(11):1384–9.
42. Dougados M. Synovial fluid cell analysis. Baillieres Clin Rheumatol. 1996;10(3):519–34.
43. Shmerling RH. Synovial fluid analysis. A critical reappraisal. Rheum Dis Clin N Am. 1994;20(2):503–12.
44. Sorlin P, Mansoor I, Dagyaran C, Struelens MJ. Comparison of resin-containing BACTEC plus aerobic/F* medium with conventional methods for culture of normally sterile body fluids. J Med Microbiol. 2000;49(9):787–91.
45. Sharp JT, Lidsky MD, Duffy J, Duncan MW. Infectious arthritis. Arch Intern Med. 1979;139(10):1125–30.
46. Coakley G, Mathews C, Field M, Jones A, Kingsley G, Walker D, et al. BSR & BHPR, BOA, RCGP and BSAC guidelines for management of the hot swollen joint in adults. Rheumatology. 2006;45(8):1039–41.
47. Kaandorp CJ, Van Schaardenburg D, Krijnen P, Habbema JD, van de Laar MA. Risk factors for septic arthritis in patients with joint disease. A prospective study. Arthritis Rheum. 1995;38(12):1819–25.
48. Martinez-Castillo A, Nunez C, Cabiedes J. Synovial fluid analysis. Reumatol Clin. 2010;6(6):316–21.
49. Harrison BJ, Symmons DP, Barrett EM, Silman AJ. The performance of the 1987 ARA classification criteria for rheumatoid arthritis in a population based cohort of patients with early inflammatory polyarthritis. American Rheumatism Association. J Rheumatol. 1998;25(12):2324–30.
50. Shmerling RH. Diagnostic tests for rheumatic disease: clinical utility revisited. South Med J. 2005;98(7):704–11; quiz 12-3, 28

4

Treatment of Systemic Rheumatic Diseases: Drug Categories

Layla Borham and Waleed Hafiz

4.1 Introduction

Over the past two decades, better understanding of the immunopathophysiologic basis of various rheumatic diseases led to the discovery of variety of drugs that are now approved and widely used in clinical practice. These drugs are categorized into the following categories: nonsteroidal anti-inflammatory drugs (NSAIDs), synthetic disease-modifying anti-rheumatic drugs (sDMARDs), biological disease-modifying anti-rheumatic drugs (bDMARDs), corticosteroids and drugs used in crystal-induced arthritis. Few other drugs are also used by rheumatologists. These include anti-resorptive drugs and symptom-specific drugs.

4.2 Learning Objectives

By the end of this chapter, you should be able to:

- Recall the main drug categories used in the treatment of systemic rheumatic diseases
- Explain the mechanism of action, dosages, indications, adverse effects, cautions, contra-indications and pregnancy category of each drug

4.3 Nonsteroidal Anti-Inflammatory Drugs (NSAIDs)

Nonsteroidal anti-inflammatory drugs (NSAIDs) are effective anti-inflammatory, antipyretic and analgesic drugs. Although they differ widely in their chemical class, they share the property of blocking the production of prostaglandins (PGs). This is achieved by inhibiting the activity of the enzyme prostaglandin G/H synthase (PGHS), also called *cyclooxygenase* (COX).

There are two different COX isoforms, COX-1 and COX-2. Inhibition of COX-2 by NSAIDs blocks PG production at sites of inflammation, while inhibition of COX-1 in certain other tissues, most importantly platelets and the gastroduodenal mucosa, can lead to common adverse effects of NSAIDs such as bleeding, bruising and gastrointestinal ulceration [1].

In addition to their use in rheumatoid arthritis and osteoarthritis, NSAIDs are widely used in the symptomatic management of other rheumatic diseases characterized by chronic musculoskeletal pain and diverse forms of acute pain.

L. Borham
Clinical Pharmacology Department
Faculty of Medicine, Umm Al-Qura and Cairo University, Makkah, Saudi Arabia
e-mail: borhaml@hotmail.com

W. Hafiz (✉)
Faculty of Medicine, Umm Al-Qura University, Makkah, Saudi Arabia
e-mail: wahafiz@uqu.edu.sa

NSAIDs are associated with elevated cardiovascular disease risk and risk for gastrointestinal bleeding and ulceration [2, 3]. For that, it is important to identify patients with these risks, and if present, avoiding NSAIDs or using intermittent, low-dose and short half-life drugs is advisable. It is also important to know that use of NSAIDs together with aspirin, which is an NSAID too, can increase gastrointestinal toxicity and lead to aspirin resistance [4].

Patients who take regular doses of NSAIDs should undergo periodic assessment of blood pressure, haemoglobin level, electrolytes and renal and liver function tests.

Complete details about different NSAIDs are shown in Table 4.1

4.4 Synthetic Disease-Modifying Anti-Rheumatic Drugs (sDMARDs)

This category consists of drugs that have been used as first-line therapies in the majority of systemic rheumatic diseases. Although their precise mechanism of action is still incompletely understood, they have both anti-inflammatory and immunomodulatory effects.

Generally, the choice of a sDMARD therapy should be decided for each patient individually. This should also give attention to patient's age, fertility plans, comorbid conditions and other concomitant drugs. Adverse effects from sDMARDs may cause significant morbidity and mortality. So, appropriate dosing and monitoring for toxicity are required.

4.4.1 Methotrexate

Over the past 25 years, methotrexate has become the sDMARD of choice in the treatment of rheumatoid arthritis and is used in many other rheumatic diseases as well (psoriasis, psoriatic arthritis, polymyositis, dermatomyositis, granulomatosis with polyangiitis, giant cell arteritis, subacute lupus erythematosus, scleroderma and vasculitis).

Methotrexate increases the concentration of adenosine, which is a potent inhibitor of inflammation. It also inhibits the enzyme dihydrofolic acid reductase [5].

The effects of methotrexate can be enhanced by using the subcutaneous form instead of the oral form or by splitting the oral dose (within 12-h window) when doses greater than 15 mg weekly are given [6]. Doses should be adjusted based on renal and hepatic function.

A weekly oral dose of folic acid 5–10 mg given 48–72 h post methotrexate dose protects against mucosal ulceration and keeps folic acid levels optimum [7].

4.4.2 Leflunomide

Leflunomide is approved for the treatment of rheumatoid arthritis. It has both anti-inflammatory and immunomodulatory effects. It inhibits the enzyme dihydroorotate dehydrogenase and pyrimidine synthesis [8].

Loading doses are not used in clinical practice due to gastrointestinal toxicity. Leflunomide is found to have a very long half-life because of its enterohepatic recirculation [9]. It is absolutely contraindicated in pregnancy.

4.4.3 Azathioprine

It is an imidazolyl derivative of mercaptopurine. It antagonizes purine metabolism and may inhibit the synthesis of DNA, RNA and proteins. It also inhibits cellular metabolism [10].

Azathioprine can be effective as a glucocorticoid-sparing agent in remission maintenance therapy, particularly in systemic lupus erythematosus and necrotizing vasculitis.

Table 4.1 Nonsteroidal anti-inflammatory drugs (NSAIDs)

<table>
<tr><th>Mechanism of action</th><th>Indication and doses</th><th>Adverse effects and caution</th><th>Pregnancy and lactation</th></tr>
<tr><td></td><td>Ibuprofen</td><td></td><td>Ibuprofen</td></tr>
<tr><td rowspan="5">Inhibit COX-1 and COX-2 isoenzymes, thus inhibiting prostaglandin synthesis and release of inflammatory mediators</td><td>Pain: 300–800 mg PO q6hrs
Fever: 100–200 mg PO q4–6hrs PRN
Inflammatory diseases: 400–800 mg PO q6–8hrs
Osteoarthritis: 300 mg, 400 mg, 600 mg or 800 mg PO q6–8hrs; not to exceed 3.2 g/day
Rheumatoid arthritis: 300–800 mg PO q6–8hrs; not to exceed 3.2 g/day</td><td rowspan="5">May cause elevated creatinine or liver enzymes in patients with active SLE.
Gastrointestinal complaints like erosion, ulceration or bleeding
Hepatotoxicity, asthma, rashes, itchiness, tinnitus, dizziness, headache and aseptic meningitis (particularly in patients with systemic lupus erythematosus)
Fluid retention and renal toxicity occur less frequently
Drug interactions:
1. Concomitant administration with aspirin will antagonize the irreversible platelet inhibition induced by aspirin
2. Reduce the natriuretic effect of furosemide and thiazides in some patients
3. May also increase lithium plasma levels due to decreased renal clearance
4. Use of NSAIDs with ACE inhibitors may potentiate renal disease states
5. Concomitant administration with prednisone may increase the risk of GIT ulceration</td><td>Pregnancy category: C or D at 30 weeks of gestation or more
May cause premature closure of ductus arteriosus
Lactation: Excreted into breast milk, use not recommended</td></tr>
<tr><td>Naproxen</td><td>Naproxen</td></tr>
<tr><td>Pain: 500 mg PO initially followed by 250 mg PO q6–8hrs PRN; alternatively, 500 mg q12hr. Not to exceed 1250 mg/day PO
Rheumatoid arthritis, ankylosing spondylitis or osteoarthritis:500–1000 mg PO divided q12hrs. Not to exceed 1500 mg/day PO</td><td>Pregnancy category: B or D if used for prolonged periods or near term
Lactation: Excreted into breast milk, use should be carefully evaluated</td></tr>
<tr><td>Meloxicam</td><td>Meloxicam</td></tr>
<tr><td>Rheumatoid arthritis, osteoarthritis or ankylosing spondylitis:
7.5–15 mg PO daily; not to exceed 15 mg/day</td><td>Pregnancy category: C or D at 30 weeks of gestation or more
May cause premature closure of ductus arteriosus
Lactation: Excretion into breast milk is unknown, use not recommended</td></tr>
<tr><td></td><td>Celecoxib</td><td></td><td>Celecoxib</td></tr>
<tr><td>Inhibits COX-2 isoenzymes (does not affect COX-1), thus inhibiting synthesis of prostaglandin and release of the inflammatory mediators</td><td>Rheumatoid arthritis, osteoarthritis or ankylosing spondylitis:
200 mg PO once daily or divided Q12hr</td><td>Headache, hypertension, abdominal pain, nausea and vomiting
Fluid retention and renal toxicity occur less frequently
Increased risk of cardiovascular events and gastrointestinal toxicity</td><td>Pregnancy category: C or D at 30 weeks of gestation or more
May cause premature closure of ductus arteriosus
Lactation: Excreted into breast milk, use should be carefully evaluated</td></tr>
</table>

It can induce severe myelosuppression in patients with low or absent thiopurine methyltransferase (TPMT) activity that is affected by a polymorphism that can be identified by genetic screening [11]. Severe myelosuppression can also occur in patients with normal TPMT activity, and regular monitoring of white blood cell counts is recommended.

Azathioprine interacts with allopurinol and this can lead to fatal myelosuppression. Concomitant use of these two drugs should be avoided.

4.4.4 Hydroxychloroquine

It is an anti-malarial drug and a well-tolerated sDMARD that is now used as a cornerstone therapy in patients with systemic lupus erythematosus and in combination therapy regimens for rheumatoid arthritis [12].

Hydroxychloroquine is more commonly used than chloroquine. It has a very long half-life, attributed to its affinity for melanin-containing cells in the skin. Doses of hydroxychloroquine should not exceed 6.5 mg/kg/day in chronic therapy to minimize the risk of retinal toxicity [13]. Although routine laboratory monitoring is not required, ophthalmologic screening is an essential component of toxicity monitoring.

Diabetic patients initiating hydroxychloroquine should be instructed to follow blood sugars closely because of the hypoglycaemic effects of the drug.

Hydroxychloroquine is considered safe in pregnancy; it is recommended that most pregnant patients with SLE remain on the drug to improve pregnancy outcomes.

4.4.5 Sulfasalazine

It is a sDMARD that has both antimicrobial and anti-inflammatory properties. The exact mechanism of action is unknown. However, it is a 5-aminocyclic acid derivative that inhibits leukotriene synthesis [14].

Sulfasalazine is commonly used as part of combination therapy for rheumatoid arthritis. Its dose should be increased gradually with regular laboratory monitoring to minimize the risk of adverse effects and drug intolerance.

Gastrointestinal intolerance and rash are common side effects. Monitoring complete blood counts, liver transaminases and creatinine levels should be done periodically during therapy [15].

4.4.6 Mycophenolate Mofetil

It is a powerful inhibitor of lymphocyte proliferation that has a potential glucocorticoid-sparing effect. It is used for the treatment of patients with various rheumatic diseases. It inhibits inosine monophosphate dehydrogenase enzyme which decreases T- and B-cell proliferation and antibody production [16].

Mycophenolate mofetil can be used as ā remission induction agent in lupus nephritis and is now increasingly used for remission maintenance treatment of systemic lupus erythematosus and necrotizing vasculitis [17].

It is generally well tolerated, although diar rhoea and leucopenia may necessitate its discontinuation. Complete blood counts should be performed within the first 2 weeks of therapy and then once every 6–8 weeks thereafter if no cytopenia is noted [18].

4.4.7 Cyclophosphamide

It is an alkylating agent and one of the most potent immunosuppressive therapies available. It is a pro-drug which prevents and inhibits cell division [19].

The indications for its use include induction of remission in lupus nephritis. It is also used to treat rheumatoid vasculitis, interstitial lung disease associated with connective tissue diseases and many types of systemic vasculitides.

Although very effective, it has the potential for devastating toxicity both in the short and long term. Its toxicities include myelosuppression, infection, ovarian failure, haemorrhagic cystitis and malignancy including bladder cancer, especially with high cumulative doses.

The intermittent intravenous doses given every 3–4 weeks are associated with less bladder toxicity compared to oral daily doses [20]. To further minimize bladder toxicity, intravenous fluids, anti-emetics and MESNA (2-mercatpoethanesulfonic acid) may be used.

4.4.8 Tofacitinib

Tofacitinib is a targeted sDMARD that is now approved for the treatment of rheumatoid arthritis. It inhibits the enzymes janus kinase 1 (JAK1) and janus kinase 3 (JAK 3) and thus prevents the phosphorylation and activation of signal transducers and activators of transcrip tion (STATs), which transmit extracellular information into the cell nucleus, influencing DNA transcription [21].

The most commonly reported adverse effects which occur in less than 5% of patients treated with tofacitinib are upper respiratory tract infections, headache, diarrhoea and nasopharyngitis. Neutropenia and lymphopenia are also reported in less than 1% of patients and laboratory monitoring is recommended.

4.4.9 Apremilast

This sDMARD is now approved for the treatment of psoriatic arthritis and psoriasis. It is a small molecule inhibitor of phosphodiesterase-4 (PDE4), which breaks down cyclic adenosine monophosphate (cAMP) in inflammatory cells. This results in down-regulation of the expression of a number of the pro-inflammatory factors like tumour necrosis factor alpha (TNFα), interleukin-17, interleukin-23 and many others and up-regulation of the anti-inflammatory interleukin-10.

Headache, back pain, nausea, diarrhoea, fatigue, nasopharyngitis, upper respiratory tract infections and weight loss are common adverse effects and are reported in up to 10% of patients taking apremilast [22].

Complete details about different sDMARDs are shown in Table 4.2.

4.5 Biological Disease-Modifying Anti-Rheumatic Drugs (bDMARDs)

The bDMARDs target specific components of the immune response that are dysregulated and are thought to be the cause of the disease process. These components are called pro-inflammatory cytokines. Tumour necrosis factor (TNF), interleukin-1 (IL-1), interleukin-6 (IL-6) and others

Table 4.2 Synthetic disease-modifying anti-rheumatic drugs (sDMARDs)

Drug name	Mechanism of action	Indication and doses	Adverse effects and caution	Pregnancy and lactation
Methotrexate (Trexall)	Inhibits the enzyme dihydrofolic acid reductase	**Rheumatoid arthritis:** 10–25 mg weekly in single PO dose, not to exceed 30 mg 15–25 mg SC weekly if tablets are not tolerable **Juvenile rheumatoid arthritis:** 10 mg/m^2 PO/IM weekly, then 5–15 mg/m^2 weekly in single dose or in 3 divided doses given q12hrs **Dosing modifications:** Renal impairment 1. CrCl 61–80 mL/min: Give 75% of dose 2. CrCl 51–60 mL/min: Give 70% of dose 3. CrCl 10–50 mL/min: Give 30–50% of dose at normal dosing interval 4. CrCl<10 mL/min: Avoid use Hepatic impairment 1. Bilirubin 3.1–5.0 mg/dL or AST >180 international units/L: Give 75% of dose 2. Bilirubin >5.0 mg/dL: Avoid use	Most commonly ulcerative stomatitis, leucopenia, nausea and abdominal distress A weekly dose of folic acid 5–10 mg given 48–72 h post methotrexate dose protects against mucosal ulceration and keeps folic acid levels optimum High doses can cause severe haematologic and gastrointestinal toxicity Progressive dose-related hepatotoxicity in the form of enzyme elevation occurs frequently, but cirrhosis is rare (< 1%) A rare "hypersensitivity" lung reaction with acute shortness of breath *Drug interactions*: NSAIDs and salicylate administered concomitantly with lower doses of methotrexate, reduce the tubular secretion of methotrexate and may enhance its toxicity Trimethoprim antibiotic may increase the toxicity of methotrexate	Pregnancy category: X Lactation: Excreted into breast milk, do not nurse **Methotrexate toxicity** Leucovorin is an antidote that restores folate and displaces intracellular methotrexate Oral, IV, or IM 15 mg (approximately 10 mg/m^2) every 6 h until methotrexate concentration declines to <0.005 mcg/mL (0.01 μM) If 24-h S_{cr} increases 50% over baseline, 24-h methotrexate concentration is >2.27 mcg/mL (5 μM, or 48-h methotrexate concentration is >0.409 mcg/mL (0.9 μM); increase leucovorin dosage immediately to 150 mg (approximately 100 mg/m^2) IV every 3 h until methotrexate concentration declines to <0.005 mcg/mL (0.01 μM)
Leflunomide (Arava)	Reversibly inhibits pyrimidine synthesis	**Rheumatoid arthritis:** 10–20 mg PO daily Dosing modifications: Can be used safely in renal impairment Cholestyramine 8 g PO TID for 11 days to wash out drug's active metabolite prior to conceive	Diarrhoea, respiratory infections, alopecia, hypertension, skin rash, gastrointestinal symptoms and liver injury are common **Contraindicated in:** 1. Active liver disease (ALT is double) 2. Active infections 3. Myelosuppressive diseases	Pregnancy category: X Lactation: Excretion into breast milk is unknown; do not nurse

Azathioprine (Imuran)	A 6-mercaptopurine derivative, inhibits the synthesis of both DNA and RNA Also inhibits cellular metabolism	**Rheumatoid arthritis:** Initial: 1 mg/kg IV/PO daily or divided BID, may increase as follows: 1. By 0.5 mg/kg/day after 6–8 weeks 2. By 0.5 mg/kg/day q4Weeks, no more than 2.5 mg/kg/day 3. Maintenance: Reduce dose by 0.5 mg/kg q4Weeks until lowest effective dose reached **Lupus nephritis:** Induction and maintenance therapy: 2 mg/kg/day PO with or without low-dose corticosteroids	Bone marrow suppression, anaemia, skin rashes, fever, nausea, diarrhoea and some increase in infection risk Rarely, fever, rash and hepatotoxicity signal acute allergic reactions **Drug interactions:** Allopurinol will decrease the metabolism of azathioprine	Pregnancy category: D Lactation: Excreted into breast milk at low levels, use not recommended
Hydroxychloroquine (Plaquenil)	Suppresses response of T lymphocyte mitogens Decreases WBC chemotaxis Stabilizes lysosomal enzymes Inhibits DNA and RNA synthesis. Traps free radicals	**Rheumatoid arthritis and systemic lupus erythematosus:** 200–400 mg daily. Not to exceed 6.5 mg/kg/day	Dizziness, nightmares, rash, itching, aplastic anaemia, leucopenia, alopecia, thrombocytopenia, nausea, vomiting, diarrhoea and abdominal cramps Corneal changes or deposits and retinal damage with long-term use Skin and musculoskeletal pigmentation	Pregnancy category: C Lactation: Compatible with nursing
Cyclosporine (Neoral)	Calcineurin inhibitor that suppresses both cellular and humoral immunities	**Rheumatoid arthritis:** 3–5 mg/kg/day divided into two doses	Nephrotoxicity. Drugs that inhibit CYP3A like diltiazem and potassium-sparing diuretics increase nephrotoxicity. So, serum creatinine should be closely monitored Other toxicities include hypertension, hyperglycaemia, gum hyperplasia, gingival hyperplasia, hyperkalaemia, hepatotoxicity and hirsutism	Pregnancy category: C Lactation: Excreted into breast milk, use not recommended
Sulfasalazine (Azulfidine)	5-Aminocyclic acid derivative inhibits leukotriene synthesis	**Rheumatoid arthritis:** Enteric coated: 2–3 g/day divided into 3 doses. Dose should be increased gradually	Tinnitus, hearing loss, hepatotoxicity and gastrointestinal complaints like erosion, ulceration or bleeding and drug rash	Pregnancy category: B or D if used for prolonged periods or near term. Increases kernicterus risk Lactation: Excreted into breast milk, used with care

(continued)

Table 4.2 (continued)

Drug name	Mechanism of action	Indication and doses	Adverse effects and caution	Pregnancy and lactation
Mycophenolate (Cellcept)	Inhibits inosine monophosphate dehydrogenase Inhibits T and B-cell proliferation and antibody production	**Class III/IV lupus nephritis:** Induction: 1 g PO q12hrs for 6 months Maintenance: 0.5–3 g/day or 1 g PO BID Administer with initial IV corticosteroid pulse for 3 days and then prednisone 0.5–1 mg/kg/day PO; after a few weeks, taper prednisone to lowest effect dose	Hyperglycaemia, hyperkalaemia, increased urea, hypertension, various infections, hypocalcaemia, hypercholesterolaemia and hypomagnesaemia Vomiting and diarrhoea are common Hepatic toxicities are infrequent but must be monitored	Pregnancy category: D Lactation: Excretion into breast milk is unknown, use not recommended
Cyclophosphamide (Cytoxan)	Immunosuppressive, a pro-drug which prevents and inhibits cell division	**Juvenile idiopathic arthritis/ vasculitis:** 10 mg/kg IV every 2 weeks **Lupus nephritis:** Induction therapy is by one of the following: 1. Low dose: 500 mg IV every 2 weeks for 6 doses plus corticosteroids, then maintenance with mycophenolate mofetil or azathioprine 2. High dose: 500–1000 mg/m^2 IV monthly for 6 doses plus corticosteroids **Dosing modifications:** Hepatic impairment: Give 75% of normal dose if transaminase levels are >3 times upper limit of normal or bilirubin is 3.1–5 mg/dL Renal impairment: CrCl<10 mL/min, give 75% of normal dose; CrCl>10 mL/min, give full dose	Can cause significant dose-related infertility in both men and women Nausea and vomiting, bone marrow suppression, alopecia, haemorrhagic cystitis and, rarely, bladder carcinoma	Pregnancy category: D Lactation: Excreted into breast milk, use not recommended

Tofacitinib (Xeljanz)	Inhibits the JAK-STAT signalling pathway	**Rheumatoid arthritis:** 5 mg PO Q12hrs or 11 mg of the extended-release tablet daily **Dosing modifications:** Co-administration with cytochrome P450 3A4 inhibitors: Not to exceed 5 mg daily Moderate renal or hepatic impairment: Reduce dose to less than 5 mg daily It has not been studied in patients with severe haptic impairment or in patients with CrCl <40 mL/min	Upper respiratory tract infections, headache, diarrhoea, nasopharyngitis, neutropenia and lymphopenia No contraindications have been listed	Pregnancy category: C Lactation: Excretion into breast milk is unknown, use not recommended
Apremilast (Otezla)	Small molecule inhibitor of PDE-4	**Active psoriatic arthritis or plaque psoriasis (moderate to severe):** Day 1: 10 mg PO in AM Day 2: 10 mg AM and PM Day 3: 10 mg AM and 20 mg PM Day 4: 20 mg AM and PM Day 5: 20 mg AM and 30 mg PM Day 6 and thereafter: 30 mg BID **Dosing modifications:** Mild to moderate renal or hepatic impairment, no adjustment required CrCl <30 mL/min: Reduce dose to 30 mg daily	Headache, back pain, nausea, diarrhoea, fatigue, nasopharyngitis, upper respiratory tract infections and weight loss Worsening depression, suicidal thoughts and other mood changes may also occur Concurrent use of strong cytochrome P450 enzyme inducers can result in loss of apremilast efficacy	Pregnancy category: C Lactation: Excretion into breast milk is unknown, use not recommended

are the pro-inflammatory cytokines found in the rheumatoid synovium. Few other bDMARDs target B and T cells. These agents have considerable efficacy in the treatment of patients with rheumatoid arthritis and other systemic inflammatory disorders.

4.5.1 TNF-α Blockers

Five TNF-α inhibitors are approved for the treatment of selected rheumatic disease by the United States Food and Drug Administration. These are adalimumab, etanercept, infliximab, golimumab and certolizumab.

A 2008 systematic review of synthetic and biologic DMARD therapy for rheumatoid arthritis concluded that anti-TNF monotherapy was similar in efficacy to treatment with methotrexate alone, while the combination of an anti-TNF agent with methotrexate reduced disease activity more and slowed radiographic progression to a greater extent than did anti-TNF monotherapy or methotrexate alone [23].

Most patients with rheumatoid arthritis respond to treatment with TNF inhibitors, with significant improvements in signs and symptoms of disease, significant decrease in radiographic damage and significant improvement in quality of life and functional status.

They have also proved to be highly effective in treating patients with ankylosing spondyli tis, psoriatic arthritis, psoriasis, Crohn's disease and juvenile idiopathic arthritis. However, they were ineffective in patients with scleroderma or vasculitis.

4.5.2 Rituximab

Rituximab is a chimeric monoclonal antibody that binds to CD20 antigen and leads to B-cell inhibition [24]. It is an effective biologic therapy for rheumatoid arthritis with a greatest benefit in seropositive patients. If given as two infusions of 1 gram each, it slows the radiographic progression in rheumatoid arthritis.

Rituximab is considered as a safe drug in rheumatoid arthritis, but infusion reactions can occur; most are mild to moderate. Pre-medication with methylprednisolone, diphenhydramine and acetaminophen can reduce these reactions.

Rituximab therapy carries a risk of hepatitis B reactivation amongst patients who have positive hepatitis B surface antigen (HBsAg) or hepatitis B core antibody (anti-HBc). All patients should be screened for HBsAg and anti-HBc prior to starting treatment [25].

4.5.3 Abatacept

It is a fully human fusion protein that inhibits co-stimulation (an essential step in the induction of adaptive immune responses) and inhibits T-cell activity [26].

Abatacept can be used when sDMARDs and/or other biologic drugs have failed to control inflammatory arthritis. Infection risk with abatacept is higher compared to other biologics [26].

It is administered as a 30-min intravenous infusion that is usually achieved without complications. Subcutaneous administration is equally effective and is now approved.

Abatacept is used to treat rheumatoid arthritis and polyarticular juvenile idiopathic arthritis. Clinical trials on abatacept in psoriatic arthritis and scleroderma have shown promising results [27].

4.5.4 Tocilizumab

It is a humanized monoclonal antibody that antagonizes the cytokinetic effect of IL-6. It has been approved for treatment of rheumatoid arthritis [28] and systemic onset juvenile idiopathic arthritis. It was recently granted a breakthrough designation status by the United States Food and Drug Association for giant cell arteritis based on positive results from a phase 3 clinical trial [29].

A dose of 4 mg/kg is started initially and then increased to 8 mg/kg based on clinical response. It is administered intravenously every 4 weeks. Administration through the subcutaneous route is also available. It may cause dyslipidemia but is generally well tolerated. Periodic monitoring of lipid profile along with other routine investigation is required.

4.5.5 Ustekinumab

Ustekinumab is a humanized monoclonal antibody that binds to and interferes with the biological effects of IL-12 and IL-23. It is approved for the treatment of psoriatic arthritis and moderate to severe plaque psoriasis [30].

It is administered at a dose of 45 mg subcutaneously at week zero, followed by a second dose at week 4 and then every 12 weeks. Nasopharyngitis, upper respiratory tract infections and nausea are common side effects.

4.5.6 Secukinumab

Secukinumab is a humanized IgG1 monoclonal antibody that selectively binds to IL-17A and inhibits its pro-inflammatory action. It is approved for the treatment of active ankylosing spondylitis, psoriatic arthritis and moderate to severe plaque psoriasis [31].

Nasopharyngitis, upper respiratory tract infections and diarrhoea are common side effects. If administered with a loading dose, 150 mg subcutaneously is given at weeks 0, 1, 2, 3 and 4 followed by 150 mg every 4 weeks. Without a loading dose, 150 mg subcutaneously is administered every 4 weeks.

Complete details about different bDMARDs are shown in Table 4.3.

4.6 Glucocorticoids

Glucocorticoids exert both anti-inflammatory and immunosuppressive effects. They inhibit prostaglandin and leukotriene synthesis, reduce macrophage phagocytosis and inhibit the release of collagenase and lysosomal enzymes [32].

Generally, five types of glucocorticoids are used in rheumatology daily practice. These are hydrocortisone, prednisolone, methylprednisolone, triamcinolone and dexamethasone. They differ considerably in potency and biologic half-life as shown in Table 4.4. They are used in the majority of systemic rheumatic diseases.

The chronic use of low-dose glucocorticoids can cause multiple adverse events [33]. For that, the dose of glucocorticoids should be tapered as quickly as possible to the lowest effective dose when chronic use is anticipated. Serum glucose, lipid profile and bone mineral density to prevent glucocorticoid-induced osteoporosis should be performed to monitor toxicity. Patients should also be screened frequently for polydipsia, oedema and shortness of breath, visual changes, weight gain and changes in blood pressure during therapy.

Complete details about different glucocorticoids are shown in Table 4.4.

Table 4.3 Biological disease-modifying anti-rheumatic drugs (bDMARDs)

<table>
<tr><th>Drug name</th><th>Mechanism of action</th><th>Indication and doses</th><th>Adverse effects and caution</th><th>Pregnancy and lactation</th></tr>
<tr><td>Infliximab (Remicade)</td><td>Chimeric monoclonal antibody against TNF-α</td><td>Rheumatoid arthritis, psoriatic arthritis and ankylosing spondylitis:
Initially: IV infusion at a dose of 5 mg/kg at weeks 0, 2 and 6
Maintenance: 5 mg/kg IV infusions every 8 weeks. Dose may be increased to 10 mg/kg</td><td rowspan="5">Common:
Infusion reactions (itching, hives, rash, nausea, headache) and upper respiratory infections (colds, sinusitis, bronchitis, etc.)
Rare and serious:
Serious bacterial infections, unusual infections (tuberculosis and fungal), worsening of CHF, hepatitis B reactivation, hepatotoxicity, possible malignancies, haematologic and neurologic events, lupus-like syndrome</td><td>Pregnancy category: B
Lactation: Excretion into breast milk is unknown, use not recommended</td></tr>
<tr><td>Adalimumab (Humira)</td><td>Humanized monoclonal antibody against TNF-α</td><td>Rheumatoid arthritis, psoriatic arthritis and ankylosing spondylitis:
40 mg SC once every other week</td><td>Pregnancy category: B
Lactation: Excretion into breast milk is unknown, use not recommended</td></tr>
<tr><td>Etanercept (Enbrel)</td><td>TNF receptor fusion protein</td><td>Rheumatoid arthritis, psoriatic arthritis and ankylosing spondylitis:
50 mg SC once weekly or 25 mg SC twice weekly</td><td>Pregnancy category: B
Lactation: Excretion into breast milk is unknown, use not recommended</td></tr>
<tr><td>Certolizumab (Cimzia)</td><td>Humanized monoclonal antibody against TNF-α</td><td>Rheumatoid arthritis, psoriatic arthritis and ankylosing spondylitis:
Initially: 400 mg SC at weeks 0, 2 and 4
Maintenance: 200 mg SC every other week</td><td>Pregnancy category: B
Lactation: Excretion into breast milk is unknown, use not recommended</td></tr>
<tr><td>Golimumab (Simponi)</td><td>Humanized monoclonal antibody against TNF-α</td><td>Rheumatoid arthritis, psoriatic arthritis and ankylosing spondylitis:
50 mg SC once monthly</td><td>Pregnancy category: B
Lactation: Excretion into breast milk is unknown, use not recommended</td></tr>
<tr><td>Rituximab (MabThera)</td><td>Monoclonal antibody, binds to CD20 antigen
B-cell inhibitor</td><td>Rheumatoid arthritis:
1000 mg IV infusion for 2 doses 2 weeks apart (one cycle)
Repeat cycle every 24 weeks or based on clinical evaluation
Systemic lupus erythematosus, granulomatosis with polyangitis and Microscopic polyangitis:
375 mg/m^2 IV every week for 4 weeks</td><td>Common toxicity:
Infusion reactions, nausea, upper respiratory tract infections, hypertension, arthralgias, pruritus and pyrexia
Rare and serious:
Fatal infusion reactions
Severe mucocutaneous reactions
Progressive multifocal leucoencephalopathy
Hepatitis B reactivation with fulminant hepatitis
Neurologic events
Lupus-like syndrome</td><td>Pregnancy category: C
Lactation: Excretion into breast milk is unknown, use not recommended</td></tr>
</table>

Table 4.3 (continued)

Drug name	Mechanism of action	Indication and doses	Adverse effects and caution	Pregnancy and lactation
Abatacept (Orencia)	Human fusion protein, inhibits co-stimulation T-cell inhibitor	**Rheumatoid arthritis:** According to body weight: < 60 kg = 500 mg IV 60–100 kg = 750 mg IV > 100 kg = 1000 mg IV At weeks 0, 2 and 4 Then repeated every 4 weeks thereafter or may be given as weight-based IV loading dose, then 125 mg SC once weekly	**Common:** Infusion reactions, headaches, upper respiratory tract infections, nausea and nasopharyngitis **Rare and serious:** Serious bacterial infections Possible malignancies COPD exacerbation	Pregnancy category: C Lactation: Excretion into breast milk is unknown, use not recommended
Tocilizumab (Actemra)	Interleukin-6 (IL-6) antagonist	**Rheumatoid arthritis:** 4 mg/kg IV every 4 weeks initially, may be increased to 8 mg/kg IV every 4 weeks based on clinical response SC: 162 mg every week	**Common:** Infusion reactions, dyslipidemia, headaches, upper respiratory tract infections, nausea and nasopharyngitis **Rare and serious:** Serious bacterial infections	Pregnancy category: C Lactation: Excretion into breast milk is unknown, use not recommended
Ustekinumab (Stelara)	Interleukin-12 and 23 (IL-12, IL-23) antagonist	**Psoriatic arthritis:** 45 mg SC at weeks 0 and 4, then every 12 weeks	**Common:** Infusion reactions, upper respiratory tract infections, nausea and nasopharyngitis **Rare and serious:** Serious infections and malignancies	Pregnancy category: B Lactation: Excretion into breast milk is unknown, use not recommended
Secukinumab (Cosentyx)	Interleukin-17A (IL-17A) antagonist	**Psoriatic arthritis and ankylosing spondylitis:** With a loading dose: 150 mg SC at weeks 0, 1, 2, 3 and 4 followed by 150 mg every 4 weeks Without a loading dose: 150 mg SC every 4 weeks	Nasopharyngitis, upper respiratory tract infections and diarrhoea	Pregnancy category: B Lactation: Excretion into breast milk is unknown, use not recommended

Table 4.4 Glucocorticoids

Mechanism of action	Indication and doses	Adverse effects and caution	Pregnancy and lactation
Anti-inflammatory and immunosuppressive drugs	**Methylprednisolone:** Used as a pulse dose in various severe systemic rheumatic diseases: Severe lupus nephritis, severe vasculitis: 1 g IV over 1 h ×3 days **Prednisolone:** Used as a high dose (1 mg/kg/day) for some active severe forms of vasculitis and then tapered slowly. Or initial dose can be started and then increased or decreased based on clinical response. Dose must be tapered slowly **Hydrocortisone:** Used as pre-medication or during the perioperative period	Fat redistribution on the face (moon face), oedema, fluid retention, hypokalaemia, hypertension, aggravation of diabetes, muscular atrophies and weakness, fatigability, menstrual cycle disturbances, peptic ulcer and increase in the risk of infections Adrenal insufficiency at rapid withdrawal of the treatment Bone disorders: Glucocorticoid-induced osteoporosis Neuropsychiatric disorders, nervousness, insomnia, depression, aggravation of epilepsy, increase in intracranial pressure in children Ocular disorders: Glaucoma, cataract Haematological effects: Leucocytosis and thrombocytosis, decrease of T-cell lymphocytes	Pregnancy category: C Lactation: Compatible with nursing but use with caution
Drug name	**Duration of action**	**Anti-inflammatory potency**	**Equivalent dose**
Hydrocortisone	Short acting	Potency is 1 for a 20 mg dose	20 mg oral dose
Prednisolone	Intermediate acting	4 times more potent than hydrocortisone	5 mg oral dose is equivalent to 20 mg hydrocortisone
Methylprednisolone	Intermediate acting	5 times more potent than hydrocortisone	4 mg oral dose is equivalent to 20 mg hydrocortisone
Triamcinolone	Intermediate acting	5 times more potent than hydrocortisone	4 mg oral dose is equivalent to 20 mg hydrocortisone
Dexamethasone	Long acting	30 times more potent than hydrocortisone	1 mg oral dose is equivalent to 20 mg hydrocortisone

4.7 Anti-Resorptive Drugs

4.7.1 Bisphosphonates

Alendronate, risedronate, ibandronate and zoledronic acid are effective for the treatment of osteoporosis. These drugs inhibit bone resorption, increase bone mass and reduce the incidence of fractures. They are considered as first-line therapy for osteoporosis in post-menopausal women and men because of their efficacy, favourable cost and the availability of safety data. For those who cannot tolerate oral bisphosphonates; who have difficulty with dosing requirements, including the inability to sit upright for 30–60 min; or who have relative contraindications to bisphosphonates (achalasia, scleroderma oesophagus, oesophageal strictures), intravenous zoledronic acid is the choice of therapy. Bisphosphonates should be avoided in renal impairment. They are also avoided in women of childbearing age due to foetal risk. Bisphosphonates cross the placenta and accumulate in the foetal bones [34].

4.7.2 Raloxifene

It is a selective oestrogen receptor modulator that inhibits bone resorption and reduces the risk of vertebral fracture. It is suggested for those who cannot tolerate or are not candidates for bisphosphonate therapy [35]. It is also usually chosen for osteoporosis when there is an independent need for breast cancer prophylaxis.

4.7.3 Teriparatide

It is a recombinant formulation of endogenous parathyroid hormone. It stimulates osteoblast function, increases gastrointestinal calcium absorption and increases renal tubular reabsorption of calcium. In postmenopausal women, teriparatide has been shown to decrease osteoporosis-related fractures. This drug is also suggested for those who cannot tolerate or are not candidates for bisphosphonates therapy [36].

4.7.4 Denosumab

It is a fully human monoclonal antibody that specifically binds to receptor activator of nuclear factor kappa B ligand (RANKL). It reduces the formation, function and survival of osteoclasts, which results in decreased bone resorption and increased bone density. It is suggested for those who cannot tolerate or are not candidates for bisphosphonate therapy [37].

Complete details about different anti-resorptive drugs are shown in Table 4.5.

Table 4.5 Anti-resorptive drugs

Drug name	Mechanism of action	Indication and doses	Adverse effects and caution	Pregnancy and lactation
Alendronate (Fosamax)	Bisphosphonate, inhibits resorption of bones Increases density of bones	**Osteoporosis (treatment and prevention), osteoporosis in men, glucocorticoid-induced osteoporosis:** 70 mg PO once weekly If CrCl is <35, not recommended Reduces hip and spinal fracture risk by 50%	Hypocalcaemia, hypophosphataemia, abdominal pain, nausea, diarrhoea, acid regurgitation, esophagitis and bony pain Must be taken at early morning with plain water on empty stomach. Then must stay in upright position for 30 min. Ensure adequate use of calcium and vitamin D	Pregnancy category: C Lactation: Excretion into breast milk is unknown; use caution

(continued)

Table 4.5 (continued)

Drug name	Mechanism of action	Indication and doses	Adverse effects and caution	Pregnancy and lactation
Ibandronate (Boniva)	Bisphosphonate, inhibits resorption of bones Increases density of bones	**Osteoporosis in postmenopausal women (treatment and prevention):** 150 mg PO every month. Or 3 mg IV every 3 months If CrCl is <30, not recommended No efficacy in non-vertebral fractures	Upper respiratory infections, back pain, dyspepsia, esophagitis and bony pain Must be taken at early morning with plain water on empty stomach. Then must stay in upright position for 30 min. Ensure adequate use of calcium and vitamin D	Pregnancy category: C Lactation: Excretion into breast milk is unknown; use caution
Risedronate (Actonel)	Bisphosphonate, inhibits resorption of bones Increases density of bones	**Osteoporosis (treatment and prevention), osteoporosis in men, glucocorticoid-induced osteoporosis:** 5 mg PO once daily, or 35 mg PO once weekly, or 150 mg PO once monthly If CrCl is <30, not recommended Reduces vertebral fracture risk by 41% and non-vertebral fracture risk by 39% over 3 years	Bony pain, diarrhoea, headache, abdominal pain, esophagitis and dysphagia Must be taken at early morning with plain water on empty stomach. Then must stay in upright position for 30 min Ensure adequate use of calcium and vitamin D	Pregnancy category: C Lactation: Excretion into breast milk is unknown; avoid using
Zoledronic acid (Aclasta)	Bisphosphonate, inhibits resorption of bones Increases density of bones	**Osteoporosis (treatment and prevention), osteoporosis in men, glucocorticoid-induced osteoporosis:** 5 mg IV every year for treatment and every 2 years for prevention If CrCl is <30, not recommended Reduces hip fracture risk by 41%, spinal fracture risk by 71% and non-vertebral fracture risk by 25% over 3 years	Bony pain, diarrhoea, headache, abdominal pain, nausea, fever, fatigue and anaemia Ensure adequate use of calcium and vitamin D	Pregnancy category: D Lactation: Excretion into breast milk is unknown; avoid using

Table 4.5 (continued)

Drug name	Mechanism of action	Indication and doses	Adverse effects and caution	Pregnancy and lactation
Teriparatide (Forteo)	Recombinant parathyroid hormone stimulates osteoblasts Increases density of bones	**Osteoporosis (treatment and prevention), osteoporosis in men, glucocorticoid-induced osteoporosis:** 20 mg SC once daily into thigh or abdominal wall Reduces spinal fracture risk by 65% and non-spinal fracture risk by 54%	Hypercalcaemia, bony pain, flulike illness, nausea and orthostatic hypotension Ensure adequate use of calcium and vitamin D	Pregnancy category: C Lactation: Safe
Raloxifene (Evista)	Selective oestrogen receptor modulator Increases density of bones	**Osteoporosis in postmenopausal women:** 60 mg PO once daily Reduces spinal fracture risk by 30–55%	Hot flashes, headache, flu syndrome, sinusitis, arthralgias and infection Increased risk of thrombosis and embolism. Thus, contraindicated in patients with history of thrombosis	Pregnancy category: X Lactation: Contraindicated
Denosumab (Prolia)	Monoclonal antibody, inhibits resorption of bones Increases density of bones	**Osteoporosis (treatment and prevention), osteoporosis in men:** 60 mg SC every 6 months	Bony pain, hypercholesterolaemia, cystitis, upper respiratory infections, sciatica and hypocalcaemia Ensure adequate use of calcium and vitamin D	Pregnancy category: X Lactation: Excretion into breast milk is unknown; avoid using
Strontium ranelate	Musculoskeletal agent Increases density of bones	**Osteoporosis (treatment and prevention), osteoporosis in men:** 2 g/day dissolved in water, prior to bedtime, 2 h after eating (preferably) If CrCl is <30, not recommended	Diarrhoea, nausea, headache, dermatitis and eczema	Pregnancy category: NA Lactation: Excretion into breast milk is unknown; avoid using

4.8 Drugs Used in Crystal Arthropathy

4.8.1 Colchicine

It is a uricosuric agent that prevents activation, degranulation and migration of neutrophils associated with mediating some gout symptoms. It can be used for both acute flare and prophylaxis against recurrent attacks of gouty arthritis [38].

Common adverse effects of colchicine may include diarrhoea and abdominal cramping. It is contraindicated in severe renal or hepatic impairment. Colchicine treatment may also benefit patients with acute episodes of pseudogout and arthritis due to other crystals.

4.8.2 Allopurinol

It is a xanthine oxidase inhibitor that inhibits its conversion to uric acid. It is considered as the first-line urate-lowering agent for the treatment of chronic gout. The dose of allopurinol should

Table 4.6 Drugs used in crystal arthropathy

Drug name	Mechanism of action	Indication and doses	Adverse effects and caution	Pregnancy and lactation
Colchicine	Uricosuric agent, prevents activation and migration of neutrophils	**Acute gout flare:** 1.2 mg PO at first sign of flare, then 0.6 mg PO 1 h later. Do not exceed 1.8 mg in 1-h period **Gout prophylaxis:** 0.6 mg PO once or twice daily. Do not exceed 1.2 mg/day	Gastrointestinal symptoms, fatigue and headache	Pregnancy category: C Lactation: Excreted into breast milk, use caution
Allopurinol	Xanthine oxidase inhibitor, inhibits its conversion to uric acid	**Chronic gout:** 100 mg/day initially, increase weekly to reach 200–300 mg/day. Do not exceed 600 mg/day in severe cases If CrCl is <40, 150 mg/day If CrCl is <20, 100 mg/day If CrCl is <10, 100 mg/2 days	Nausea, rash, vomiting, arthralgias and rarely Steven-Johnson syndrome	Pregnancy category: C Lactation: Excreted into breast milk, use caution
Febuxostat	Xanthine oxidase inhibitor, inhibits its conversion to uric acid	Chronic gout: Initial: 40 mg PO once daily. Maintenance: 40–80 mg PO once daily	Nausea, rash, vomiting, arthralgias and liver function abnormalities	Pregnancy category: C Lactation: Excretion into breast milk is unknown

be adjusted based on the stage of renal disease. Febuxostat is another urate-lowering agent that can be used if allopurinol is to be avoided [39]. Allopurinol decreases the metabolism of azathioprine.

Complete details about different drugs used in crystal arthropathy are shown in Table 4.6.

4.9 Symptom-Specific Drugs

Systemic rheumatic diseases are multi-system diseases that can affect different body organs. These disease cause symptoms that can be either due to the immunopathologic changes or adverse effects from the DMARD therapy. Most of these rheumatic symptoms are effectively treated with different DMARDs. However, few other symptoms require additional specific drugs. For example, Raynaud's phenomenon, fatigue, generalized aches and pains and acid reflux are common symptoms that patients describe to their rheumatologists. Table 4.7 provides a list of common symptom-specific medications that rheumatologists prescribe during their daily clinical practice. Table 4.8 defines the pregnancy categories for pharmacological agents.

Table 4.7 Common symptom-specific drugs

Drug name	Mechanism of action	Indication and doses	Adverse effects and caution	Pregnancy and lactation
Dihydropyridine calcium channel blockers	Inhibit influx of extracellular calcium ions across myocardial and vascular smooth muscle cell membranes, resulting in vasodilation of main coronary and systemic arteries	**Raynaud's phenomenon:** **Nifedipine:** 30–120 mg (extended release) PO daily **Amlodipine:** 5–10 mg PO daily	Peripheral oedema, dizziness, flushing and headache	Pregnancy category: C Lactation: Excreted into breast milk, discontinue drug or refrain from nursing
Sildenafil	Inhibits phosphodiesterase-5, thus increasing cyclic guanosine monophosphate to allow smooth muscle relaxation and vasodilation	**Raynaud's phenomenon:** 5 or 20 mg PO 3 times daily	Dizziness, flushing, headache and epistaxis	Pregnancy category: B Lactation: Excretion into breast milk is unknown
Pilocarpine	Cholinergic parasympathomimetic with muscarinic action, increases secretion of exocrine glands	**Xerostomia associated with Sjogren's syndrome:** 5 mg PO up to 4 times daily	Sweating, headache, flushing, dizziness, nausea, urinary frequency and diaphoresis	Pregnancy category: C. Lactation: Excretion into breast milk is unknown.
Amitriptyline	Anticholinergic, serotonin and norepinephrine reuptake inhibitor.	**Fibromyalgia:** 10–50 mg PO at bedtime, dose can be escalated up to 200 mg daily.	Dizziness, headache and dry mouth	Pregnancy category: C Lactation: Excreted into breast milk, discontinue drug or refrain from nursing
Duloxetine	Serotonin and norepinephrine reuptake inhibitor	**Fibromyalgia:** 30 mg PO daily initially for 1 week, then increase to 60 mg daily	Dizziness, headache, dry mouth and somnolence	Pregnancy category: C Lactation: Excreted into breast milk, discontinue drug or refrain from nursing
Proton pump inhibitors	Bind to hydrogen-potassium-exchanging adenosine triphosphatase in gastric parietal cells, resulting in suppression of acid secretion	**Heart burn or gastritis:** **Omeprazole:** 20–40 mg PO daily **Esomeprazole:** 20–40 mg PO daily	Headache, flatulence, indigestion, nausea and abdominal pain	Pregnancy category: C Lactation: Excretion into breast milk is unknown, discontinue drug or refrain from nursing

Table 4.8 Pregnancy category definitions

Category	Definition
A	Generally acceptable. Controlled studies in pregnant women show no evidence of foetal risk
B	May be acceptable. Either animal studies show no risk but human studies not available or animal studies showed minor risks and human done and showed no risk
C	Use with caution if benefits outweigh risks. Animal studies show risk and human studies not available or neither animal nor human studies done
D	Use in life-threatening emergencies when no safer drug is available. Positive evidence of human foetal risk
X	Do not use in pregnancy. Risks involved outweigh potential benefits. Safer alternative exists
NA	Information not available

Abbreviations

ACEIs	Angiotensin-converting enzyme inhibitors
ALT	Alanine amino transferase
Anti-HBc	Hepatitis B core antibody
AST	Aspartate aminotransferase
BID	Two times a day
cAMP	Cyclic adenosine monophosphate
COX	Cyclooxygenase
CrCl	Creatinine clearance
DMARDs	Disease-modifying anti-rheumatic drugs
HBsAg	Hepatitis B surface antigen
IL	Interleukin
IM	Intramuscular
IV	Intravenous
MESNA	2-Mercatpoethanesulfonic acid
NSAIDs	Nonsteroidal anti-inflammatory drugs
PDE-4	Phosphodiesterase-4
PGHS	Prostaglandin G/H synthase
PGs	Prostaglandins
PO	Orally (by mouth)
PRN	As needed (pro re nata)
q6hrs	Every 6 hours
QID	Four times a day
RANKL	Receptor activator of nuclear factor kappa B ligand
SC	Subcutaneous
SLE	Systemic lupus erythematosus
STATs	Signal transducers and activators of transcription
TID	Three times a day
TNF	Tumour necrosis factor
TPMT	Thiopurine methyltransferase

References

1. Meade EA, Smith WL, DeWitt DL. Differential inhibition of prostaglandin endoperoxide synthase (cyclooxygenase) isozymes by aspirin and other non-steroidal anti-inflammatory drugs. J Biol Chem. 1993;268:6610.
2. Trelle S, Reichenbach S, Wandel S, et al. Cardiovascular safety of non-steroidal anti-inflammatory drugs: network meta-analysis. BMJ. 2011;342:c7086.
3. Blot WJ, McLaughlin JK. Over the counter non-steroidal anti-inflammatory drugs and risk of gastro-intestinal bleeding. J Epidemiol Biostat. 2000;5:137.
4. Catella-Lawson F, Reilly MP, Kapoor SC, et al. Cyclooxygenase inhibitors and the antiplatelet effects of aspirin. N Engl J Med. 2001;345:1809.
5. Morabito L, Montesinos MC, Schreibman DM, et al. Methotrexate and sulfasalazine promote adenosine release by a mechanism that requires ecto-5′-nucleotidase-mediated conversion of adenine nucleotides. J Clin Invest. 1998;101:295.
6. Hoekstra M, Haagsma C, Neef C, et al. Bioavailability of higher dose methotrexate comparing oral and subcutaneous administration in patients with rheumatoid arthritis. J Rheumatol. 2004;31:645.
7. van Ede AE, Laan RF, Blom HJ, et al. Homocysteine and folate status in methotrexate-treated patients with rheumatoid arthritis. Rheumatology (Oxford). 2002;41:658.
8. Strand V, Cohen S, Schiff M, et al. Treatment of active rheumatoid arthritis with leflunomide compared with placebo and methotrexate. Leflunomide rheumatoid arthritis investigators group. Arch Intern Med. 1999;159:2542.
9. Cohen SB, Iqbal I. Leflunomide. Int J Clin Pract. 2003;57:115.
10. Elion GB. The purine path to chemotherapy. Science. 1989;244:41.

11. Black AJ, McLeod HL, Capell HA, et al. Thiopurine methyltransferase genotype predicts therapy-limiting severe toxicity from azathioprine. Ann Intern Med. 1998;129:716.
12. Wallace DJ, Gudsoorkar VS, Weisman MH, Venuturupalli SR. New insights into mechanisms of therapeutic effects of antimalarial agents in SLE. Nat Rev Rheumatol. 2012;(8):522.
13. Wolfe F, Marmor MF. Rates and predictors of hydroxychloroquine retinal toxicity in patients with rheumatoid arthritis and systemic lupus erythematosus. Arthritis Care Res (Hoboken). 2010;62:775.
14. Smedegård G, Björk J. Sulphasalazine: mechanism of action in rheumatoid arthritis. Br J Rheumatol. 1995;34(Suppl 2):7.
15. Saag KG, Teng GG, Patkar NM, et al. American College of Rheumatology 2008 recommendations for the use of nonbiologic and biologic disease-modifying antirheumatic drugs in rheumatoid arthritis. Arthritis Rheum. 2008;59:762.
16. Allison AC, Eugui EM. Mycophenolate mofetil and its mechanisms of action. Immunopharmacology. 2000;47:85.
17. Riskalla MM, Somers EC, Fatica RA, McCune WJ. Tolerability of mycophenolate mofetil in patients with systemic lupus erythematosus. J Rheumatol. 2003;30:1508.
18. Ong LM, Hooi LS, Lim TO, et al. Randomized controlled trial of pulse intravenous cyclophosphamide versus mycophenolate mofetil in the induction therapy of proliferative lupus nephritis. Nephrology (Carlton). 2005;10:504.
19. Haubitz M, Bohnenstengel F, Brunkhorst R, et al. Cyclophosphamide pharmacokinetics and dose requirements in patients with renal insufficiency. Kidney Int. 2002;61:1495.
20. Haubitz M, Schellong S, Göbel U, et al. Intravenous pulse administration of cyclophosphamide versus daily oral treatment in patients with antineutrophil cytoplasmic antibody-associated vasculitis and renal involvement: a prospective, randomized study. Arthritis Rheum. 1998;41:1835.
21. Ghoreschi K, Jesson MI, Li X, Lee JL, Ghosh S, Alsup JW, Warner JD, Tanaka M, Steward-Tharp SM, Gadina M, Thomas CJ, Minnerly JC, Storer CE, Labranche TP, Radi ZA, Dowty ME, Head RD, Meyer DM, Kishore N, O'Shea JJ. Modulation of Innate and Adaptive Immune Responses by Tofacitinib (CP-690,550). J Immunol. 2011;186(7):4234–43.
22. Schafer P. Apremilast mechanism of action and application to psoriasis and psoriatic arthritis. Biochem Pharmacol. 2012;83(12):1583–90.
23. Donahue KE, Gartlehner G, Jonas DE, et al. Systematic review: comparative effectiveness and harms of disease-modifying medications for rheumatoid arthritis. Ann Intern Med. 2008;148:124.
24. Rituximab (Rituxan) for rheumatoid arthritis. Med Lett Drugs Ther. 2006;48:34.
25. Mitka M. FDA: increased HBV reactivation risk with ofatumumab or rituximab. JAMA. 2013;310:1664.
26. Salliot C, Dougados M, Gossec L. Risk of serious infections during rituximab, abatacept and anakinra treatments for rheumatoid arthritis: meta-analyses of randomised placebo-controlled trials. Ann Rheum Dis. 2009;68:25.
27. Mease P, Genovese MC, Gladstein G, et al. Abatacept in the treatment of patients with psoriatic arthritis: results of a six-month, multicenter, randomized, double-blind, placebo-controlled, phase II trial. Arthritis Rheum. 2011;63:939.
28. Smolen JS, Beaulieu A, Rubbert-Roth A, et al. Effect of interleukin-6 receptor inhibition with tocilizumab in patients with rheumatoid arthritis (OPTION study): a double-blind, placebo-controlled, randomised trial. Lancet. 2008;371:987.
29. Stone JH, Tuckwell K, Dimonaco S, Klearman M, Aringer M, Blockmans D, Brouwer E, Cid MC, Dasgupta B, Rech J, Salvarani C, Spiera RF, Unizony SH, Collinson N. Efficacy and safety of Tocilizumab in patients with Giant cell arteritis: primary and secondary outcomes from a phase 3, randomized, double-blind, placebo-controlled trial [abstract]. Arthritis Rheumatol. 2016;68
30. McInnes IB, Kavanaugh A, Gottlieb AB, et al. Efficacy and safety of ustekinumab in patients with active psoriatic arthritis: 1 year results of the phase 3, multicentre, double-blind, placebo-controlled PSUMMIT 1 trial. Lancet. 2013;382:780.
31. McInnes IB, Sieper J, Braun J, et al. Efficacy and safety of secukinumab, a fully human anti-interleukin-17A monoclonal antibody, in patients with moderate-to-severe psoriatic arthritis: a 24-week, randomised, double-blind, placebo-controlled, phase II proof-of-concept trial. Ann Rheum Dis. 2014;73:349.
32. Buttgereit F, Straub RH, Wehling M, Burmester GR. Glucocorticoids in the treatment of rheumatic diseases: an update on the mechanisms of action. Arthritis Rheum. 2004;50:3408.
33. Saag KG, Koehnke R, Caldwell JR, et al. Low dose long-term corticosteroid therapy in rheumatoid arthritis: an analysis of serious adverse events. Am J Med. 1994;96:115.
34. Patlas N, Golomb G, Yaffe P, et al. Transplacental effects of bisphosphonates on fetal skeletal ossification and mineralization in rats. Teratology. 1999;60:68.
35. Silverman S, Christiansen C. Individualizing osteoporosis therapy. Osteoporos Int. 2012;23:797.

36. National Osteoporosis Foundation (NOF). Clinician's guide to prevention and treatment of osteoporosis. Washington, DC, 2013.
37. Cummings SR, San Martin J, McClung MR, et al. Denosumab for prevention of fractures in postmenopausal women with osteoporosis. N Engl J Med. 2009;361:756.
38. Khanna D, Fitzgerald JD, Khanna PP, et al. 2012 American College of Rheumatology guidelines for management of gout. Part 1: systematic nonpharmacologic and pharmacologic therapeutic approaches to hyperuricemia. Arthritis Care Res (Hoboken). 2012;64:1431.
39. Becker MA, Schumacher HR Jr, Wortmann RL, et al. Febuxostat compared with allopurinol in patients with hyperuricemia and gout. N Engl J Med. 2005;353:2450.

5

Diagnosis of Rheumatic Disorders: Radiological Modalities

Nizar Al Nakshabandi, Ehab Joharji, and Hadeel El-Haddad

5.1 Introduction

This chapter addresses different modalities of imaging in approaching the common musculoskeletal diseases (explaining the radiological part of diagnosis), we included: infectious arthritis (septic, tuberculous, and brucellosis), metabolic arthritis (gout and CPPD), rheumatoid arthritis, spondyloarthropathies (ankylosing spondylitis, psoriasis, and reactive arthritis), and degenerative bone diseases like osteoarthritis; it also addresses the role of the musculoskeletal interventional radiologist in the management of rheumatological diseases.

5.2 Learning Objectives

By the end of this chapter, you should be able to:

- Identify the radiological modalities used to diagnose different rheumatological disorders and their appropriate utilization.
- Emphasize on the importance of early radiological detection of infectious arthritis.
- Address the role of the radiologist in the prevention of the long-term rheumatological disabilities.
- Define the proper interpretation of the different musculoskeletal radiological modalities.

N. Al Nakshabandi (✉)
Professor of Radiology, King Saud Medical City, College of Medicine, King Saud University, Riyadh, Saudi Arabia
e-mail: nizar.nakshabandi@ksu.edu.sa

E. Joharji
Umm Al-Qura University, Mecca, Saudi Arabia

H. El-Haddad
Department of Medicine, Dr. Soliman Fakeeh Hospital, Jeddah, Saudi Arabia
Hematology Fellow, King Abdulaziz Medical City, Jeddah, Saudi Arabia

5.3 Infectious Arthritis

5.3.1 Septic Arthritis

Septic arthritis is an emergency and a type of destructive infectious arthropathy; it can cause significant mortality and morbidity, if unrecognized and left untreated. Irreversible joint destruction to a joint can be prevented by early diagnosis and prompt and effective treatment [1]. It is well-known that the definite diagnostic method is arthrocentesis by identification of an organism in the synovial fluid. The presence of painful, swollen joint and fever should raise clinical suspicion. Radiological studies play a significant role especially in cases where synovial fluid cannot be retrieved. In these cases, ultrasound- or fluoroscopic-guided joint aspiration demonstrates their importance in reaching the diagnosis. In general, imaging has an adjunct role to arthrocentesis in diagnosing septic arthritis. Effusion and inflammation in some joints like the hip and sacroiliac

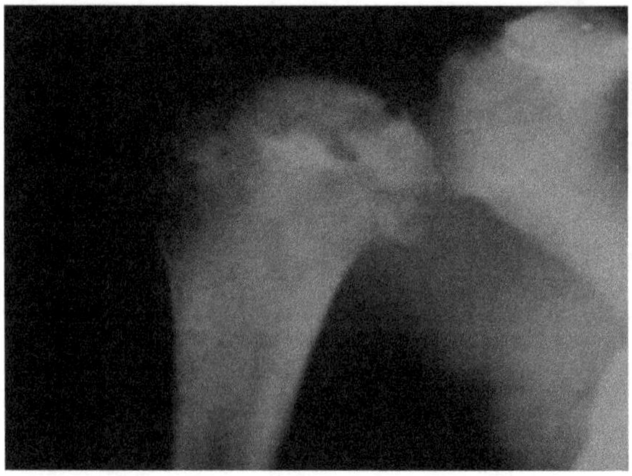

Fig. 5.1 AP view of the right shoulder demonstrates widening of the glenohumeral joint indicative of an effusion with sclerotic changes present on both sides of the sacroiliac joint

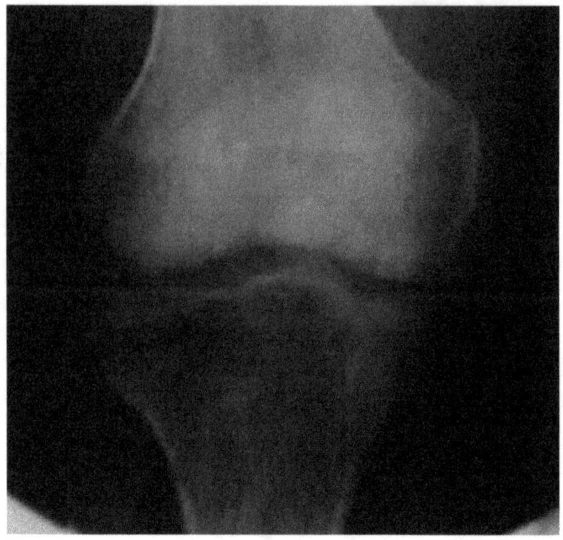

Fig. 5.2 AP view of the right knee demonstrates sclerotic changes present in the distal femur with periarticular osteopenia present in the tibia indicative of hyperemia

joints are difficult to examine clinically but can be detected by scintigraphy, CT scan, or MRI for defining extent of infection. MRI is a useful modality, while CT-guided bone biopsy or aspiration is the test of choice for defining the extent of bone involvement [2]. In rare cases, associated osteomyelitis or concurrent joint disease may be present, so radiographs should be obtained for an infected joint. In addition, it is useful to have a baseline radiograph to follow the response to therapy. In cases of failure to respond to intravenous antibiotics therapy, imaging should not be underestimated as it may change the line of management and guide intervention.

The following demonstrates the imaging modalities used to diagnose septic arthritis and characteristic findings in each one.

5.3.1.1 Radiographs

Conventional radiography should always be the first imaging technique used, although results are usually normal at presentation and generally lack sensitivity and specificity. The radiological findings vary according to the stage of the disease, for example, in the very early stage of the disease, X-ray may be normal, joint effusion may be seen Fig. 5.1, hyperemia may cause juxta-articular osteoporosis (Fig. 5.2), joint space may narrow due cartilage destruction in the acute phase, subchondral bone destruction may be evident on both sides of a joint, reactive juxta-articular sclerosis may develop if left untreated, and, in severe cases, ankylosis may develop (Fig. 5.3). In acute osteomyelitis, the early finding is osteopenia and then cortical destruction and periosteal new bone formation. Subacute and chronic osteomyelitis have different imaging features than marginal sclerosis and osteopenia, which indicate areas of healing. In chronic osteomyelitis, the most specific finding is a sequestrum (a fragment of dead bone surrounded by inflammatory tissue), which radiographically appears as a focal area of sclerotic bone within an area of lucency [1].

5.3.1.2 Ultrasonography

A noninvasive and inexpensive technique, it is considered an improved method for the early diagnosis of septic arthritis, with joint effusion and echoes inside being the characteristic finding of a septic joint. Clearly, it is superior to radiographs in detecting joint effusions as it can detect minor effusions, as small as 1–2 ml, and this allows ultrasound-guided arthrocentesis to be performed in patients with suspected septic arthritis. Furthermore, it is useful for examining inaccessible joints such as the hip. It can also show increased perisynovial vascularity using color Doppler. Echogenic debris may be present; it is very helpful in differentiating between tran-

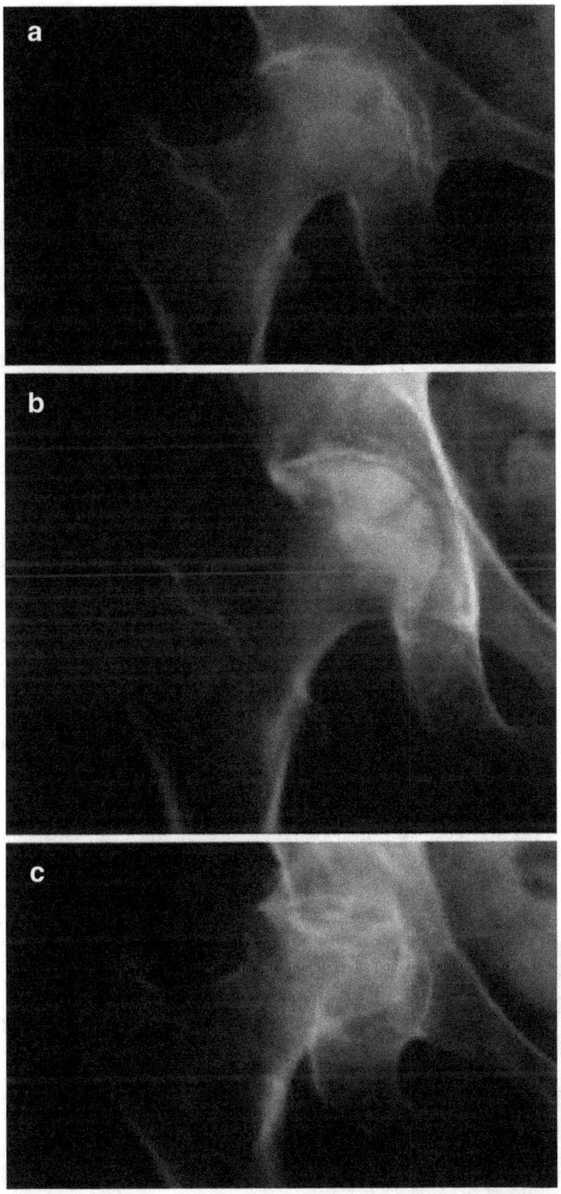

Fig. 5.3 Septic arthritis of the hip, (**a**) moderate osteoarthritic changes with concentric joint space narrowing early, (**b**) demonstrates sclerotic changes in the femoral head indicative of avascular necrosis after 4 months, (**c**) end stage after 8 months demonstrates flattening of the femoral head with osteolysis

sient synovitis and fresh hemorrhagic effusions. Echo-free image is seen in transient synovitis and fresh hemorrhagic effusions, while clotted hemorrhagic collections and septic arthritis do not have an echo-free image. This means that a negative sonogram will exclude fluid collection and the presence of echo-free effusion will virtually rule out septic arthritis [3]. However, for joints with non-distensible capsules (e.g., sacroiliac, sternoclavicular, and acromioclavicular joints), septic arthritis cannot be excluded in the absence of a visible joint effusion, and, if suspected, MR (or CT) imaging together with guided joint aspiration should be undertaken [4]. As mentioned earlier, on ultrasound, the hallmark of septic arthritis is the presence of a joint effusion in a patient with clinical signs and symptoms of joint infection. Ultrasound allows early diagnosis and treatment of septic arthritis, by enabling recognition and guiding the aspiration of joint fluid at an early stage [4]. Joint fluid in septic arthritis may be hypoechoic and clearly demarcated from joint synovium and capsule or hyperechoic and less clearly demarcated from joint synovium or capsule [4].

There are numerous advantages of clinical application of ultrasonography for the diagnosis of septic arthritis. Ultrasound is very sensitive in detecting the joint effusion of septic arthritis. The pathological extent of septic arthritis, in addition to the joint effusion and the joint surrounding subperiosteal abscess and cortical erosion, can be clearly defined and may indicate a concurrent osteomyelitis, which will help clinicians to treat by appropriate surgical debridement. Ultrasound can also help the clinicians avoid unnecessary needle joint aspiration by differentiating soft tissue abscess or tenosynovitis from septic arthritis [5].

5.3.1.3 CT Scan

CT features of septic arthritis are similar to the radiograph features; a fat-fluid level can be a specific sign in the absence of trauma. CT is better for visualizing local edema, bone erosions, osteitis foci, and sclerosis.

CT scan is also an imaging modality which may contribute to the decision of treatment, whether medical or surgical, not in septic arthritis itself but in concurrent osteomyelitis, and is able to detect some radiological features that indicate the need for surgical intervention and cannot be detectable by conventional imaging, for example, sequestra, medullary involvement, and the extent of sinus tracts; from this point, the value of CT scan in planning medical and surgical treatment of chronic osteomyelitis is appreciated [6].

5.3.1.4 MRI

In general, MRI is the most powerful modality used for the evaluation of musculoskeletal joint infections and provides better resolution than radiography or CT scan for detecting joint effusion and for differentiating between bone and soft tissue infection. When IV gadolinium contrast is used with MRI showing the synovial enhancement, the sensitivity and specificity increase to 100% and 77%, respectively [7].

Joint effusion, cartilage and bone destruction, soft tissue abscesses, bone edema, and cortical interruption all are MRI findings of septic arthritis with or without osteomyelitis; MRI also can differentiate acute from chronic osteomyelitis. In acute infections, there is no sharp zone of transition between normal and abnormal bone marrow, and there is no cortical thickening or sequestrum (Figs. 5.4–5.6).

The presence of bone erosions is a good indicator for an infected joint, but it can also be a finding of non-septic inflamed joint. The same findings can be present in both infected and inflamed joint, so no single sign can be considered as pathognomonic for a septic joint or help

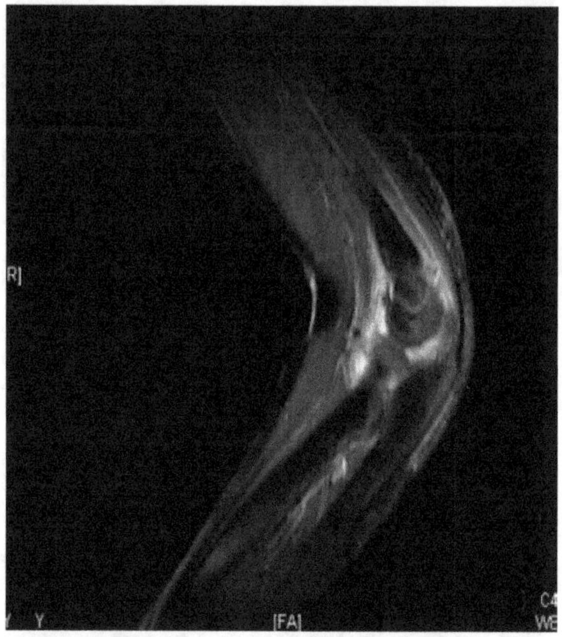

Fig. 5.5 T1-weighted images on your right demonstrate no effusion

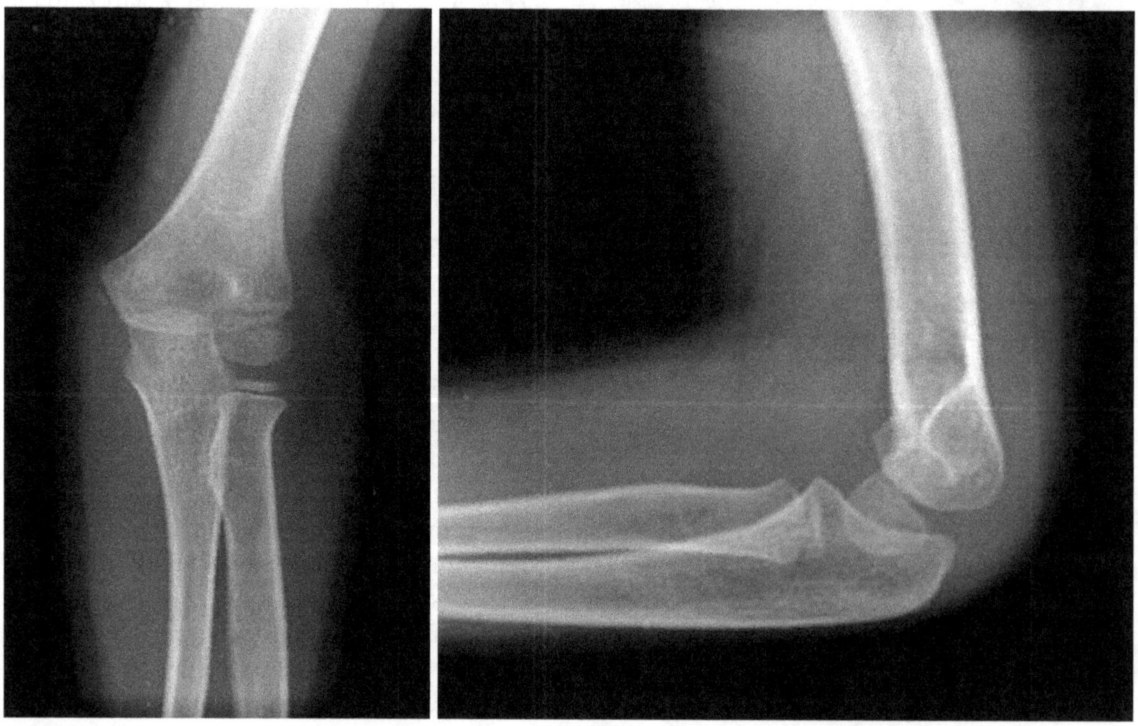

Fig. 5.4 AP and lateral radiographs of the left elbow demonstrate no specific abnormality

exclude its presence. Therefore, MRI is unable to differentiate between infective and other inflammatory arthritis [8].

5.3.1.5 Scintigraphy

This imaging modality can be helpful when evaluating suspected septic arthritis, particularly in the setting of prosthetic joint. Leukocyte-labeled 111-In combined with 99-Tc sulfur colloid studies provides accuracy of 90% in this clinical situation. Uptake of the 111-In in an area that does not show marrow activity with sulfur colloid is considered positive for infection [7].

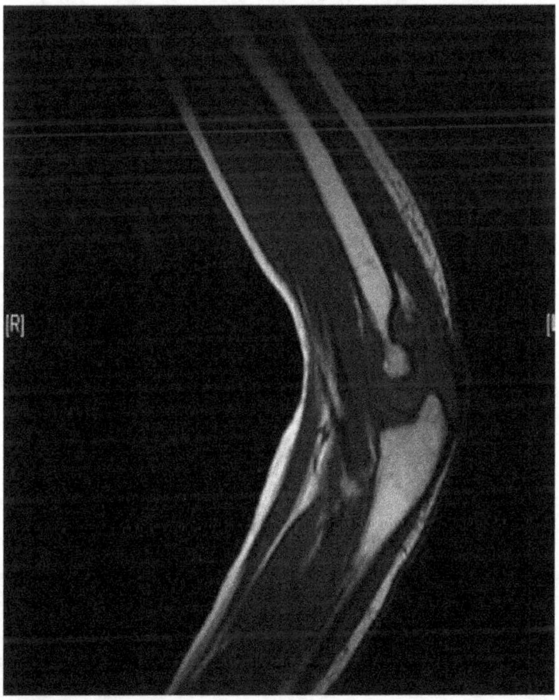

Fig. 5.6 T1 fat-suppressed images with IV gadolinium on your left demonstrate enhancement of the synovial lining of the elbow joint with some fluid present

5.3.2 Tuberculous Arthritis

Tuberculous arthritis is usually monoarticular, like other infectious joint diseases; the large joints, such as the hip and the knee, are most commonly involved, but in general, any other joint can be affected, with lower extremity joints being more affected than upper extremity joints [9]. Tuberculous arthritis is still considered a major concern for clinicians and healthcare workers, especially in developing countries. Advanced stage of the disease may be the first presentation, because of the delay in diagnosis.

In contrast to the old time when the diagnosis was made based on the clinical and basic radiological presentation alone (Table 5.1) [10], nowadays, the radiological investigations improved with more new modalities and new interventional methods, making the diagnosis of an infected joint more easy at any stage. In early stages of the disease, when plain X-rays are negative, it is considered a diagnostic dilemma, so, to avoid missing the diagnosis, the new diagnostic modalities like ultrasonography, CT, MRI, and image-guided aspiration of synovial fluid for PCR and tissue diagnosis should be used [10].

Usually, tuberculous arthritis is secondary to tuberculous osteomyelitis, in which a primarily tuberculous metaphyseal focus crosses the epiphyseal plate. One of the hallmarks of tuberculous skeletal infection is this transphyseal spread, which is not found in pyogenic arthritis,

Table 5.1 Clinico-radiological classification of tuberculosis of the hip [10]

Stages	Clinical findings	Radiologic features
Synovitis	Flexion, abduction, external rotation, apparent lengthening	Haziness of articular margins and rarefaction
Early arthritis	Flexion, adduction, internal rotation, apparent shortening.	Rarefaction, osteopenia bony erosions in femoral head, acetabulum or both No reduction in joint space
Advanced arthritis	Flexion, adduction, internal rotation, shortening	All of the above and destruction of articular surface, reduction in joint space
Advanced arthritis with subluxation/dislocation	Flexion, adduction, internal rotation with gross shortening	Gross destruction and reduction of joint space, wandering acetabulum

Source: Tuli, Tuberculosis of Skeletal system, fourth ed., 2010. p. 72.

so, without pre-existing osteomyelitis, arthritis less frequently occurs, owing to hematogenous spread of the tubercle bacillus to the synovial membrane [9].

Like any inflammatory joint, reactive hyperemia causing juxta-articular hyperemic osteoporosis, osseous erosions, and cortical and subcortical destruction on both sides of the joint space may be seen. Granulomatous inflammation can cause synovial thickening, and joint effusion may result in expansion of the joint; granulomatous synovial lesions expand inwards from the joint periphery, eroding the articular surface, with patchy cartilage destruction, erosions, and lytic bone lesions [9]. In a tuberculous joint, further extension to adjacent para-articular soft tissue with collection of cold abscess and sinus tracts may occur if not treated and discovered early, so early diagnosis is essential [9]. Radiological investigations play an important role in the diagnosis of tuberculous arthritis.

The following demonstrate the imaging modalities used to diagnose tuberculous arthritis and characteristic findings in each one:

5.3.2.1 Radiograph

Plain X-rays are reliable for detecting and for follow-up of treatment of tubercular joint.

Features are summarized in the Phemister's triad, which consists of juxta-articular osteoporosis, peripheral osseous erosions, and gradual narrowing of the joint space.

In tight or weight-bearing joints like the hip, knee, and ankle, marginal erosions are characteristic features of tuberculous arthritis.

In the early stage of tuberculous arthritis, lack of sclerosis or periostitis is another typical feature. In the end stage of tuberculous arthritis, severe joint destruction and eventually sclerosis and fibrous ankylosis may occur. Bony ankylosis may also occur, but it is less common than in pyogenic arthritis and, when present, is more likely to be secondary to previous surgical intervention [9].

5.3.2.2 Ultrasonography

The only finding is joint effusion, which is nonspecific and can occur in any joint inflammation.

5.3.2.3 CT Scan

CT scan is able to demonstrate bone destruction, sequestration, as well as extension of infection to the surrounding soft tissue or any sinus tract formation (Fig. 5.7) [9].

5.3.2.4 MRI

To detect early changes, MRI is the study of choice. On T2-weighted images, joint effusion appears hyperintense, loose bodies, calcifications and hemosiderin deposits due to bleeding may be hypointense; therefore, tuberculous arthritis should be considered in the differential; when an articular lesion with low- or intermediate-signal intensity on T2-weighted images is seen, marrow changes are of low-signal intensity on T1-weighted images and of high-signal intensity on T2-weighted images.

MRI is better than CT to detect associated soft tissue abnormalities, such as cellulitis, myositis, sinus tract formation, and para-articular collections. With IV gadolinium contrast, sinus

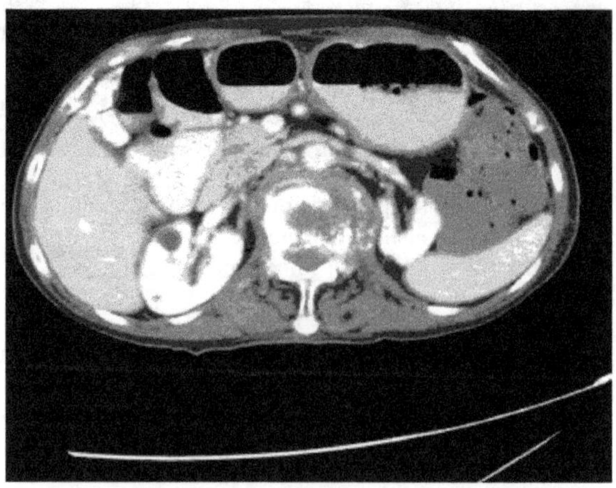

Fig. 5.7 CT scan of the abdomen and the level of the T12 demonstrate a destructive lesion of the body of T12 on the left side extending into the left parapelvic region with some calcification and enhancement peripherally

tracts display a linear high-signal intensity on T2-weighted images with marginal "tram track enhancement" on T1-weighted images. Tuberculous collections may be slightly hyperintense on T1-weighted images, in contrast to collections originating from many other infections (Fig. 5.8).

Precontrast T1-weighted images show a hyperintense rim around these collections, which enhances after administration of gadolinium contrast [9].

For differentiation of tuberculous arthritis and pyogenic arthritis, MR imaging of bone abnormalities, extra-articular lesions, and associated abscesses provides useful information [11].

5.3.3 *Brucella* Arthritis

Brucellosis is still considered a major health and economic issue in many parts of the world, and it can affect different parts of the body. Radiological investigations play an important role in the diagnosis and management of brucellosis [12]. Any joint in the body can be affected by *Brucella*, including sternoclavicular joints and sacroiliac joints, with large joints having more affinity to be involved. In long standing and neglected cases of *Brucella*, avascular necrosis of the femoral head can occur [12]. A favorite location for *Brucella* septic arthritis and osteomyelitis is the sacroiliac joint, and its involvement can extend to bone and muscle involvement in the region [8]. It also affects both joint spaces in the sacroiliac joint and causes erosive and bony destruction of the sacroiliac joint, with enhancement, which is one of the hallmarks of *Brucella* septic arthritis [12]. The radiologic features of the affected joints are indistinguishable from those of tuberculous or pyogenic arthritis; thus, differentiation depends on laboratory findings [13].

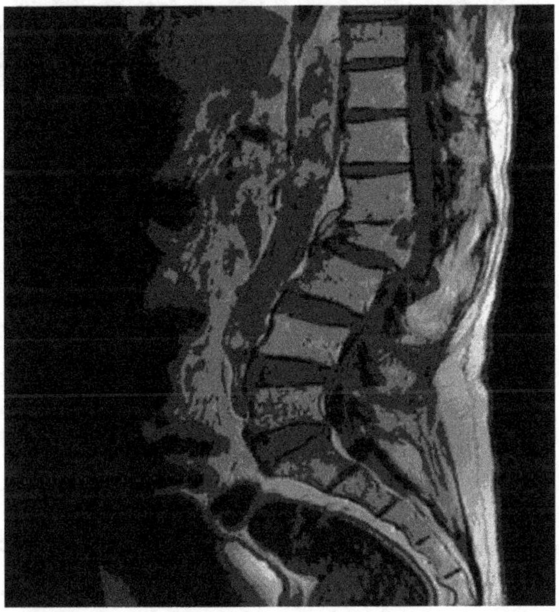

Fig. 5.8 Sagittal MRI T1-weighted of the lumbar spine demonstrates kyphotic deformity of L2 with destructive lytic lesions of the body of L2 and L5 from tuberculous involvement

5.3.3.1 Radiograph

The radiographic findings in a *Brucella* arthritis are not specific and range from poorly defined joints, joint space narrowing or widening, ankylosis, sclerosis, subchondral erosions, to no visible abnormalities [14].

5.3.3.2 Ultrasonography

Like any joint inflammation or infection, ultrasound can detect joint effusion, which is a nonspecific finding, and guide aspiration of synovial fluid to help in the diagnosis.

5.3.3.3 CT Scan

One of the hallmarks of *Brucella* septic arthritis is that it affects both joint spaces in the sacroiliac joint and causes erosive and bony destruction of the sacroiliac joint, with enhancement [12].

5.3.3.4 MRI

In *Brucella* sacroiliitis, bone marrow edema and intra-articular synovial fluids are important clues for early diagnosis. Sclerosis and ankylosis are observed in late phase of the disease.

Peripheral joint involvement can be diagnosed by the presence of bone marrow edema, joint derangement, enhancement of synovium, and periarticular soft tissues after intravenous injection of gadolinium (Figs. 5.9 and 5.10) [15].

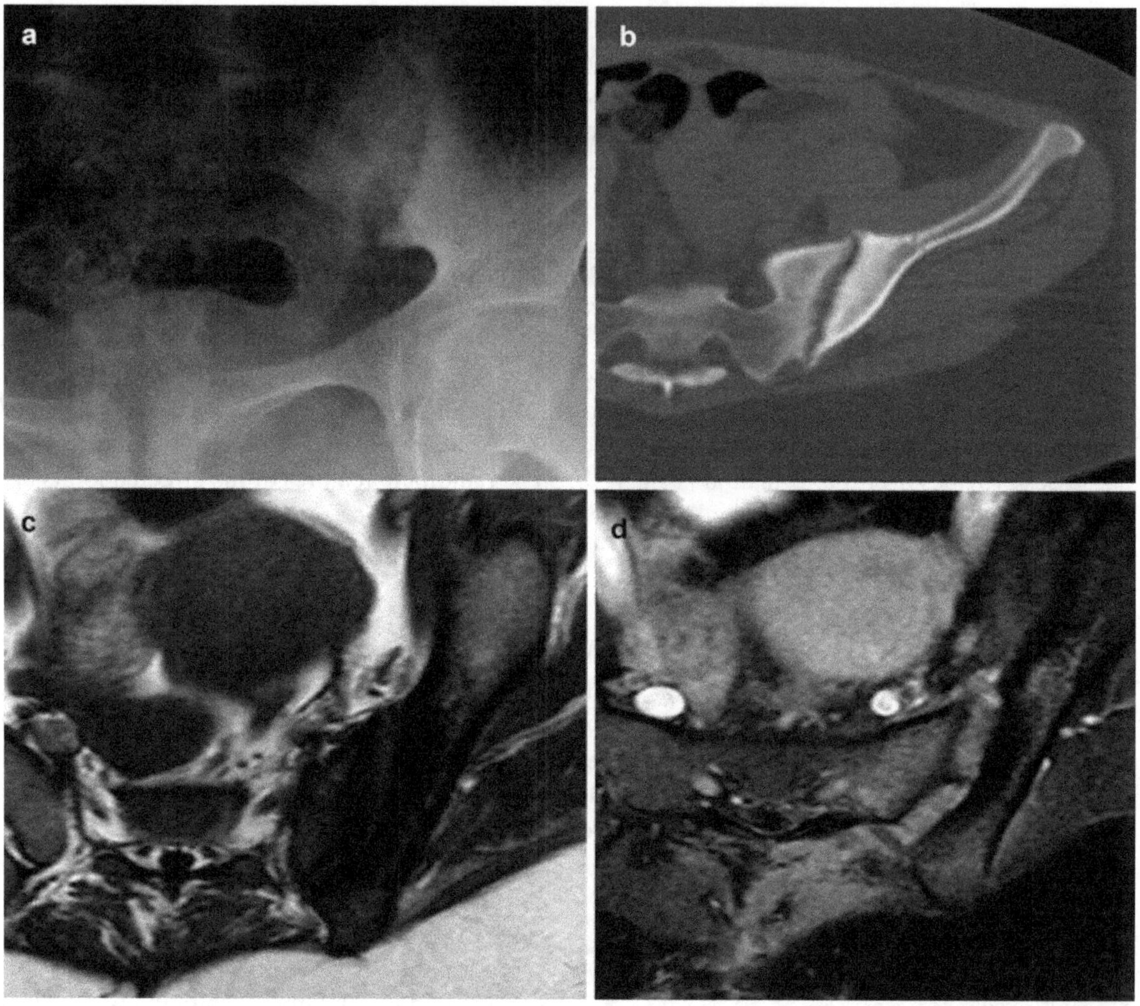

Fig. 5.9 (**a**) Plain radiograph of the left sacroiliac joint demonstrates sclerotic changes on the iliac side of the sacroiliac joint and widening of the sacroiliac joint on the left side. (**b**) demonstrates sclerotic changes of the left sacroiliac joint on the iliac side with widening of the sacroiliac joint. (**c**) Axial T1-weighted image demonstrates sclerotic changes of the sacroiliac joints with some widening. (**d**) demonstrates widening of the left sacroiliac joint with marked enhancement following gadolinium administration that extends into the left paraspinal muscles and subcutaneous tissue

5.3.3.5 Scintigraphy

Joints involved in a vast majority of patients show an increased uptake on bone scans.

5.4 Metabolic Arthritis

5.4.1 Gouty Arthritis

Gout is a common cause of arthritis; it can be diagnosed by expert clinician based on clinical picture and laboratory findings, with little or even no benefit from imaging, but still imaging is needed in cases where deep structures like the spine or sacroiliac joints are affected or when the gouty joint mimics mass lesion or infection. However, many patients with gout visit non-specialized physician, and in such cases, imaging may have an adjunctive role in gout diagnosis and management. Different radiological findings can be found in gout, for example, erosions, synovial proliferation, tophus, bone marrow edema, cartilage involvement, and joint effusion, all these findings need different imaging modalities, with

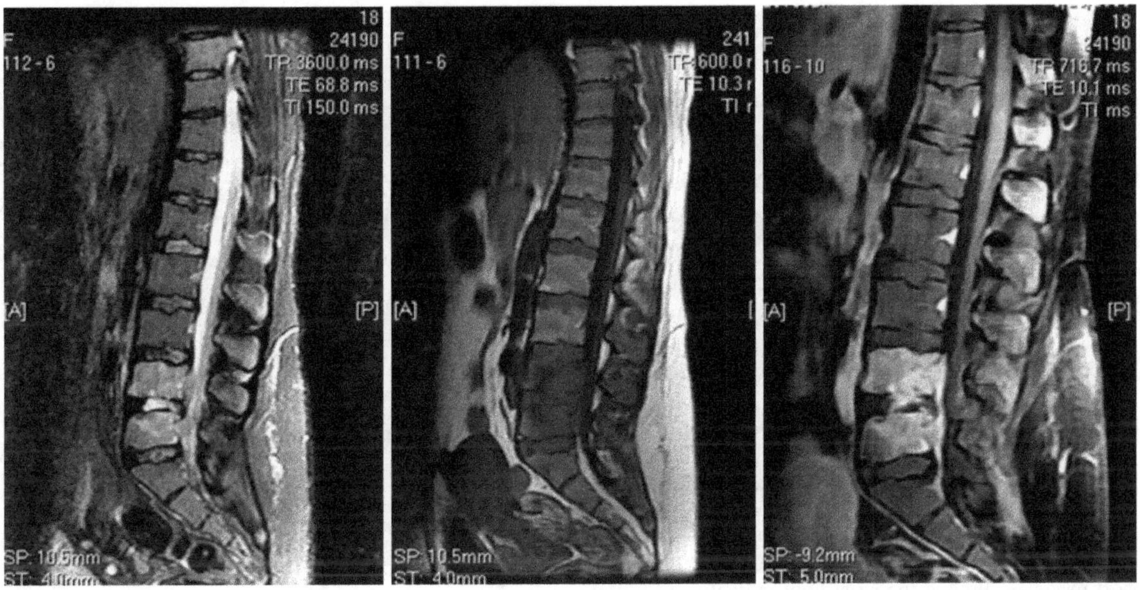

Fig. 5.10 First image on your left demonstrates high signal changes in the L4 and L5 vertebral bodies on this T2-weighted sagittal MRI of the lumbar spine. Middle image is a sagittal T1-weighted image of the lumbar spine with extensive low-signal changes of L4 and L5 with involvement of the disc space. The third image on the right is a sagittal MRI T1-weighted image with gadolinium enhancement and demonstrates marked enhancement of the L4 and L5 vertebral body with enhancement of the L4-L5 disc space

Table 5.2 Comparative utility of X-ray, US, CT, and MRI in the diagnosis of gout [16]

	X-ray	US	CT	MRI
Erosion	+	++	+++	++
Effusion	+	+++	++	+++
Synovial proliferation	–	+++	+	+++
Tophus	+	+++	++	+++
Joint space narrowing	+++	–	+++	+++
Tendon pathology	–	+++	++	+++
Bone marrow edema	–	–	+	+++
Tophus or synovial vascularity	–	+++	–	+++

Source: Review Article, Imaging Appearances in Gout, Volume 2013 (2013), Article ID 673401, 10 pages.

different utilities for each, based on sensitivity (Table 5.2) [16].

5.4.1.1 Radiographs

It is usually a late finding, underestimating the degree of involvement; first MTP involvement is a characteristic finding of gout, juxta-articular erosions with sclerotic margins and overhanging edges, and preservation of joint spaces and periarticular bony density until the disease process is late. The gouty deposits around the joint can be juxta-articular, intra-articular, and subchondral and usually not symmetric (Fig. 5.11). The hallmark of chronic gout is the formation of tophus, which is a soft tissue nodule that represents the granulomatous immune reaction of the body to monosodium urate (MSU) crystals. Tophus calcification is a late finding and may be associated with calcium metabolism disturbance. Erosions are often located next to a tophus (Figs. 5.12 and 5.13) [16].

5.4.1.2 Ultrasonography

Without contrast agent, sonography can detect tophaceous deposits in the soft tissues, joints, cartilage, as well as synovitis, erosions, and

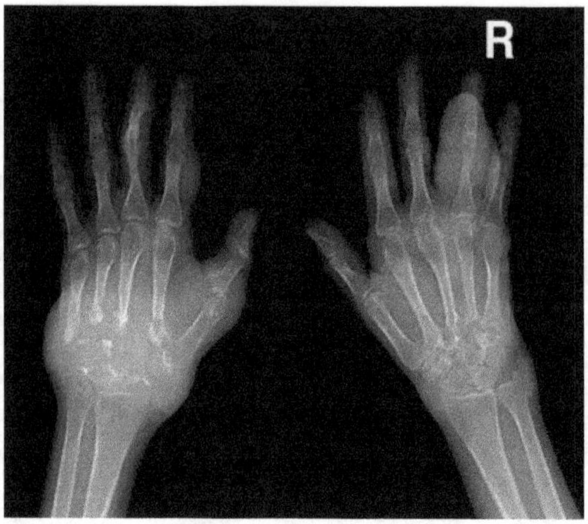

Fig. 5.11 AP view of both hands demonstrates punched out erosions of the left carpal bones along with marked soft tissue swelling at the wrist joint indicative of tophus formation

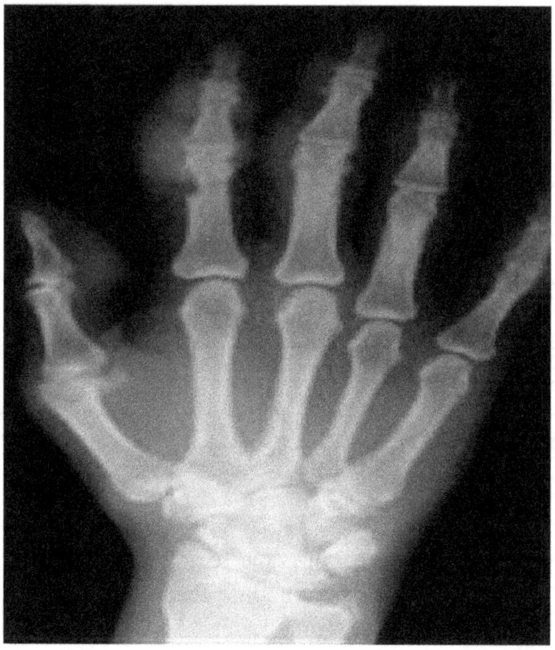

Fig. 5.12 AP view of the right hand demonstrates marked soft tissue swelling at the first metacarpophalangeal joint, second PIP along with punched out erosion of the proximal second phalanx

increased vascularity. It has a good role in the early diagnosis and monitoring the response of the treatment of gouty arthritis. In patients with an acute gout flare, or patients with history of prior gout attacks, or even patients with asymptomatic hyperuricemia, the "double contour sign" is a sign that can be seen by ultrasound, an irregular echogenic line, caused by urate deposition over the most superficial layer of hyaline cartilage, with a sensitivity ranging from 25% to 95% in patients with gout [16].

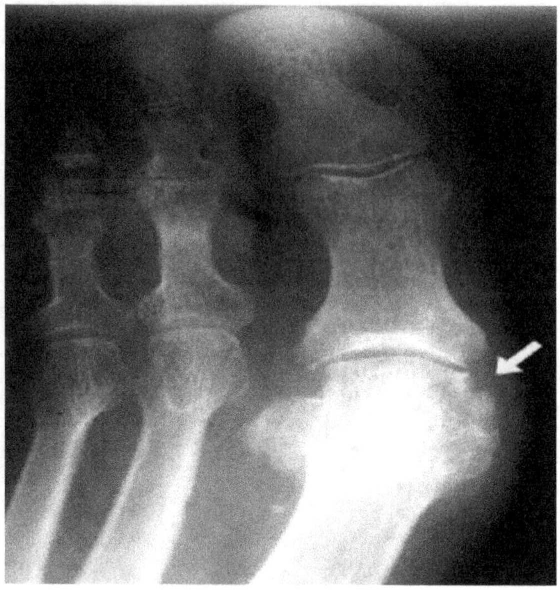

Fig. 5.13 AP radiograph of the left first toe demonstrates punched out erosion of the first metatarsophalangeal joint and first metatarsal head. Notice that the joint space is preserved

The tophus on ultrasonography appears as an anechoic halo and hyperechoic heterogeneous center. Tophi by ultrasound appearance could be either soft or hard tophi, based on sonolucency (soft tophi), and difficulty to image the structure below them (hard tophi), which are usually long-standing tophi [16]. Synovitis in gout by ultrasound shows mixed echogenicity, predominantly hyperechoic with associated increased vascularity. Some cases show hyperechoic foci which represent microtophi, resulting in "snow storm appearance."

Ultrasonography is excellent for identifying bursitis, intratendinous deposition, enthesitis, and subcutaneous nodules seen with gout [16].

5.4.1.3 CT Scan

Dual-energy computed tomography (DECT) has a promising role in diagnosing gout. Based on the spectral dual-energy properties, unique color-coded aggregates of urate crystal can be seen. This distinguishes gout from other crystal deposition disease, such as hydroxyapatite crystal deposition disease. Characteristic gout erosions and tophi are very sensitive to be detected by conventional CT, but its use is limited by cost. Gouty tophus can be intra-articular or extra-articular, or located in tendons and subcutaneous tissues, with pressure points preponderance. CT and MRI are very accurate in following up response to treatment, as tophi are known to decrease in size, but ultrasonography is more practical for follow-up studies as it is more available at lower cost with less ionizing radiation [16].

5.4.1.4 MRI

When gout affects deep tissues like the spine or locations not amenable to clinical examination like interosseous deposits in the midfoot, MRI is very helpful. It is also accurate in diagnosing the extent of gout involvement of the bursae and tendons and any associated tendon tears. On MRI, tophi appear as low signal on T1-weighted MRI and mostly intermediate signal on T2-weighted MRI [16].

5.4.2 Calcium Pyrophosphate Dehydrate (CPPD) Deposition Disease or Pseudogout

CPPD or pseudogout is a syndrome that manifests as arthritis clinically and as chondrocalcinosis radiographically or as an arthropathy that resembles that of degenerative joint disease. Most likely joints to be involved are the knee, symphysis pubis, and triangular cartilage of the wrist, and they should be examined in suspected patients. CPPD crystals can be found in any cartilage and in the soft tissues where it may mimic calcific tendinitis [17].

5.4.2.1 Radiograph

Arthropathy of CPPD crystal deposition is characterized by sclerosis, joint space narrowing, and osteophyte formation which is difficult to distinguish from degenerative joint disease except by the affected sites which are different than the sites of true degenerative joint disease. For example, pseudogout should be considered if radiocarpal joint, the elbow, or only the patellofemoral compartment of the knee joint is showing degenerative joint disease (Figs. 5.14 and 5.15) [17].

5.4.2.2 Ultrasonography

Based on studies, ultrasonography is more useful in cases of chondrocalcinosis than radiograph which is not sensitive nor specific [18], and it is better than radiograph and CT scan in diagnosing chondrocalcinosis in CPPD cases [19].

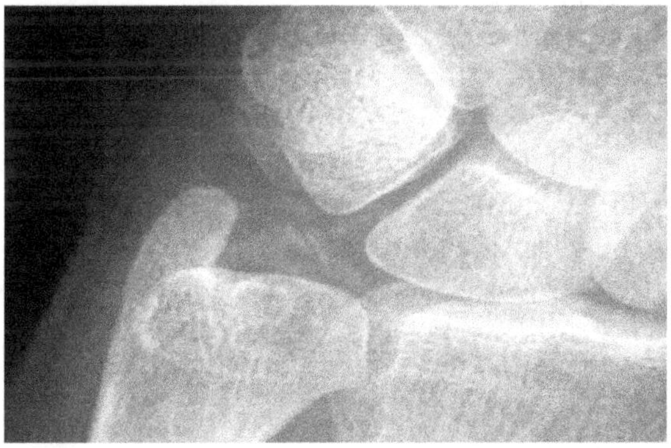

Fig. 5.14 AP oblique view of the right wrist demonstrates chondrocalcinosis of the triangular fibrocartilage complex

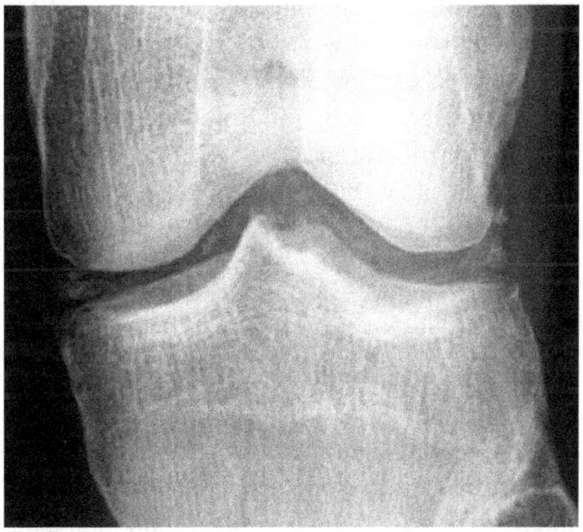

Fig. 5.15 AP view of the right knee demonstrates calcification of the articular lining of the knee. Consistent with chondrocalcinosis and related to calcium pyrophosphate dehydrate deposition disease

5.4.2.3 CT Scan

CT scan and conventional radiography are almost equal in the detection of chondrocalcinosis [19]. The pattern of CPPD on CT scans may show a calcific mass with a lobulated configuration, typically in the ligamentum flavum or within the joint capsule, and within the mass are septum like low-density areas. In addition, pressure erosions may be noted with disruption of adjacent bony cortex. Fine granular calcifications may also be noted. Subchondral cysts or erosions, as well as fractures, may be observed [20].

5.4.2.4 MRI

In detecting the CPPD deposits presence, MRI is not as sensitive as radiography, but 4 T MRI holds better promise in detecting CPPD crystals [21]. Calcifications of chondrocalcinosis are present on MRI as a signal void or decreased signal intensity. High-field MRI is especially effective for visualization of CPPD deposits. Because MRI does not visualize calcific structures well, CT scanning or radiographic confirmation is required; it has low sensitivity for visualization of CPPD deposits but can display massive deposition [20].

Rheumatoid arthritis (RA): It is the most common chronic inflammatory joint disease [22]. It is characterized by joint swelling, joint tenderness, and destruction of the synovial joints, leading to severe disability and premature mortality [23]. The hallmark of RA is bilateral symmetric arthritis of more than three joints (polyarthritis) [3]. Over 60% of patients initially present with symmetric arthritis of multiple small hand joints [3]. Typically, the second and third metacarpophalangeal (MCP) and the third proximal interphalangeal (PIP) joints are involved early in the course of the disease; the ulnar and radial aspects of the radiocarpal joint and the intercarpal, carpometacarpal, metacarpophalangeal, and proximal interphalangeal joints are other common sites [3]. Simultaneous synovitis of tendon sheaths of the wrists and hands is another distinct finding [3]. Bilateral and symmetric involvement of foot joints is another typical manifestation of RA [3]. The metatarsophalangeal and the interphalangeal (great toe) joints are favored sites [3]. All midfoot joints may be involved [3]. The talonavicular, subtalar, and tarsometatarsal joints are specific target areas [24].

Later in the course of the disease, large extremity joints and cervical spine joints could be insulted.

The role of radiology in RA is to either diagnose the disease or assess the disease status and progression.

5.4.2.5 Radiographs

Conventional radiography (CR) has been considered the gold standard for imaging in RA, its sensitivity for structural damage in RA diagnosis is low, and disease activity cannot be assessed [25]. When there is diagnostic doubt, CR, ultrasound, or MRI can be used to improve the certainty of a diagnosis of RA above clinical criteria alone [25]. CR of the hands and feet should be used as the initial imaging technique to detect damage. However, ultrasound and/or MRI should be considered if CR do not show damage and may be used to detect damage at an earlier time point (especially in early RA) [25]. The periodic evaluation of joint damage, usually by radiographs of the hands and feet, should be considered [25]. Monitoring of functional instability of the cervical spine by lateral radiograph obtained in flexion and neutral should be performed in patients with clinical suspicion of cervical involvement. When the radiograph is positive or specific neurological symptoms and signs are present, MRI should be performed [25].

Erosion: It is discontinuity of the white cortical line (marginal erosions) and subsequently become projection-like (Figs. 5.16 and 5.17).

Subcortical cysts: These are cystic changes in the subcortical bone which are easily identified as translucent lesions [24].

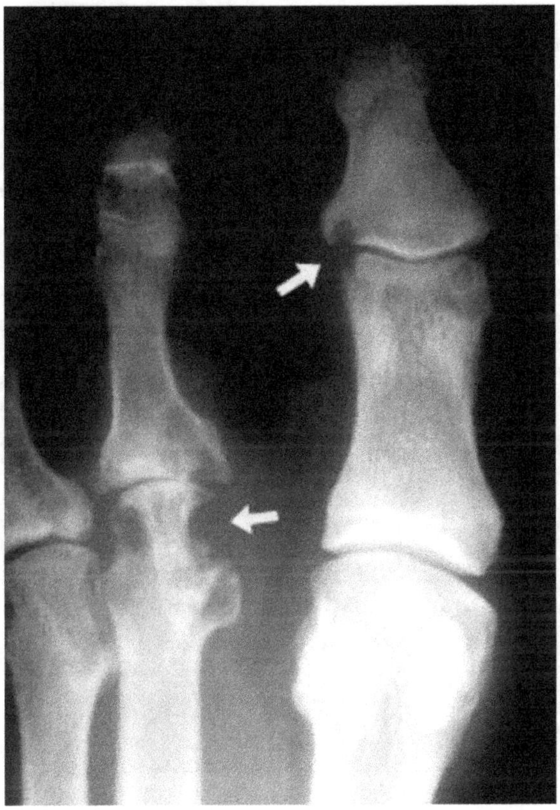

Fig. 5.16 PA view of the forefoot shows erosive changes (arrow)

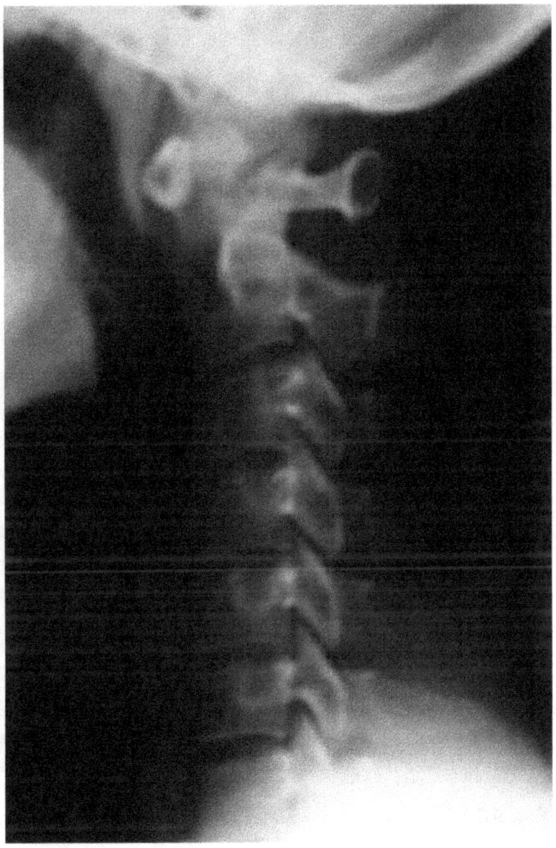

Fig. 5.17 Flexed lateral view of the cervical spine shows straightening of the cervical spine with atlantoaxial subluxation

Joint spacc narrowing: It is a latc finding of RA and can be detected by CR (Fig. 5.18).

Periarticular osteopenia: This refers to non-sharp cortical end plates [3]. This finding is important especially radiographs are used as the first-line imaging tool.

Effusion: Plain radiographs demonstrate indirect signs of effusion such as joint space widening and soft tissue swelling as well as shifting of fat pads [24].

5.4.2.6 Ultrasonography/Magnetic Resonance Imaging (MRI)

Over the past decade, there have been significant advances in the field of musculoskeletal imaging, especially in the application of ultrasound (US) and magnetic resonance imaging (MRI) to the management of rheumatoid arthritis (RA). Both modalities offer significant advantages over the previous standards of clinical examination and radiography and allow direct visualization of both joint inflammation and structural damage. Although measuring similar pathology, each of these imaging tools has its own benefits and limitations, understanding of which can help researchers and clinicians to determine the appropriate role for these tools in RA joint assessment [22].

Ultrasound and/or MRI should be considered if CR do not show damage and may be used to detect damage at an earlier time point (especially in early RA) [25].

Synovitis: Cytokines mediate capillary leakage and edema in the acute phase. This facilitates syno-

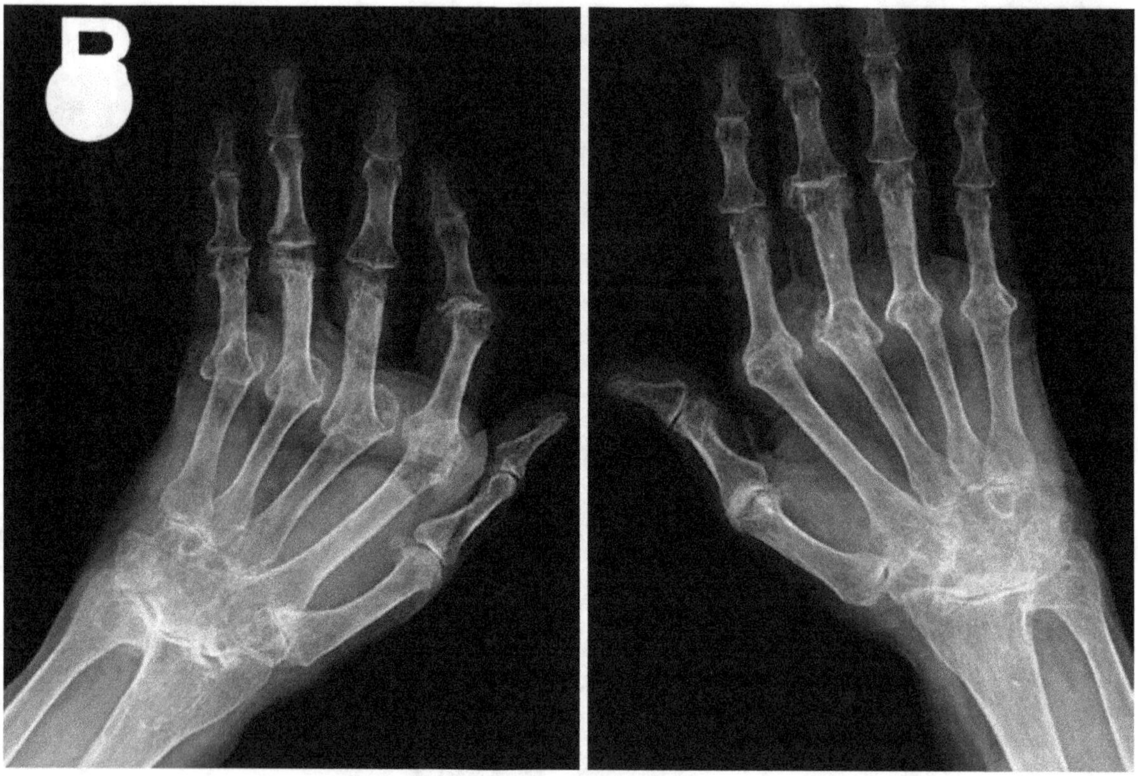

Fig. 5.18 PA view of the hands shows joint space narrowing, erosions, and diffused osteoporosis

vial swelling and leads to widening of the joint space, which may well be exaggerated by effusion [24]. Synovitis initially starts at bare areas.

Subcortical cysts: A number of more than three, in an eccentric location, and non-sharp margins increase the likelihood that the subcortical cyst is the result of an inflammatory joint process [3]. On MRI, arthritic cysts usually do not contain fat or trabecular bone [3]. When subcortical cysts are detected by MRI or US, they are considered pre-erosive changes.

Effusion: Both US and MRI can detect small effusion in small joints.

Periarticular osteopenia: This finding is a secondary indirect sign of synovitis.

Bone marrow edema (BME): MRI is the only modality of choice which can detect this finding. BME is a very useful prognostic indicator in RA. Affected marrow will readily show significant uptake of contrast material [24]. It is associated with disease activity.

Erosions: Naturally, erosions arise at the bare areas first due to the lack of the protecting cartilage layer. The diagnosis of erosions is very important as it may well influence therapy. MR imaging demonstrates erosions clearly [24]. US can detect them too.

Computed tomography (CT): It detects all bony changes and pathology; however, its use is limited due to high radiation.

Scintigraphy: Baseline inflammatory disease measured by scintigraphy appears to be associated with radiographic progression. In addition, multiple regression analysis has demonstrated that progression of radiographic joint destruction was primarily predicted by 99mTc-IgG scintigraphy, while joint swelling and erythrocyte sedimentation rate (ESR, IgM rheumatoid factor (RF)) are not predictive. This suggests that scintigraphy may be superior to conventional clinical and laboratory measurements in the prediction of joint destruction [25].

5.5 Summary

The diagnosis of RA is based on history, clinical examination, and laboratory results. If there is a doubt about RA diagnosis, the radiologic modalities take place to improve the diagnosis. CR is the gold standard modality for imaging in RA. MRI and/or US should be considered if the CR does not show any abnormality.

Assessment and follow-up periodic radiographs should be obtained for follow-up. MRI and/or US assesses the disease progression.

Spondyloarthropathies (SpA): They are a group of diseases that have a strong association with human leukocyte antigen B27 (HLA-B27), are characterized by inflammation of sacroiliac joints (sacroiliitis), and affect axial and appendicular skeleton. They include ankylosing spondylitis (AS), psoriatic arthritis (PsA), reactive arthritis known as Reiter's syndrome, and other uncommon arthritic diseases.

Ankylosing Spondylitis (AS): It is a disease that affects young age group, is rarely seen after the age of 40, and is more predominant in male gender. The inflammation affects the axial skeleton in symmetrical way and starts at sacroiliac joint in almost all cases. Spondylitis occurs in 50% of patient with AS and starts at the thoracolumbar and lumbosacral spines. Cervical spine joints are rarely seen affected alone. AS is easy to diagnose as it has a unique pattern of distribution and clear clinical picture.

Radiography: CR is still the first imaging modality and should be obtained for the diagnosis of AS. Anteroposterior (AP) pelvic, AP, and lateral spine X-ray should be ordered when AS is suspected. Other radiologic modalities are used to detect the disease in earlier stage or to determine the prognosis. CR can detect many changes in AS but not at early stage as compared to MRI and CT scan.

Erosions: Small erosions resembling the serrated edges of the postage stamp typically start at iliac side of the joint early in the disease course [26]. In the spine, the earliest change is enthesitis at the insertion of annulus fibrosis fibers. This process is a result of erosions and reactive sclerosis which occur at vertebral corner (Romanus lesions) (shiny corners) and cause vertebral squaring. AS is the least erosive spondyloarthropathy.

Ossification: The ossification of the ligaments at sacroiliac joints may appear as star shape, and complete joint fusion may be seen in advanced stage. As the disease progresses in the spines, the ossification starts developing at annulus fibrosis (**syndesmophytes**). When the ossification continues through the apophyseal joint, complete spinal fusion occurs (**bamboo spine**). In advance disease, **dagger sign** (Fig. 5.19) appears which is the ossification of supra- and interspinous ligaments and can be detected by radiograph as slim ossified streak. When the ligamentous ossification occurs together with ossification of apophyseal joint capsules, there are three vertical

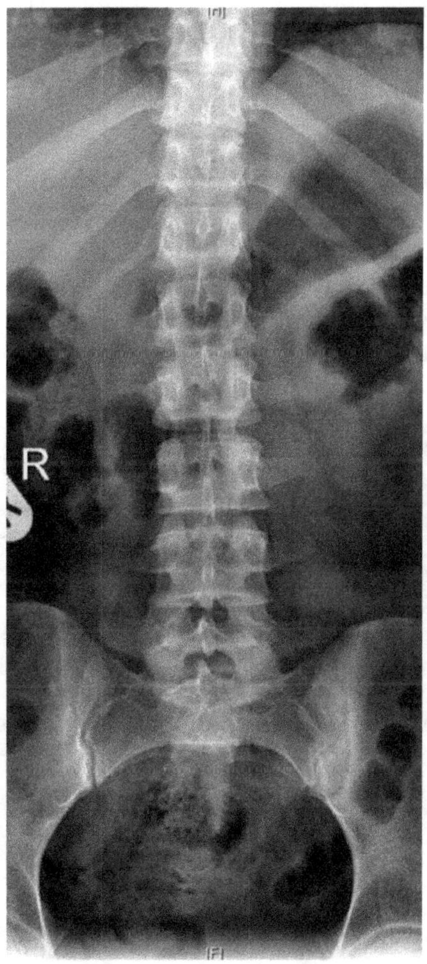

Fig. 5.19 PA view of the pelvis and spines shows bone fusion at sacroiliac joint (ankylosed) and spine fusion (dagger sign)

radiodense lines on frontal radiography (**trolley-track sign**) [27].

Ultrasonography: It has some utility for the evaluation of sacroiliitis when it is very active by using Doppler ultrasonography to assess blood flow and synovitis [26]. It may be useful in some cases in young children as an initial study but is limited to the evaluation of soft tissues surrounding the joint and not the joint itself [26]. Ultrasound may be used for diagnostic and therapeutic injections into the sacroiliac joints as an alternative to fluoroscopy in some cases [26].

Magnetic Resonance Imaging (MRI): MRI has become the gold standard imaging modality for the diagnosis of SpA of sacroiliac joints and spine [26]. It is very sensitive and specific to detect inflammatory changes in and around the sacroiliac joints and spine. Therefore, MRI findings are divided into active and chronic inflammatory findings.

5.5.1 Active Inflammatory Findings

Bone Marrow Edema (BME): It can appear in the sacroiliac joints and spine. It is strongly associated with disease activity and reflects the response to the treatment (Fig. 5.20).

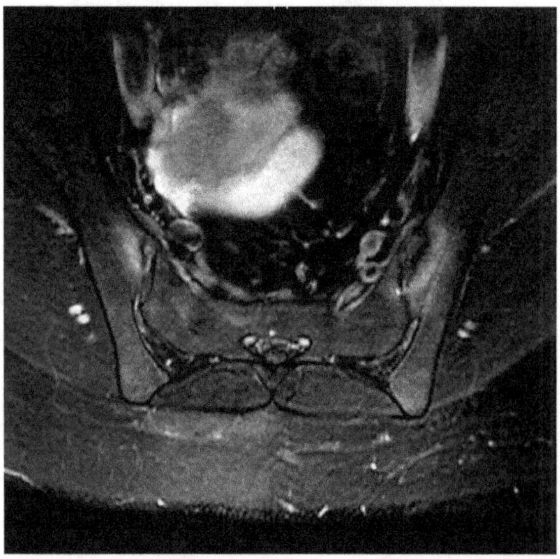

Fig. 5.20 MRI of the sacroiliac joints shows reduced bilateral sacroiliac joint space with symmetrical focal bone marrow edema along the iliac side of both joints

Synovitis/Capsulitis: These findings rarely occur without the occurrence of other findings in AS.

Enthesitis: This finding almost always occurs at muscle insertion and is considered a transient feature.

5.5.2 Chronic Inflammatory Findings

Sclerosis: This appears as low intensity on MRI and mainly develops at joint margins.

Fat deposition: This occurs at bone marrow area in the sacroiliac joint and at vertebral corners in the spine.

Bone bridging: This results from the ossification of ligaments which further lead to the formation of bone bridging and ankylosis as a final result.

Erosions: They are bony defects that can be seen as irregular shapes at joint margins.

Computed tomography (CT): CT is superior to MRI in detecting erosions. It is also used in case of trauma and emergency if fracture is suspected.

Psoriatic arthritis (PsA): PsA is a chronic systemic disease characterized by inflammatory joint changes and is accompanied with skin psoriasis. PsA affects joints asymmetrically. It involves the hands (no sparing joint), feet, and axial skeleton and rarely affects large joints. PsA develops in 7% of patients with skin psoriasis [26]. Axial psoriatic arthritis occurs in approximately 40% of patients with peripheral PsA [26].

Radiography: Radiographs are the first radiologic modality that should be obtained. The radiographic hallmark of PsA is the combination of destructive changes and bone proliferation.

Erosion: It is discontinuity of the white cortical line. Marginal erosion is an early PsA sign which then becomes irregular and ill-defined because of bone formation adjacent to erosions. This sign is also called "pencil in cup" (Fig. 5.21).

Joint space narrowing: Dramatic joint space narrowing may lead to serious disability.

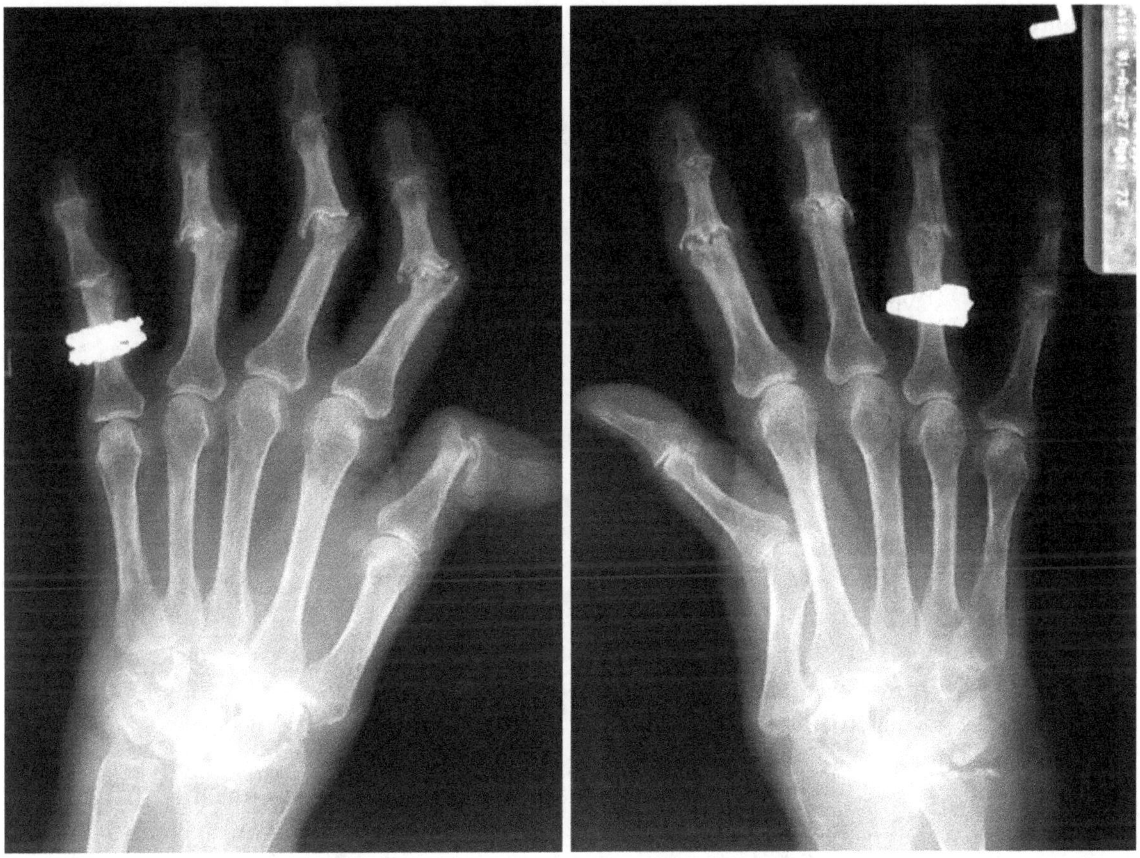

Fig. 5.21 AP view of the hand shows aggressive erosions (pencil in cup) which appear in all PIP joint of both hands; bone proliferation appears at distal part of metacarpal bones. Pan-carpal bone involvement. MCP joints are spared

Bone proliferation: This is a feature of PsA involving particularly metaphysis and diaphysis of the hands and feet.

Ultrasonography: Ultrasound (US) in conjunction with power Doppler (PD) indicative of degree of inflammatory activity has an increasing important role in the evaluation of PsA. In fact, US is useful mainly for its ability to assess musculoskeletal (joints, tendons, entheses) and cutaneous (skin and nails) involvement, to monitor efficacy of therapy and to guide steroid injections at the level of inflamed joints, tendon sheaths, and entheses [28].

Synovitis: Asymptomatic US synovitis and enthesopathy may indicate subclinical musculoskeletal involvement [28].

Erosions: These can also be detected by US.

Tenosynovitis: US findings indicative of tendon involvement include fusiform swelling and focal derangement of tendon echotexture [28]. Achilles tendon, plantar fascia, patellar tendon, and tenosynovial sheaths of the hand and ankle are frequently affected in patients with PsA [28].

Enthesitis: US signs of enthesitis include hypoechoic swelling of the tendon insertion, enthesophytes, and possible bursal enlargement [28].

Magnetic resonance imaging (MRI): This modality is mainly used when the axial skeleton is affected. MRI is the most sensitive imaging for the detection of subtle bilateral changes, which can be important in distinguishing PsA from septic sacroiliitis. The spondylitic changes in PsA and reactive arthritis appear more randomly than those in AS. Large chunky-appearing paravertebral ossification is commonly seen in the thoracolumbar junction. These ossifications do not bridge the intervertebral discs as seen in AS. Ankylosis, squaring of vertebral bodies, and spinal fusion are very rare in PsA.

Computed tomography (CT): CT has little role in the assessment of peripheral joints but may be useful in assessing elements of spine disease [28]. The accuracy of CT is similar to MRI in the assessment of erosions in sacroiliac joints; however, CT has radiation and is not effective in detecting synovial inflammation [28].

Reactive Arthritis (ReA): It is previously known as Reiter's syndrome. It is usually accompanied by conjunctivitis and urethritis. It affects males between the ages of 15 and 35 years. Arthritis might be the only clinical manifestation of ReA. The radiographic features are identical to those in PsA, but the difference is in the pattern of distribution which begins in the feet and then hand. History and clinical examination are helpful in differentiating ReA from PsA.

Osteoarthritis (OA): OA is the most common arthropathy in elderly. It impacts the quality of life, and it has a major implication on public healthcare. OA asymmetrically affects joints of the hands (sparing MCP joints), shoulders, feet, knees, hip, and spine.

Radiography: CR is the gold standard radiologic modality in detecting OA. It detects many OA features. Radiographic progression appears specific (91%) but not sensitive (23%) for cartilage loss [29].

Joint space narrowing: Non-uniform narrowing of the joint spaces occurs in OA.

Osteophytes: These are joint spurs that occur along joint margins. Osteophytes can also be observed on the joint line (Fig. 5.22). The definition of OA relies on the presence of osteophytes on anteroposterior weight-bearing radiographs [29].

Sclerosis: It is seen as an increased density on radiograph [30].

Cyst formation: This is seen as a loss of trabecular structure [30].

Ultrasonography: US is widely used in RA and has been accepted to be used in OA too. US has the advantage of assessing and visualizing many OA features without exposing the patient to radiation. One limitation of US is that it cannot penetrate the bony parts to visualize the structures beyond them. The use of US is more common for hand and knee OA and has very limited usage in the assessment of other joints.

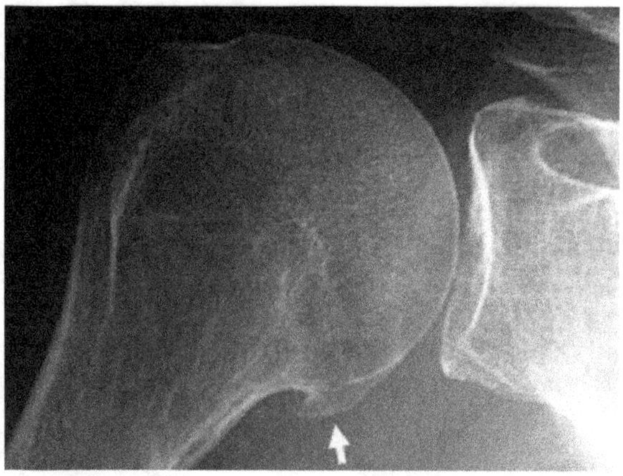

Fig. 5.22 AP view of the shoulder joint shows osteophyte formation (arrow)

Osteophyte: They can be seen as a disturbed acoustic window.

Synovitis: This appears as thickening of synovial membrane.

Erosions: They can be detected in erosive OA.

Magnetic resonance imaging (MRI): MRI is widely used in knee OA and spondylolisthesis as it has the ability of providing a multiplanar image of all compartments. MRI can assess all features of OA, osteophytes, synovitis, effusion, joint spaces, bone marrow lesions, ligaments, cartilage, and vertebral height, as it decreases with degenerative diseases.

Computed tomography (CT): This test is of limited use as it exposes the patient to radiation. It still has its main role emergencies and in cases of suspected fracture.

Acknowledgments The authors would like to thank Dr. Waleed Hafiz for his assistance in the development of this chapter.

References

1. DS C. Septic arthritis and tuberculosis arthritis. J Arthritis. 2012;27(1):526–35
2. Zimmermann B 3rd, Mikolich DJ, Lally EV. Septic sacroiliitis. Semin Arthritis Rheum. 1996;26(3):592–604.
3. Manoj AS, Patel AM. A brief review on calcium pyrophosphate deposition disease pseudogout. Journal of PharmaSciTech. 2014;4:7–11.

4. Chau C, Griffith J. Musculoskeletal infections: ultrasound appearances. Clin Radiol. 2005;60(2):149–59.
5. Tien Y-C, Chih H-W, Lin G-T, Hsien S-H, Lin S-Y. Clinical application of ultrasonography for detection of septic arthritis in children. Kaohsiung J Med Sci. 1999;15(9):542–9.
6. Seltzer SE. Value of computed tomography in planning medical and surgical treatment of chronic osteomyelitis. LWW. 1984;8:482.
7. Christian S, Kraas J, Conway WF, editors. Musculoskeletal infections. Seminars in roentgenology: WB Saunders; 2007.
8. Graif M, Schweitzer M, Deely D, Matteucci T. The septic versus nonseptic inflamed joint: MRI characteristics. Skelet Radiol. 1999;28(11):616–20.
9. De Vuyst D, Vanhoenacker F, Gielen J, Bernaerts A, De Schepper AM. Imaging features of musculoskeletal tuberculosis. Eur Radiol. 2003;13(8):1809–19.
10. Saraf SK, Tuli SM. Tuberculosis of hip: a current concept review. Indian J Orthop. 2015;49(1):1.
11. Hong SH, Kim SM, Ahn JM, Chung HW, Shin MJ, Kang HS. Tuberculous versus pyogenic arthritis: MR imaging evaluation 1. Radiology. 2001;218(3):848–53.
12. Al-Nakshabandi NA. The spectrum of imaging findings of brucellosis: a pictorial essay. Can Assoc Radiol J. 2012;63(1):5–11.
13. Al-Shahed MS, Sharif HS, Haddad MC, Aabed MY, Sammak BM, Mutairi MA. Imaging features of musculoskeletal brucellosis. Radiographics. 1994;14(2):333–48.
14. Geyik MF, Gur A, Nas K, Cevik R, Sarac J, Dikici B, et al. Musculoskeletal involvement of brucellosis in different age groups: a study of 195 cases. Swiss Med Wkly. 2002;132(7-8):98–105.
15. Bozgeyik Z, Aglamis S, Bozdag PG, Denk A. Magnetic resonance imaging findings of musculoskeletal brucellosis. Clin Imaging. 2014;38(5):719–23.
16. Girish G, Melville DM, Kaeley GS, Brandon CJ, Goyal JR, Jacobson JA, et al. Imaging appearances in gout. Arthritis. 2013;2013:673401.
17. Helms CA, Vogler JB III, Simms DA, Genant HK. CPPD crystal deposition disease or pseudogout. Radiographics. 1982;2(1):40–52.
18. Zhang W, Doherty M, Bardin T, Barskova V, Guerne P-A, Jansen T, et al. European league against rheumatism recommendations for calcium pyrophosphate deposition. Part I: terminology and diagnosis. Ann Rheum Dis. 2011;70(4):563–70.
19. Barskova VG, Kudaeva FM, Bozhieva LA, Smirnov AV, Volkov AV, Nasonov EL. Comparison of three imaging techniques in diagnosis of chondrocalcinosis of the knees in calcium pyrophosphate deposition disease. Rheumatology. 2013:kes433.
20. Rothschild B, Bruno M. Imaging in calcium pyrophosphate deposition disease. 2015.
21. Suva MA, Patel AM. A brief review on calcium pyrophosphate deposition disease (pseudogout). Journal of PharmaSciTech. 2014;4:7–11.
22. Tan YK, Ostergaard M, Bird P, Conaghan PG. Ultrasound versus high field magnetic resonance imaging in rheumatoid arthritis. Clin Exp Rheumatol. 2013;32(1 Suppl 80):S99–105.
23. Aletaha D, Neogi T, Silman AJ, Funovits J, Felson DT, Bingham CO, et al. 2010 rheumatoid arthritis classification criteria: an American College of Rheumatology/European League Against Rheumatism collaborative initiative. Arthritis Rheum. 2010;62(9):2569–81.
24. Sommer OJ, Kladosek A, Weiler V, Czembirek H, Boeck M, Stiskal M. Rheumatoid arthritis: a practical guide to state-of-the-art imaging, image interpretation, and clinical implications 1. Radiographics. 2005;25(2):381–98.
25. Colebatch AN, Edwards CJ, Østergaard M, Van Der Heijde D, Balint PV, D'Agostino M-A, et al. EULAR recommendations for the use of imaging of the joints in the clinical management of rheumatoid arthritis. Ann Rheum Dis. 2013;72(6):804–14.
26. Amrami KK. Imaging of the seronegative spondyloarthopathies. Radiol Clin N Am. 2012;50(4):841–54.
27. Jurik AG. Imaging the spine in arthritis—a pictorial review. Insights Imaging. 2011;2(2):177–91.
28. Spadaro A, Lubrano E. Psoriatic arthritis: imaging techniques. Reumatismo. 2012;64(2):99–106.
29. Roemer FW, Crema MD, Trattnig S, Guermazi A. Advances in imaging of osteoarthritis and cartilage. Radiology. 2011;260(2):332–54.
30. Haugen IK, Bøyesen P. Imaging modalities in hand osteoarthritis-status and perspectives of conventional radiography, magnetic resonance imaging, and ultrasonography. Arthritis Res Ther. 2011;13(6):248.

Part II

Patients with Rheumatic Diseases and their Medical Issues: A Diagnostic Approach

6

Diagnosis and Assessment of LBP

Khaled Albazli, Manal Alotaibi, and Hani Almoallim

6.1 Introduction

Low-back pain (LBP) is mainly managed in primary health care. It is a symptom that is commonly belittled and misdiagnosed. This chapter aims to present a simple approach for the diagnosis and assessment of LBP according to the latest clinical recommendations. This content will discuss in details the definition and prevalence of LBP and the important stepwise approach to reach a diagnosis and start treatment. This approach starts from history-taking, physical examination, and radiological studies and, finally, concludes with the management and referral guidelines. Also, inflammatory back pain will be explained thoroughly in an easy to digest way.

A major advantage of this chapter is that carefully designed tables, diagrammatic presentations, and illustrations were used to help practicing clinicians perform proper and adequate work up for patients with LBP.

6.2 Learning Objectives

By the end of this chapter, you should be able to:

1. Present a comprehensive approach for the diagnosis and assessment of low-back pain in accordance with updated clinical guidelines.
2. Recognize the red flags of LBP and the proper time for referral.
3. Prevent the delay of the diagnosis and management of inflammatory back pain (IBP) to avoid the long-term disabilities.

6.3 Definition

LBP is defined as pain or stiffness in the area between the costal margin and the inferior gluteal folds; this pain could also extend to the lower limbs [1]. LBP can also be classified as acute or chronic; this would be helpful for prognostic and management purposes. Acute

K. Albazli
Department of Medicine, Faculty of Medicine in Al-Qunfudhah, Umm Al-Qura University, Makkah, Saudi Arabia

The George Washington University School of Medicine and Health Sciences, Washington, D.C., USA

M. Alotaibi
Northwestern University Feinberg School of Medicine, Chicago, IL, USA

Internal Medicine Department, College of Medicine, Umm Al-Qura University, Makkah, Saudi Arabia

H. Almoallim (✉)
Medical College, Umm Al-Qura University (UQU), Makkah, Saudi Arabia
e-mail: hmmoallim@uqu.edu.sa

LBP is considered if the symptom was present for less than 6 weeks, while sub-acute and chronic would be considered if the pain lasts from 6 to 12 weeks and more than 12 weeks, respectively [2]. Table 6.1 shows some important definitions for some terminologies used while dealing with patients complaining of LBP.

6.4 Prevalence

LBP is a worldwide problem that is more commonly found in females and those aged between 40 and 80 years [3–5]. Lifetime prevalence of LBP has increased significantly to become as high as 84%, while chronic LBP has reached 23%. Of this population, 11–12% will develop some form of impairment or disability.

6.5 Differential Diagnosis

Back pain is a frequently encountered symptom that could be caused by many specific and non-specific underlying causes, as shown in Table 6.2 However, mechanical low-back pain represents 97% of the causes [6].

6.6 Approach to Diagnosis

When assessing a patient presenting with LBP, it is important to rule out neurologic deficits or other serious inflammatory or medical conditions with a focused history and physical examination. Thorough assessments are also important to aid physicians in screening the patients who need further diagnostic investigations to rule out serious pathologies (see Fig. 6.1) [7, 8].

Table 6.1 Important terminologies in low-back pain

Spondylosis	A degenerative osteoarthritis of the spine. It can be seen radiographically as a narrowed disc with arthritic changes
Spondyloarthritis	Also called spondyloarthropathy is a group of inflammatory rheumatic diseases that cause arthritis. The most common is ankylosing spondylitis, which affects mainly the spine. Others include reactive arthritis, psoriatic arthritis, and enteropathic arthritis/ spondylitis associated with inflammatory bowel diseases
Spondylolisthesis	Anterior or posterior displacement of a vertebra or the vertebral column in relation to the vertebrae below. The slippage is determined by spinal X-ray and graded from grade 1 to 4 Grade 1: Less the 25% slippage Grade 2: 25%–50% slippage Grade 3: 50%–75% Grade 4: More than 75%
Spondylitis	Inflammation of vertebrae manifested by back pain and progressive stiffness of the spine. The inflamed spine can be visible in MRI
Discitis	An inflammation of the intervertebral disc space often related to infection
Radiculopathy	Impairment of a nerve root, usually causing radiating pain, numbness, tingling, or muscle weakness that corresponds to a specific nerve root

The history-taking elements for LBP include the following:

- Type of onset and character may hint at the underlying pathology:
  - Bones: dull and nagging.
  - Muscles: dull aching.
  - Nerves: sharp and lightning like.

Table 6.2 Lower-back pain causes and risk factors

Specific causes of LBP	**Musculoskeletal:** • **Musculoligamentous strain**: Experienced by up to 80% of population at some time • **Fibromyalgia:** Widespread pain in all 4 quadrants of the body, at least 3 months, 11 out of 18 positive tender points on physical exam • **Osteoarthritis:** Affects mainly the hips, knees, spine, first CMC, DIP, and PIP • **Rheumatoid arthritis:** May affect facet joints. It presents with pain, swelling, and impaired function of joints with morning stiffness for ≥1 hour and has extra-articular manifestations, positive RF, and ACPA • **Spondylolisthesis:** Dull, aching pain in the lower lumbar or upper sacral region. Pain also extends into the buttocks or posterior thigh • **Vertebral compression fracture:** Symptoms could mean compression of the nerves at the fracture site: Numbness, tingling, weakness, and incontinence • **Inflammatory:** Spondyloarthritis (ankylosing spondylitis, reactive arthritis, psoriatic arthritis) **Spinal cord**: Myelopathy **Nerve root**: Radiculopathy **Degenerative or traumatic:** Disc herniation, spondylosis, fracture **Metabolic:** Paget's disease, osteomalacia **Neoplastic:** Lung, breast, prostate, multiple myeloma, lymphoma **Infectious**: TB discitis, osteomyelitis, epidural abscess, zoster, Lyme, CMV, HIV **Referred pain:** • **Gastroenterology:** PUD, cholelithiasis, pancreatitis, pancreatic cancer • **Genitourinary:** Pyelonephritis, nephrolithiasis, uterine or ovarian cancer, salpingitis • **Vascular:** Aortic dissection, leaking aortic aneurysm
Nonspecific causes	Poor posture, sitting and standing, lifting ergonomics, unknown causes
Risk factors	Overweight, smoking, pregnancy, long-term use of medication (e.g., corticosteroids), stress, depression, occupation

CMC carpometacarpal *joint*, *DIP* distal interphalangeal joint, *PIP* proximal interphalangeal *joint*, *RF* rheumatoid factor, *ACPA* anti-citrullinated protein antibodies, *CMV* cytomegalovirus, *HIV* human immunodeficiency virus, *PUD* peptic ulcer disease

  - Nerve root: sharp and shooting.
  - Sympathetic nerve: burning, pressure like, stinging, and aching.
  - Vascular: throbbing and diffuse.
- Duration: this would help guide imaging and treatment decisions.
- The site of pain and any radiation: this would help to rule out radiculopathy.
- Intensity of the pain.
- Continuous versus on and off.
- Progressive or not.
- Factors that improve or worsen the pain: daytime vs nighttime, certain positions, activity vs rest, and response to treatments.
- Severity of pain.
- Associated symptoms: extra-axial joint pain, sciatica, paresthesias, pseudoclaudication, and bowel/bladder dysfunction.
- Assess for symptoms specific for certain diseases like spondyloarthropathies, i.e., enthesitis, dactylitis, history of psoriasis, and bowel symptoms.
- Assess for red flags (see "radiological studies"):
  - History of trauma [9].
  - Symptoms suggestive of an infection or malignancy, i.e., fever and unexplained weight loss.
  - Neurological deficits or other symptoms that may give a clue to serious underlying pathologies like cauda equine syndrome, compression fractures, spinal stenosis, herniated disc, or radiculopathy.
- Review of systems:
  - Referred pain due to underlying visceral pathologies.

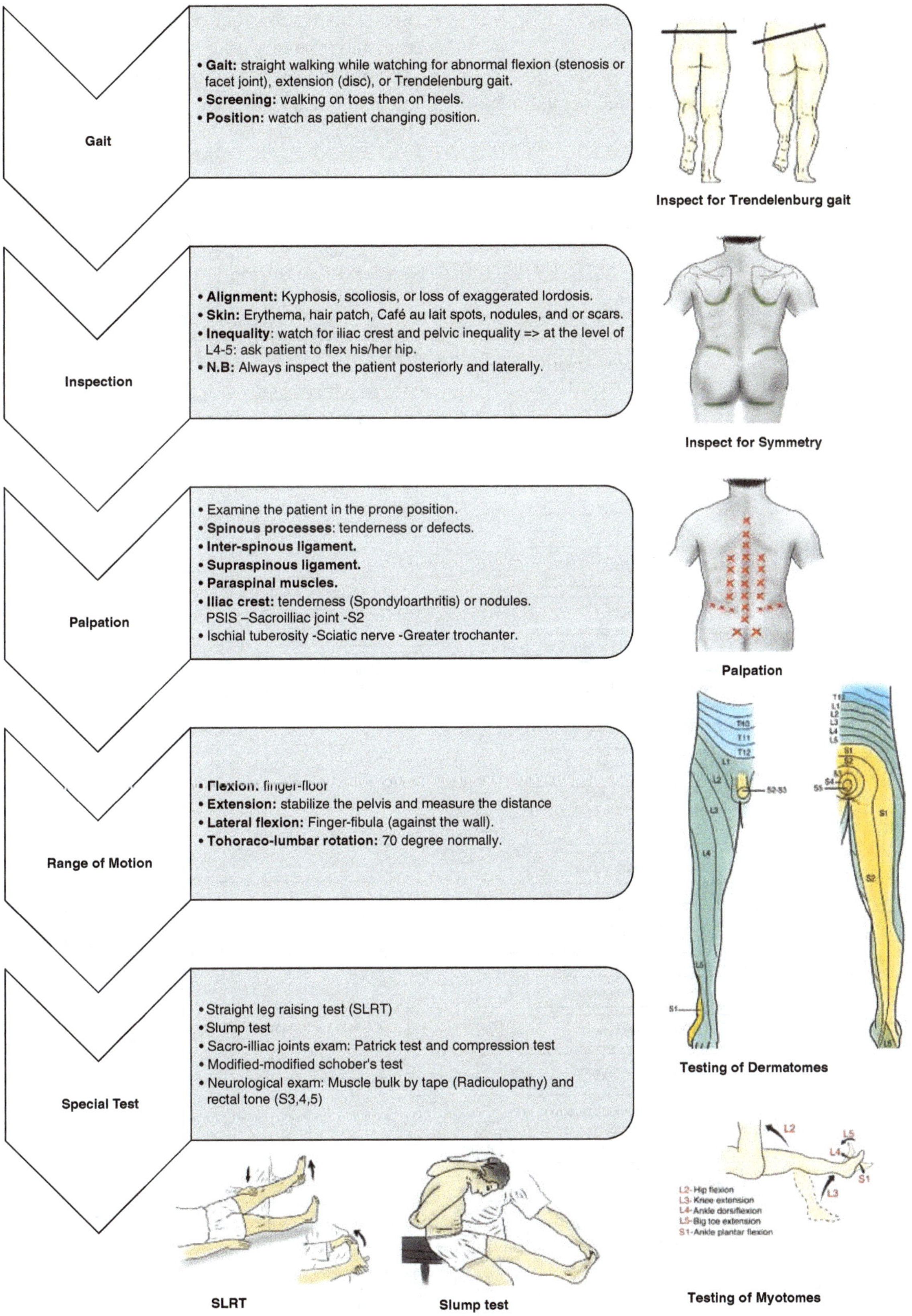

Fig. 6.1 Approach to back MSK examination

- Past medical and surgical history:
  - Previous history of cancer.
  - Medications.
  - History of osteoporosis and/or pathologic fractures.
  - Anxiety or depression.
- Social history: history of smoking, illicit drug use, and type of work.
- The physical examination steps for the assessment of LBP include the following (see Fig. 6.2):

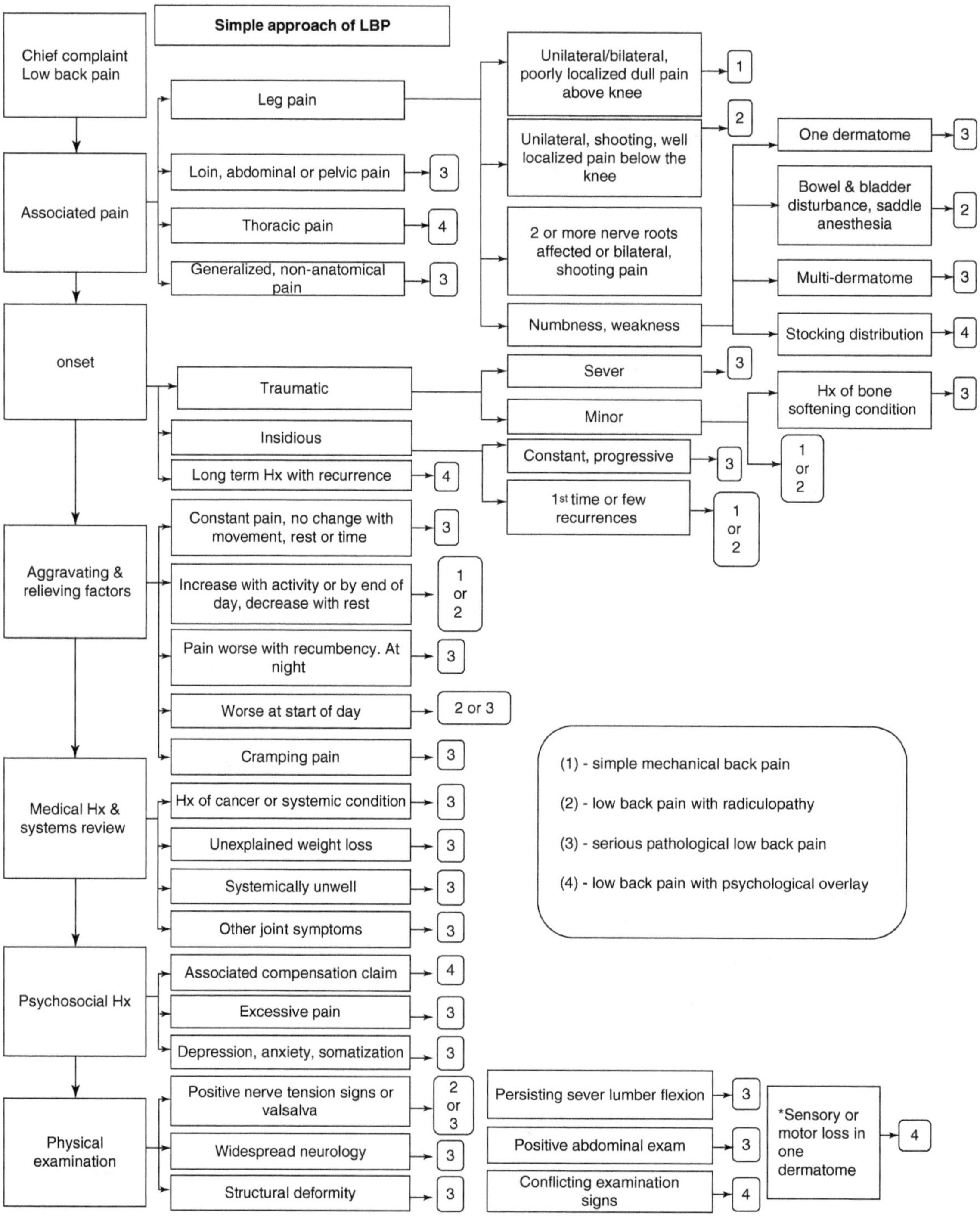

Fig. 6.2 Simple approach of LBP

- Inspection for skin changes and gait abnormalities.
- Palpation for tenderness.
- Range of motion.
- Special tests (Table 6.3).

Table 6.3 Special tests for LBP

Special test	Technique and significance
Straight leg raise test (SLRT)	• To test for the presence of a disc herniation • In supine position, flex the patient's hip while maintaining the knee in full extension • Watch for the degree of hip flexion where the patient reports pain • **Positive SLRT:** Radicular pain down the posterior portion of the tested leg at 40 degrees of hip flexion or less • Sensitivity 33%, specificity 87%
Slump test	• Ask the patient to hold hands behind his/her back while seated upright • Instruct to the patient to (slump) flex his/her spine, followed by neck flexion • With examiner's hand on top of head, the patient performs knee extension and dorsiflexion of foot • Ask the patient to return the neck to neutral (no flexion) • **Positive slump test:** The patient's symptoms are increased in the slumped position and released as the patient actively extends • Sensitivity 84%, specificity 83%
Patrick's test (FABER)	• To assess for the sacroiliac joint dysfunction or hip joint pathology • In supine position, bring the tested leg to hip flexion, abduction, and external rotation • Against the medial knee, try to bring the bent leg passively towards the table • **Positive test**: Reproduction of groin pain or buttock pain • Sensitivity 82%
Compression test	• To assess for the sacroiliac joint dysfunction • While standing behind the patient, bring him/her to sideline position • Ask the patient to flex hip at 60 degrees and knees at 90 degrees • Apply an inward/downward force on iliac crest • **Positive test:** Pain on sacroiliac joint • Sensitivity 69% and specificity 93%
Modified-modified Schober test	• Identify the PSISs by marking the inferior margins of the patient's PSISs with his or her thumbs • Mark along the midline of the lumbar spines horizontal to the PSISs • Make another mark 15 cm above the original mark • With a tape pressed firmly on the line between the two marked points, instruct the patient to bend forward into full lumbar flexion • Measure the new distance between the superior and inferior skin markings • Distance increases less than 5 cm indicates limited lower back flexion
Neurological assessment	• Measure the muscle bulk by tape • Assess for muscle power: Hip flexion (L2), knee extension (L3), ankle dorsiflexion (L4), big toe extension (L5), and ankle plantar flexion (S1) • Check knee reflex (L3 and L4) and ankle reflex (L5 and S1) • Check for skin sensory loss • Assess anal sphincter tone by digital examination (S3, 4, 5)

PSIS posterior superior iliac spine, *L* Lumbar vertebrae, *S* Sacral vertebrae

6.7 Radiological Studies for LBP

Acute LBP that is free of any red flags is generally a benign and self-limiting condition that does not warrant any further imaging evaluation. If there are any signs of complications, an MRI should be requested as it has replaced CTs and myelographies as the first-line imaging modality. MRIs are useful for detecting infections and neoplasia and for postoperative assessments. However, CTs are more useful in patients with abnormalities in bone structure and for evaluation of surgical fusion or instrumentation procedures. CTs are also useful when MRIs are contraindicated. Other imaging modalities like myelography/CT, discography/CT, and radioisotope bone scans can be used in selected patients [10, 11].

Red flags that warrant further imaging [9]:

- Onset above age 70 years old.
- Pain that has persisted for more than 6 weeks.
- History of trauma, even mild trauma in patients aged >50.
- History of surgery in the same site of pain.
- History of malignancy.
- History of IV drug abuse.
- History of osteoporosis or long-term use of steroids.
- Weight loss that is unexplained.
- Fever without an obvious source of infection.
- The presence of focal neurological deficits.
- The use of immunosuppressive medication.

Imaging studies that may be considered include:

1. **X-ray**
   - It is useful in delineating degenerative bone disease, disc prolapse, spondylolisthesis, fractures, and neoplasia and to assess prior surgical interventions.
   - Erythrocyte sedimentation rate (ESR) is a useful tool that can suggest the presence or absence of an infection or neoplasia. In patients with no more than 1 risk factor for systemic disease and an ESR less than 20, infections and malignancy would be considered less likely.
2. **CT**
   - It can help in detecting degenerative bone disease, spondylolisthesis, fractures, and malunion. It can also delineate inflammation in the sacroiliac joints.
   - It can show false-positive findings following trauma.
3. **MRI**
   - This is the optimal imaging modality for detection of soft tissue abnormalities. It should be offered to patients presenting with neurological deficits. It is a valuable tool for detecting conditions like disk herniation, spinal stenosis, osteomyelitis, discitis, spinal epidural abscess, bone metastasis, arachnoiditis, and neural tube defects.
   - It can reveal inflammatory changes in the sacroiliac joints before they start showing on plain X-rays.
4. **Electromyography (EMG)**
   - It is useful in patients complaining of radiculopathic pain with inconclusive findings on imaging modalities who may be considered for surgery.
   - It can be helpful in patients who were found to have multilevel affection on imaging.
5. **Radionuclide bone scans**
   - It is a more sensitive tool than plain X-rays, especially for the detection of hidden infections or malignancy.
   - In patient who have normal ESR values and plain radiographs, however, these will be of limited utility.

6.8 Detection of Inflammatory Back Pain

Inflammatory back pain (IBP) is usually diagnosed late especially in primary care settings. Causes for this delay may include difficulties in differentiating between mechanical and inflammatory back pain. IBP can lead to significant functional disability. The longer the diagnosis is delayed, the worse the functional outcome [11, 12].

Seronegative spondyloarthropathies are an important cause of IBP. They are a group of inflammatory diseases that are characterized by seronegative arthritis (rheumatoid factor negative) which is linked with the presence of the human leukocyte antigen HLA-B27.

The seronegative spondyloarthropathies include the following disorders:

- Undifferentiated spondyloarthritis.
- Ankylosing spondylitis: involves the spine, peripheral joints, and entheses. This disorder is a frequently underdiagnosed cause of low-back pain.
- Reactive arthritis or Reiter's syndrome: presents with conjunctivitis, urethritis, and arthritis.

- Spondyloarthritis associated with psoriasis: arthritis that is associated with psoriasis.
- Spondyloarthritis with inflammatory bowel disease: Crohn's disease and ulcerative colitis are often associated with ankylosing spondylitis or peripheral arthritis.
- Juvenile onset ankylosing spondylitis: affects children under the age of 16 years.

IBP definition criteria includes the following items [13, 14]:

- The pain has an insidious character.
- Pain increases at night.
- Pain that improves with activity and does not improve with rest.
- Onset of pain occurs in patients <40 years of age.

Four criteria out of five are required to make a diagnosis of IBP. The sensitivity and specificity of these criteria are at 77% and 91.7%, respectively. Referral to a rheumatologist should be considered if these criteria are fulfilled (Fig. 6.3) [15, 16].

6.9 Treatment of Low-Back Pain (Acute or Sub-Acute Pain) [17, 18]

- In patients with favorable prognosis, reassurance is imperative.
- Physical activity and supervised exercise regimens.
- Bed rest should not be recommended.
- Nonpharmacological therapy that can be used in an acute setting with moderate-quality evidence includes superficial heat, massage, and acupuncture. Low-quality evidence therapies include spinal manipulation.
- Second-line agents include nonsteroidal anti-inflammatory drugs, muscle relaxants, and duloxetine (as co-medications for pain control). Newer guidelines no longer support the use of acetaminophen and tricyclic antidepressants.
- Modalities such as electrotherapy should not be used.
- Medications and other therapies should only be used short term.
- There should be a multidisciplinary approach to treatment.

6.10 Treatment of Inflammatory Back Pain (IBP)

The main target for therapy is to decrease the severity of symptoms and inflammation and to halt the progression to impairment and functional disability. Nonpharmacological therapy includes exercise and patient counselling. Group exercises are favored over home exercises. Treatment of patients suffering from IBP should be tailored to each patient's individual manifestations and general condition. Factors that should be kept in mind include the patient's age, sex, presence of comorbidities, medication interactions, socioeconomic status, severity of symptoms and signs, and his overall prognosis. Certain clinical findings should be considered while formulating a therapeutic plan, such as axial or peripheral symptom predominance and entheseal and extra-articular affection.

If the patient complains of persistent symptoms, NSAIDs are used as first-line pharmacological therapy. In cases where NSAIDs are contraindicated or not tolerated, paracetamol and/or opioids can be used. Disease-modifying anti-rheumatic drugs (DMARDs) such as systemic steroids, sulfasalazine, and methotrexate were not found to be useful in axial predominant disease. However, intra-articular injections in affected sites can be beneficial.

If patients exhibit significantly active disease, anti-TNF agents can be considered. Surgery should be offered to patients suffering from pain that is refractory to all previously mentioned treatment lines. It can also be offered to patients with functional impairment and anatomical damage found on imaging [19]. Spinal corrective osteotomy can be considered in patients suffering from severe deformities and significant functional impairment. Referral to surgery should also be done in AS and acute vertebral fracture cases (Fig. 6.4).

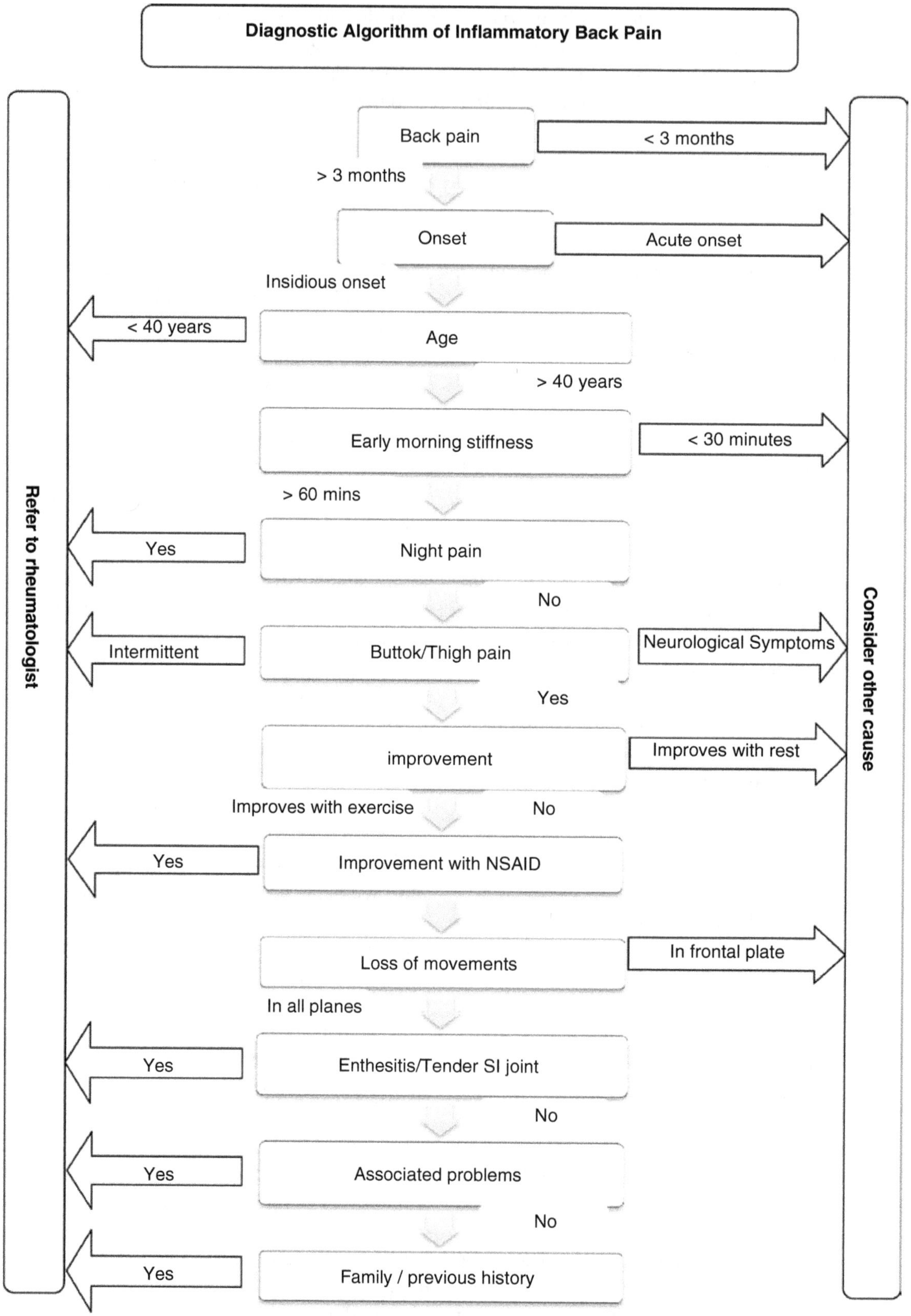

Fig. 6.3 Diagnostic algorithm of low back pain

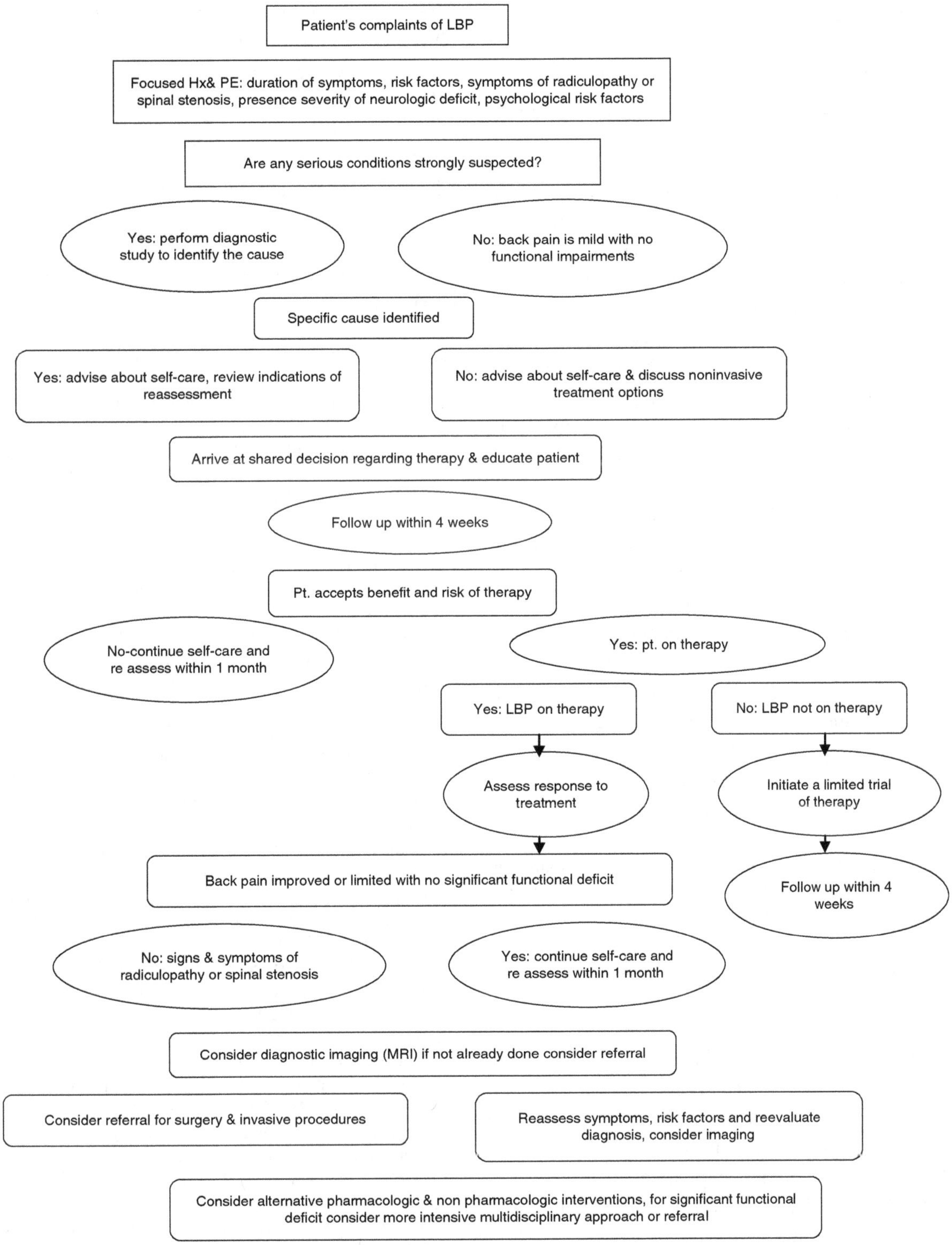

Fig. 6.4 How to approach a LBP patient in the clinic

6.11 Referral

Consultations to neurosurgery or orthopedics are needed if any of the following symptoms and/or signs occur:

1. Cauda equina syndrome: this should be suspected if the patient complains of typical features like bowel and bladder dysfunction (urinary retention), saddle anesthesia, and bilateral leg weakness and numbness.
2. Spinal cord compression: this should be suspected in cancer patients who have a risk of spinal metastasis. They may present with acute neurologic deficits and need emergent evaluation for surgical decompression or radiation therapy.
3. Progressive or severe neurologic deficits or if any neuromotor deficits that persist after 4 to 6 weeks of conservative therapy: these patients should be referred to a neurologist.
4. Sciatica, sensory deficit, or reflex loss persistent for 4–6 weeks in a patient with positive straight leg raise test, consistent clinical findings, and favorable psychosocial circumstances such as realistic expectations and absence of depression, substance abuse, or excessive somatization.

Acknowledgments The authors would like to thank Dr. Waleed Hafiz and Dr. Rola Hassan for their assistance in the development of this chapter.

Abbreviations

ACPA	Anti-citrullinated protein antibodies
AS	Ankylosing spondylitis
CMC	Carpometacarpal *joint*
CMV	Cytomegalovirus
DIP	Distal interphalangeal joint
DMARDs	Disease-modifying anti-rheumatic drugs
GI	Gastrointestinal
HIV	Human immunodeficiency virus
HLA	Human leukocyte antigen
IBP	Inflammatory back pain
L	Lumbar vertebrae
LBP	Low-back pain
NSAIDs	Nonsteroidal anti-inflammatory drugs
PIP	Proximal interphalangeal *joint*
PSIS	Posterior superior iliac spine
PUD	Peptic ulcer disease
RF	Rheumatoid factor
S	Sacral vertebrae

References

1. Balagué F, et al. Non-specific low back pain. Lancet. 2012;19(9829):1874.
2. Chou R, Qaseem A, et al. Diagnosis and treatment of low back pain: a joint clinical practice guideline from the American College of Physicians and the American pain society. Ann Intern Med. 2007;147(7):478–91.
3. Concannon M, Bridgen A. Lower back pain: a need for thorough assessment. Pract Nurs. 2011;22(9)
4. Hoy D, Bain C, Williams G, March L, Brooks P, Blyth F, et al. A systematic review of the global prevalence of low back pain. Arthritis Rheum. 2012;64(6): 2028–37.
5. Hill JC, Whitehurst DG, Lewis M, Bryan S, Dunn KM, Foster NE, et al. Comparison of stratified primary care management for low back pain with current best practice (STarT Back): a randomised controlled trial. Lancet. 2011;378(9802):1560–71.
6. Williams CM, Maher CG, Hancock MJ, McAuley JH, McLachlan AJ, Britt H, et al. Low back pain and best practice care: a survey of general practice physicians. Arch Intern Med. 2010;170(3):271–7.
7. Henschke N, Maher CG, Refshauge KM, Herbert RD, Cumming RG, Bleasel J, et al. Prognosis in patients with recent onset low back pain in Australian primary care: inception cohort study. BMJ. 2008;337:a171.
8. Bhangle SD, Sapru S, Panush RS. Back pain made simple: an approach based on principles and evidence. Cleve Clin J Med. 2009;76(7):393–9.
9. Henschke N, Maher CG, Ostelo RW, De Vet HC, Macaskill P, Irwig L. Red flags to screen for malignancy in patients with low-back pain. Cochrane Database Syst Rev. 2013;2:CD008686.
10. Dagenais S, Tricco AC, Haldeman S. Synthesis of recommendations for the assessment and management of low back pain from recent clinical practice guidelines. Spine J. 2010;10(6):514–29.
11. Sieper J, Landewé R, et al. New criteria for inflammatory back pain in patients with chronic back pain: a real patient exercise by experts from the assessment of SpondyloArthritis international society (ASAS). Ann Rheum Dis. 2009;68(4):784–8.
12. Braun J, Inman R. Clinical significance of inflammatory back pain for diagnosis and screening of

patients with axial spondyloarthritis. Ann Rheum Dis. 2011;69(7):1264–85.
13. Harper BE, John D, et al. Spondyloarthritis: clinical suspicion, diagnosis, and sports. Curr Sports Med Rep. 2009;8(1):29–34.
14. Dincer U, Cakar E, et al. Diagnosis delay in patients with ankylosing spondylitis: possible reasons and proposals for new diagnostic criteria. Clin Rheumatol. 2008;27(4):457–62.
15. Kubiak EN, Moskovich R, et al. Orthopaedic management of ankylosing spondylitis. J Am Acad Orthop Surg. 2005;13(4):267–78.
16. Braun J, Baraliakos X, et al. 2010 update of the ASAS/EULAR recommendations for the management of ankylosing spondylitis. Ann Rheum Dis. 2011;70(4):896–904.
17. Chou R, Huffman LH. Medications for acute and chronic low back pain: a review of the evidence for an American Pain Society/American College of Physicians clinical practice guideline. Ann Intern Med. 2008;148(3):247–8.
18. Perianayagam GR, Newey M, Sell P. NICE guidelines in the management of non-specific back pain in primary care: are they being used? Bone Joint J. 2013;95B(SUPP 1):184.
19. Koes W, et al. An updated overview of clinical guidelines for the management of non-specific low back pain in primary care. Eur Spine J. 2010;19(12):2075–94.

7

CTDs and their Pulmonary Manifestations

Rabab Taha and Maun Feteih

7.1 Introduction

Pulmonary manifestations cause a huge burden for patients with connective tissue diseases (CTD). It has been associated with higher rates of mortality and morbidity.

There are six CTDs which have significant pulmonary manifestations:

- Systemic sclerosis (SSc) or scleroderma.
- Rheumatoid arthritis (RA).
- Systemic lupus erythematosus (SLE).
- Sjogren syndrome (SS).
- Mixed connective tissue disease (MCTD).
- Polymyositis/dermatomyositis (PM/DM).

7.2 Chapter Objectives

- To develop a practical approach to chronic and acute dyspnea and cough for the previously mentioned CTDs' patients.
- To know when and how to screen for the pulmonary diseases related to the CTDs.
- To develop knowledge about most of the pulmonary manifestations of CTDs and how to diagnose them and treat them sufficiently.

7.3 About the Chapter

In the chapter, for every CTD, the pulmonary manifestations will be discussed according to the anatomical structure of the respiratory system as follows:

- Airways:
  - Upper airway.
  - Lower airway.
- Parenchyma:
  - Alveolar space.
  - Interstitium.
- Vasculature:
  - Pulmonary artery.
- Pleura:
  - Pleural space.
  - Pleura.
- Respiratory muscles:
  - Diaphragm.
  - Chest wall muscles.

7.4 To Get the Most of the Chapter

- In general, interstitial lung diseases (ILD) and pulmonary arterial hypertension (PAH) are the most common pulmonary manifestations of CTDs.

R. Taha (✉)
Infectious Diseases Unit, Internal Medicine Department, Doctor Soliman Fakeeh Hospital, Jeddah, Saudi Arabia

King Abdulaziz University, Jeddah, Saudi Arabia

M. Feteih
Pulmonary Medicine, King Faisal Specialist Hospital & Research Center, Jeddah, Saudi Arabia

- The most common subtypes of ILD are non-specific interstitial pneumonia (NSIP) and usual interstitial pneumonia (UIP). Furthermore, for all CTDs except SSc, NSIP, which presents with ground glass opacities (GGO) on high resolution computed tomography (HRCT), has better prognosis than UIP, which presents as reticular opacities with or without honeycombing on HRCT. That's because GGO represents an ongoing inflammatory process, while reticular opacities and honeycombing represent fibrosis.

Due to the rarity of some CTDs or some of the pulmonary manifestations, there are few or lack of large randomized control trials (RCTs) to relay on in decision making, which makes the management not standardized.

7.5 Important Information about Pulmonary Manifestations of CTDs before Going through the Chapter

Most of the pulmonary manifestations could occur before, co-exist, or after the CTD itself being clinically manifested.

- The prevalence of each entity of pulmonary manifestations related to each CTD is presented in Table 7.1.
- Screening for pulmonary complications in CTD patients is not well established. However, the following model seems to be acceptable to be applied to all CTDs, while physicians should tailor it according to their patients and the clinical context (Fig. 7.1).
- CTD-related interstitial lung disease (CTD-ILD) subtypes are similar to those in idiopathic interstitial pneumonia (IIP). Each subtype has been named according to its histological and/or radiological pattern (Table 7.2).
- Classification of pulmonary hypertension (Fig. 7.2; Table 7.3).
- The decision of when to start treatment in CTD-ILD is considered a dilemma because some patients present with respiratory symptoms and others are asymptomatic but have physiological (i.e., pulmonary function test [PFT]) or radiological (i.e. HRCT) abnormalities related to ILD. Thus, a useful stepwise approach developed by the authors of the Scleroderma lung study could be used depending on the severity of the disease on HRCT. See text below (SSc-ILD treatment) and combine it with (Fig. 7.3). We think it's appropriate to apply it to the rest of the CTD-ILD.
- The approach to screening for CTD-related pulmonary hypertension (CTD-PAH) is illustrated in Fig. 7.4 [1].
- The approach to acute dyspnea in CTDs is presented in Fig. 7.5.
- The approach to chronic dyspnea in CTDs is presented in Fig. 7.6.

Table 7.1 Connective tissue diseases and pulmonary manifestations

CTDs and common pulmonary manifestations					
	ILD	Airways	Pleura	Vascular	DAH
Systemic sclerosis	+++	–	–	+++	–
Systemic sclerosis	++	++	++	+	–
Primary Sjogren's syndrome	++	++	+	+	–
Mixed CTD	++	+	+	++	–
Polymyositis/dermatomyositis	+++	–	–	+	–
Systemic lupus erythematosus	+	+	+++	+	++

Adopted from Aryeh Fischer, Prof Roland du Bois. Interstitial lung disease in connective tissue disorders The Lancet, Volume 380, Issue 9842, Pages 689–698, 18 August 2012. The signs show prevalence of each manifestation (–, no prevalence; +, low prevalence; ++, medium prevalence; +++, high prevalence)

ILD interstitial lung disease, *DAH* diffuse alveolar hemorrhage, *CTD* connective tissue disease

Fig. 7.1 Screening of pulmonary complications of CTDs. *BNP* B-type natriuretic peptide, *CTD* Connective tissue disease, *ECG* Electrocardiogram, *Echo* Echocardiogram, *HRCT* High-resolution computed tomography, *Hx* History, *P/E* Physical examination, *PFT* Pulmonary function test

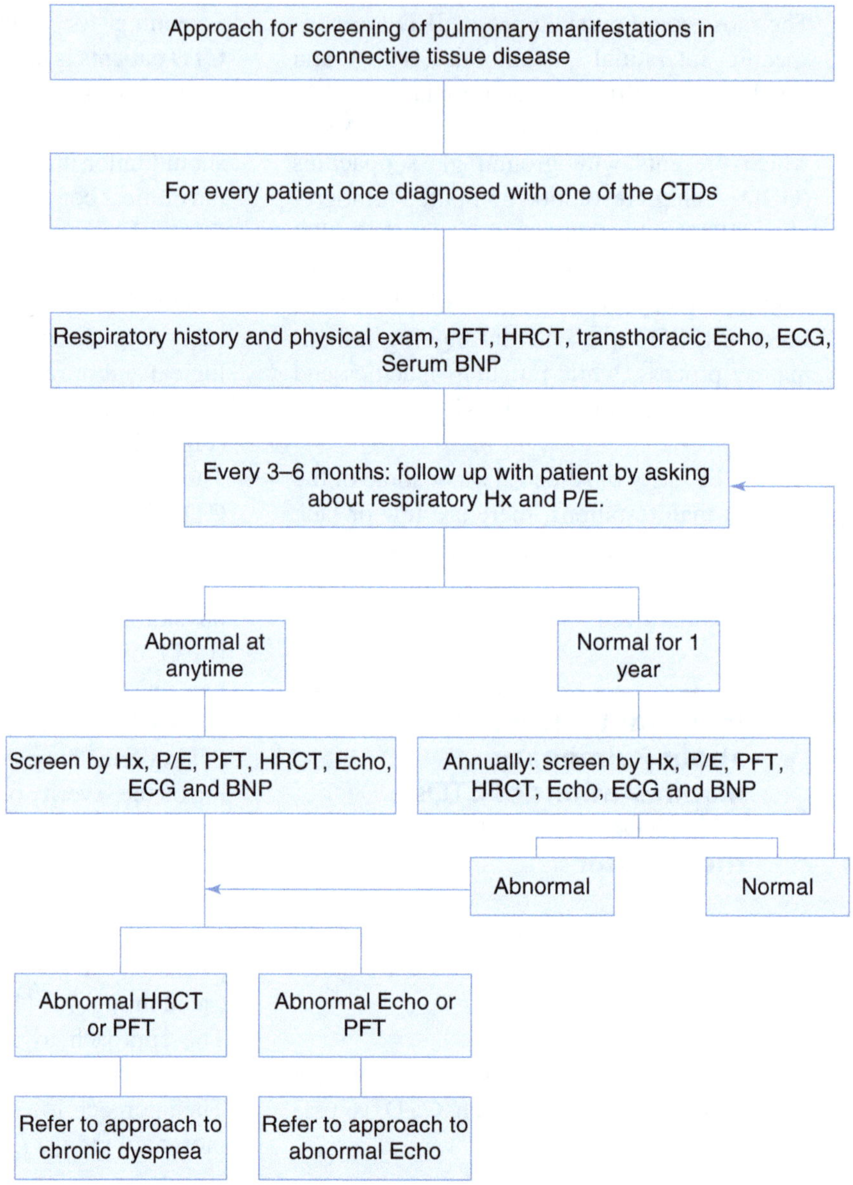

- Pleural fluid analysis for CTDs (except for PM/DM and MCTD, due to the lack of sufficient information about them) (Table 7.4).
- Although drug-induced lung injury is an uncommon complication (mostly reported in observational studies), treating physicians should consider it as one of the differential diagnoses of lung injuries. Furthermore, it's important to know the common and serious adverse events of the medications used in CTD-ILD, so it would be easier to monitor them and follow them up with patients. Once drug-induced lung injury is suspected, one should take into consideration the duration between starting the drug and the development of pulmonary manifestation in addition to the dose of the drug. Eventually, there is no single test that could help in confirming this diagnosis. However, withdrawal of the offending drug appears to be best step to diagnose it besides other findings, which are presented in Table 7.5. Moreover, a useful website established by French pulmonologists from Dijon University has been launched to provide information about drugs causing lung toxicity (www.pneumotox.com). Of

Table 7.2 Radiological and histological patterns of idiopathic interstitial pneumonias

Radiological pattern	Histological pattern
IPF	UIP
NSIP	NSIP
OP	OP
LIP	LIP
RB-ILD	RB
AIP	DAD

Adopted from American Thoracic Society/European Respiratory Society international multidisciplinary consensus classification of the idiopathic interstitial pneumonias. Am J Resp Crit Care Med 2002; 165:277
IPF Idiopathic pulmonary fibrosis, *UIP* Usual interstitial pneumonia, *NSIP* Non-specific interstitial pneumonia, *OP* Organizing pneumonia, *LIP* Lymphocytic interstitial pneumonia, *RB-ILD* Respiratory Bronchiolitis interstitial lung disease, *RB* Respiratory Bronchiolitis, *AIP* Acute interstitial pneumonia, *DAD* Diffuse alveolar damage

note, doing bronchoalveolar lavage (BAL) is a must to rule out infections (bacterial, viral, fungal, mycobacterial).

7.6 Pulmonary Manifestations According to each CTD

7.6.1 Systemic Sclerosis or Scleroderma (SSc)

Systemic sclerosis (SSc) is a rare multisystem disease that involves skin and other body organs causing fibrosis and vascular complications. It is divided into local cutaneous systemic sclerosis (lcSSc), which is more commonly associated

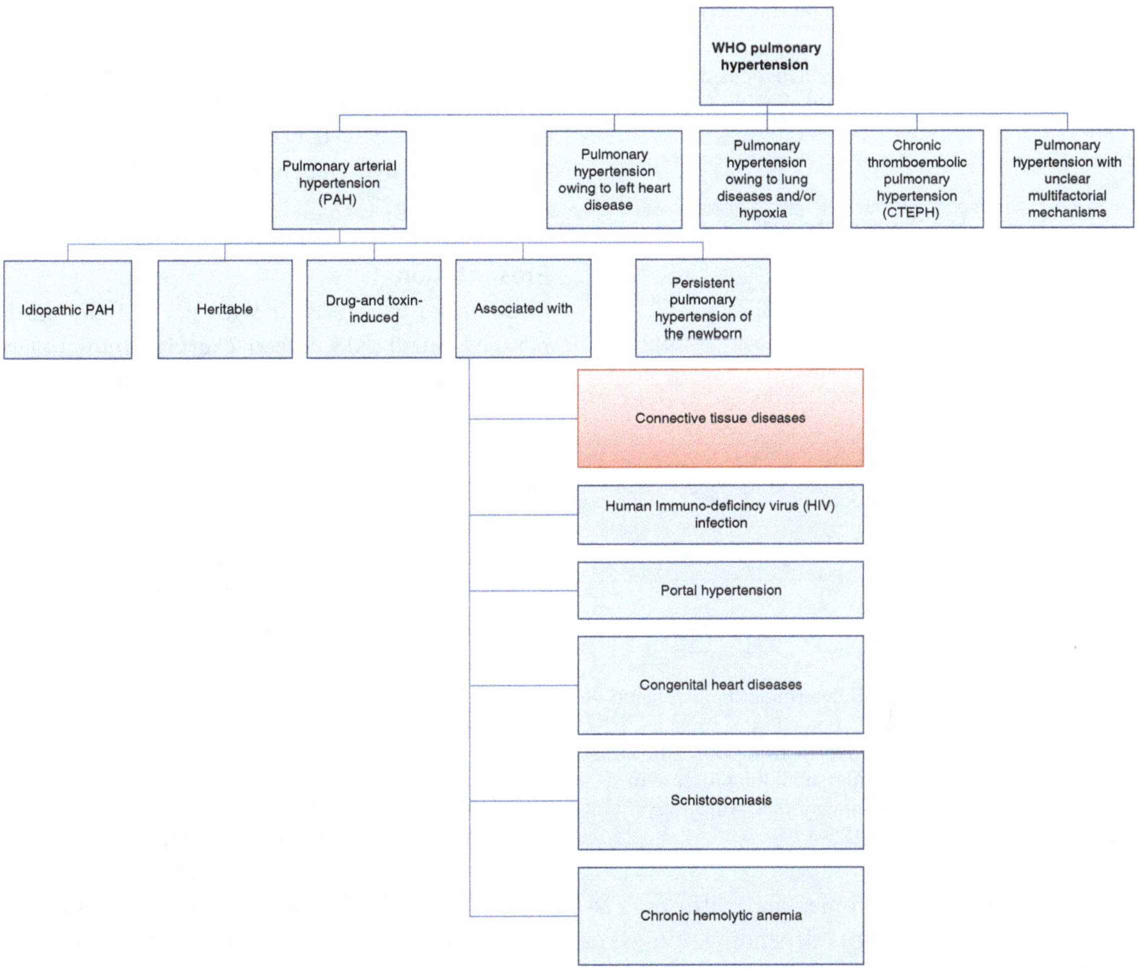

Fig. 7.2 World health organization (WHO) classification of pulmonary hypertension. (Adopted from Simonneau G, Galie N, Rubin L, et al. Clinical classification of pulmonary hypertension. J Am Coll Cardiol. 2004;43 Suppl 1:S5–12)

Table 7.3 World health organization functional classification of pulmonary hypertension

	WHO functional classification
I	Patients with pulmonary hypertension but without resulting limitations of physical activity. Ordinary physical activity does not cause undue fatigue or dyspnea, chest pain, or heart syncope
II	Patients with pulmonary hypertension resulting in slight limitation of physical activity. They are comfortable at rest. Ordinary physical activity results in undue fatigue or dyspnea, chest pain, or heart syncope
III	Patients with pulmonary hypertension resulting in marked limitation of physical activity. They are comfortable at rest. Less than ordinary physical activity causes undue fatigue or dyspnea, chest pain, or heart syncope
IV	Patients with pulmonary hypertension resulting in inability to carry on any physical activity without symptoms. These patients manifest signs of right heart failure. Dyspnea and/or fatigue may be present even at rest. Discomfort is increased by physical activity

Adopted from: Rich, S. Primary hypertension: executive summary. Evian, France. World Health Organization, 1998

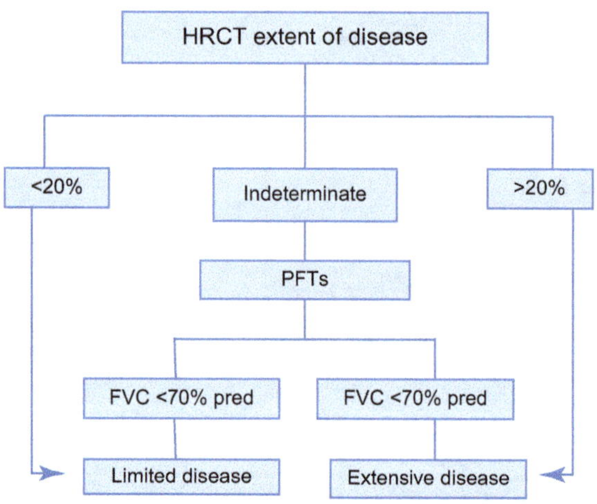

Fig. 7.3 A simple system to determine the extension of interstitial lung disease. *FVC* Forced vital capacity, *PFT* Pulmonary function test. (Adopted from Goh NS, Desai SR, Veeraraghavan S, et al. Interstitial lung disease in systemic sclerosis: a simple staging system. Am J Respir Crit Care Med 2008; 177: 1248–1254)

with the CREST syndrome, and diffuses systemic sclerosis (dcSSc) depending on skin involvement and distribution. Furthermore, lung involvement occurs in about 70% of SSc cases. Also, it is considered to be the leading cause of death in SSc patients [2]. Moreover, the most common pulmonary manifestations in SSc are ILD and PAH. While less common pulmonary involvements are pleural effusion, aspiration pneumonitis, spontaneous pneumothorax, bronchiectasis, drug-associated pneumonitis, and lung cancer.

7.6.1.1 Parenchymal Lung Diseases

SSc-associated interstitial lung disease (SSc-ILD), it occurs in about 40–52% of all SSc patients. However, the dcSSc type appears to be associated with higher risk to develop it compared with lcSSc. Risk factors are African American, gastroesophageal reflux disease (GERD), higher skin score, high level of C-reactive protein (CRP), hypothyroidism, cardiac involvement, Th/To ribonucleoprotein antibodies (anti-Th/To), and anti-topoisomerase I (Scl-70). On the other hand, anti-centromere antibody is considered protective against ILD in SSc. Of note, SSc-ILD is classified into limited versus extensive depending on HRCT finding and FVC (Fig. 7.3).

Presentation

Usually patients present with dry cough, shortness of breath, decreased exercise intolerance, fine bibasilar crackles, and, infrequently, finger clubbing.

Diagnosis

The diagnosis is made collectively by symptoms, signs, PFT (which mostly shows restrictive pattern with low diffusion lung capacity of carbon monoxide [DLCO]) and imaging (chest radiograph may appear normal at the beginning but then progresses to irregular linear opacities and marked interstitial marking). However, in HRCT, it may show GGO without honeycombing in NSIP or reticular pattern with basilar honeycombing in UIP with/without traction bronchiectasis. Furthermore, the most common subtypes of SSc-ILD are NSIP followed by UIP. Although usually the subtypes of ILD may affect the outcome of CTD-ILD, in SSc it is not the case. For that, it is enough to diagnose it as SSc-ILD without specifying the subtype. While BAL is helpful

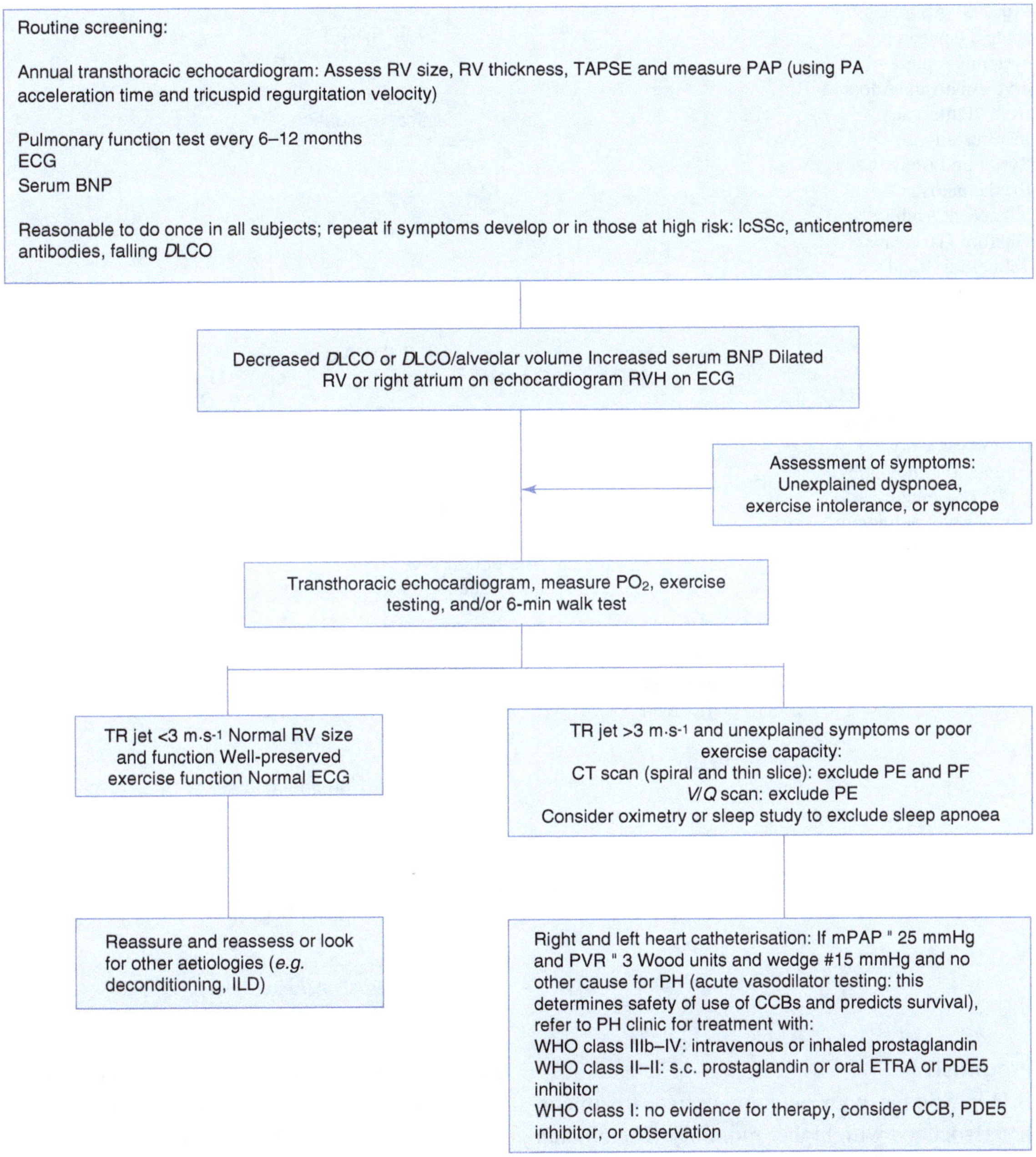

Fig. 7.4 The approach to screening for CTD-related pulmonary hypertension (CTD-PAH). *BNP* B-type natriuretic peptide, *CCBs* Calcium channel blockers, *DCLO* Diffusing capacity carbon monoxide, *ECG* Electrocardiogram, *ETRA* Endothelin receptor antagonist, *FVC* Forced expiratory vital capacity, *LcSSc* Limited cutaneous systemic sclerosis, *mPAP* mean pulmonary artery, *PDE-5 inhibitor* phosphodiesterase type 5 inhibitor, *PE* pulmonary embolism, *PF* pulmonary fibrosis, *RV* right ventricular, *RVH* right ventricular hypertrophy, *TAPSE* Tricuspid annular plane systolic excursion, *TR* Tricuspid regurgitation, *V/Q* Ventilation/perfusion, *WHO* World health organization, *WU* Wood Units. (Adopted from Sweiss NJ, Hushaw L, Thenappan T, et al. Diagnosis and management of pulmonary hypertension in systemic sclerosis. Curr Rheumatolo Rep)

in ruling out infection in the appropriate clinical context, lung biopsy is not usually required, unless such diagnosis is doubtful. Worth mentioning, the most serious complications of SSc-ILD are respiratory failure and pulmonary hypertension.

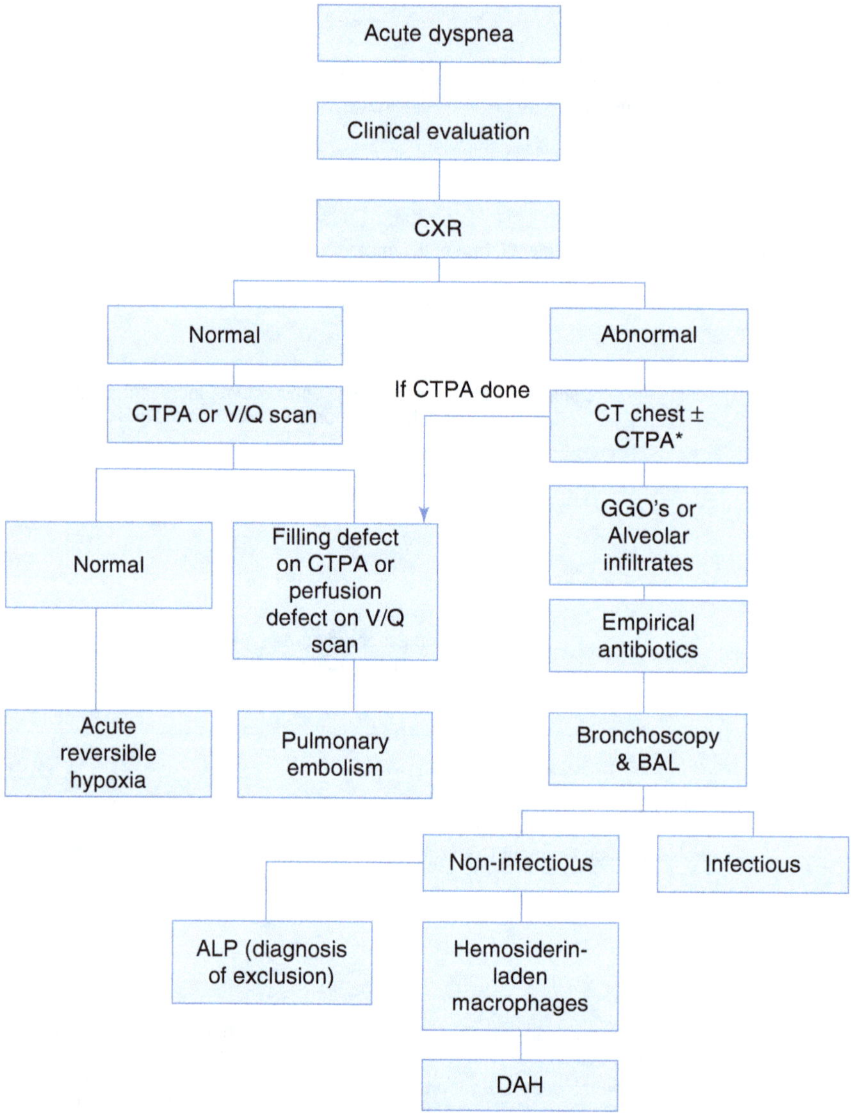

Fig. 7.5 Approach for acute dyspnea in systemic lupus erythematosus. Adopted from "Pulmonary manifestations of Systemic Lupus Erythematosus" (Chapter), Abdul Ghafoor Gari, Amr Telmesani, Raad Alwithenani, Systemic Lupus Erythematosus (Book), published by opentech. *ALP* Acute lupus pneumonitis, *BAL* bronchoalveolar lavage, *CXR* chest x-ray, *CT* computed tomography, *CTPA* computed tomography pulmonary angiogram, *DAH* diffuse alveolar hemorrhage, *GGO's* ground-glass opacities, *V/Q Scan* ventilation/perfusion lung scan

Prognosis

ILD in SSc has poor outcome despite treatment. It's associated with higher mortality. The median survival for patients is 5–8 years.

Treatment

Many issues are involved in treating SSc-ILD, which are the decision of initiation of treatment, treatment modalities, the follow-up of treatment, duration of treatment, and assessment of success of treatment and promising drugs.

It is difficult to decide whether to initiate treatment or not since treatment has a minor effect on the outcome of SSc-ILD. Physicians should balance between the benefit of treatment and the adverse drug reactions. Factos that favor starting treatment are the presence of respiratory symptoms, abnormal or declining lung functions (specially DLCO and forced vital capacity [FVC]), progressive disease, early intervention (within 12–24 months of the diagnosis of SSc-ILD), young age, GGO on HRCT, and no contraindications (such as active or suspected infection, neutropenia, history of cyclophosphamide hemorrhagic cystitis, pregnancy, and lactation) [3, 4].

When physician and patient agree to start treatment, there are three modalities available, which are drug therapy, lung transplantation, and hematopoietic stem cell transplantation. To start

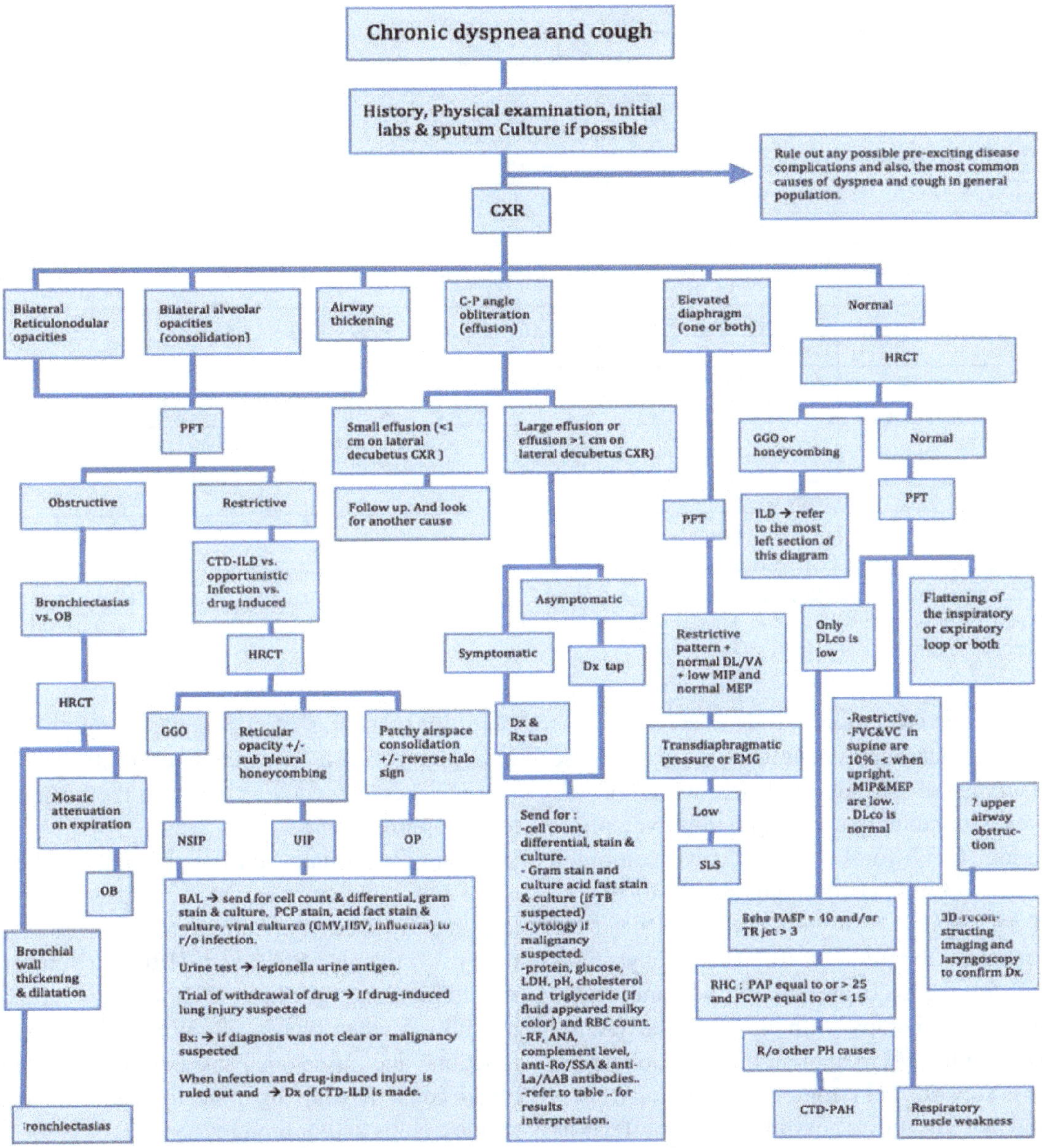

Fig. 7.6 The approach to chronic dyspnea in CTDs. *CXR* Chest X-ray, *CTD* Connective tissue disease, *C-P* Costophrenic angle, *Dx* Diagnostic, *Rx* Therapeutic, *Bx* Biopsy, *GGO* Ground glass opacity, *HRCT* High resolution computed tomography, *PFT* Pulmonary function test, *ILD* Interstitial lung disease, *NSIP* Non-specific interstitial pneumonia, *OP* Organizing pneumonia, *UIP* Usual interstitial pneumonia, *OB* Obliterative bronchiolitis, *DLco* Diffusion Lung capacity for carbon monoxide, *DL/VA* Diffusion per unit area of alveolar volume, *MIP* Maximum inspiratory pressure, *MEP* Maximum expiratory pressure, *VC* Vital capacity, *FVC* Forced vital capacity, *EMG* Electromyogram, *SLS* Shrinking lung syndrome, *PASP* Pulmonary artery systolic pressure, *TR* Tricuspid regurge, *RHC* Right heart catheterization, *PAP* Pulmonary artery pressure, *PCWP* Pulmonary capillary wedge pressure, *R/o* Role out, *PH* Pulmonary hypertension, *PCP* Pneumocystis pneumonia, *CMV* Cytomegalovirus, *HSV* Herpes simplex virus, *TB* Tuberculosis, *LDH* Lactate dehydrogenase, *RF* Rheumatoid factor, *RBC* Red blood cell, Anti-nuclear antibody

Table 7.4 Pleural fluid analysis for rheumatic diseases

	RA	SLE	Sjogren
Appearance	Variable	Clear	N/A
WBC	<5000 cells/mm^3	<5000	High lymphocytes
Glucose	Low (<1.6 mmol/L)	Normal/low	Normal
Protein	High (>30 g/L)	Low	High
Cholesterol	>5.18 mmol/L	N/A	N/A
RBC	0	0	N/A
pH	Low (< 7.3)	N/A	Normal
Cytology	Positive tadpole cells	N/A	N/A
Complement	Low	Low	Low
RF	>240 IU/mL (titer >1:320)	None	N/A
ANA	+/–	Positive (titer >1:160 is more sensitive than specific)	N/A
LDH	High (> 700 IU/L)	High	N/A
Anti-Ro/anti-La antibodies	N/A	N/A	Positive
Immune complex	High	High	N/A

ANA Anti-nuclear anti-body, *LDH* Lactate dehydrogenase, *RBC* red blood cell, *RF* rheumatoid factor, *N/A* not applicable

with, there is no drug, up to date, considered as the gold standard treatment for SSc-ILD because of lacking of strong evidence to relay on. However, commonly used regimen is cyclophosphamide (CYC) (oral or intravenous) combined with low dose glucocorticoids (equal to or less than 10 mg/day equivalent to prednisone) for 12 months duration [5–10].Then, physicians could stop the CYC and the steroids and start a maintenance therapy with azathioprine (AZA) for18 months [11]. Although oral cyclophosphamide is superior to IV route, some clinicians prefer the IV route due to possible less side effects as a result of lower cumulative dose. An alternative regimen to CYC and steroids is AZA plus low-dose prednisone [12, 13]. This regimen is inferior to CYC and steroids but could be used if patient could not tolerate CYC. Steroids are used mostly as an adjuvant therapy to cyclophosphamide with low doses (equal to or less than 10 mg/day equivalent to prednisone). That's because moderate to high doses (>15 mg/day equivalent to prednisone) could expose patients to the risk of developing scleroderma renal crisis (SRC), which presents with acute kidney injury (AKI), hypertension (including hypertensive crisis), and mild proteinuria. Of note, there are some other promising drugs such as mycophenolate mofetil [14–20], rituximab [21, 22], and imatinib [23, 24], but more trials are needed to compare their efficacy to cyclophosphamide.

Monitoring usually consists of monthly follow-up to make sure there are no drug adverse events and, then, a visit every 6 months to check for respiratory symptoms, PFT, and HRCT. Clinicians should monitor patients for CYC drug toxicity by monitoring white blood cell (WBC) count, renal function, and urine analysis (specially for red blood cells [RBCs]) in urine to predict hemorrhagic cystitis and/or proteinuria [25].

Afterward, the treatment is considered successful if stabilization (no improvement nor deterioration) of respiratory symptoms and PFT is achieved. However, mild to moderate improvement could occur.

Cyclophosphamide is associated with high toxicity profile, which is a concern for both patients and physicians. The new preferred regimen is mycophenolate mofetil (MMF) (oral or intravenous) along with glucocorticoids. Both regimens showed significant reduction in loss of pulmonary function, but mycophenolate mofetil has safer profile with less side effects, better toleration, and the improvement last longer with (MMF) than (CYC).

Table 7.5 Drug-induced lung injury in CTD

	Type of lung disease occur	Duration of drug use until symptoms occur	Dose of the drug and other risk factors	Hx and P/E	Blood work	PFT	Imaging	BAL and Biopsy	Treatment	Notice
Gold	Interstitial pneumonia (NSIP, OP or eosinophilia pneumonia.)	1 week–84 months (typically >6 months)	– 30–3000 mg total accumulative dose (specially >500 mg) – Female	Hx: Acute or chronic cough, dyspnea and fever within P/E: Crackles but no clubbing	Non-specific): Leukocytes and eosinophilia. (rarely: Leucopenia, thrombocytopenia and hypogammaglobulinemia)	– Restrictive pattern with low DLCO	CXR: Upper zone opacity (unlike in CTD_ILD which occur in the lower zone) HRCT: Non-specific: GGO or diffuse or patchy opacities	– BAL: High lymphocyte no, CD4+/CD8+ <1, also, use it to r/o infection – Biopsy: NSIP, OP or eosinophilia pneumonia	Stop the drug and start systemic corticosteroid	BO, pulmonary-renal syndrome and DAH
D-Penicillamine	OB	3–14 months	375–1250 mg/day	Subacute dyspnea on exertion and cough	N/A	Obstructive pattern with no response to bronchodilator	CXR: Normal or hyperinflation. HRCT: Mosaic attenuation	Biopsy: Typical for OB	Stop the offending drug and start prednisolone 1–1.5 mg/kg/day Using other immunosuppressive therapy (e.g., CYC or AZA) may help	N/A

NSAIDs	Eosinophilia pneumonia	N/A	N/A	Hx: Fever, cough dyspnea. P/E: Wheeze and crackles	Eosinophilia	N/A	Non-specific: Diffuse or patchy consolidations	Poorly defined granuloma + eosinophils infiltration	Stop the drug and in severe cases add systemic corticosteroid	N/A
MTX	ILD, acute lung injury (ALI) with DAD, pleurisy, pleural effusion, nodulosis, bronchitis, airway hyper-sensitivity and cough	12 weeks-18 years	– Minimum of <20 mg/week. – Age > 60 -rheumatoid pleuro-pulmonary involvement – Previous use of DMARD – Hypoal-buminemia – DM	Dyspnea, dry cough, fever +/– chest pain	Eosinophilia	– Restrictive – Low DLCO – High A-a gradient	Non-specific: Interstitial infiltrate	Cellular interstitial infiltrates, eosinophils, granuloma, DAD	Stop the drug and in severe cases add corticosteroid or other immuno-suppressive therapy like CYC or AZA. Folinic acid may be used (not fully studied)	Reusing the medication after the treatment of its adverse event is not recommen-ded
Lefluno-mide	Fatal exacerbation of previously diseased lung, diffuse nodulosis, pulmonary alveolar proteinosis and DAD	12 weeks	Previous lung disease or MTX pneumonitis	– Hx: Dyspnea, cough fever P/E: Crackles.	High C-reactive protein and KL-6	N/A	HRCT: GGO, reticular opacities and honey-combing or airspace disease	Bx: Pneumonitis with eosinophils, OP or DAD	Systemic steroids + Cholestyramine (8 g/day for 3 days)	Avoid using it when patients already have ILD. If new patients with no known ILD, screen by PFT and HRCT before starting the drug

(continued)

Table 7.5 (continued)

	Type of lung disease occur	Duration of drug use until symptoms occur	Dose of the drug and other risk factors	Hx and P/E	Blood work	PFT	Imaging	BAL and Biopsy	Treatment	Notice
TNF-a (etanercept, infliximab and adali-mumab)	Exacer-bation of ILD, UIP and OP	8 weeks	N/A	Dyspnea, cough and fever	N/A	N/A	Reticular opacities or airspace disease	Bx: Reticular opacities or airspace disease	Stop the drug and any DMARD added with it + systemic steroid (e.g., 40 mg/day)	N/A
CYC	NISP or fibrosis.	– Early onset: 1–6 months. – Late onset: >6 months	– 150 mg–81 g – Risk factors: If used with other drugs cause lung toxicity, e.g., bleomycin, busulfan and amiodarone	Dyspnea, cough +/– fever	N/A	– Restrictive pattern with low DLCO	– Early onset: GGO on HRCT. – Late onset: Reticular opacities with honey-combing (in the mid to upper zone, unlike in CTD-ILD)	Bx: Non-specific. But granuloma and hemosiderin could be present	– Early onset: Atop medication + systemic corticosteroids (prednisone 60 mg/day) – Late onset: Stop medication only. Steroid showed no effectiveness	N/A
AZA	OP and UIP	1 week–1 month	Total dose of 2300–28,600 mg	Dyspnea, cough and fever	N/A	N/A	N/A	To r/o infections	Stop medication and start systemic steroid	It's very rare for AZA to cause lung toxicity especially in CTD population

MMF	Acute respiratory failure, fibrosis and DAH	After 6 days	2 g/day	Dyspnea and cough	N/A	N/A	Diffuse airway opacity (could be in unilateral)	To r/o infections.	Stop the drug and start systemic corticosteroids (methyl-prednisolone 125 mg 4 time/day)	It's a rare compli-cation of MMF

AZA Azathioperine, *CYC* Cyclophosphamide, *MTX* Methotrexate, *MMF* Mycophenolate Mofetil, *DM* Diabetes mellitus, *NSAIDs* Non-steroidal anti-inflammatory drugs, *ILD* Interstitial pneumonia, *DAH* Diffuse alveolar hemorrhage, *DAD* Diffuse alveolar damage, *NSIP* Non-specific interstitial pneumonia, *TNF-a* Tumor necrosis factor –alpha, *Hx* History, *P/E* Physical examination, *KL-6* Human Kerbs Von Den Lungem 6, *DLCO* diffusion lung capacity for carbon monoxide, *A-a gradient* Alveolar-arterial gradient, *CXR* chest radiography, *GGO* graound glass opacity, *R/o* Rule out, *BAL* Bronchoalveolar lavage, *PFT* Pulmonary function test, *Bx* Biopsy, *DMARD* disease-modifying anti-rheumatic drugs, *N/A* Not applicable

Although the MMF duration in the last study was for 2 years, most of expertise recommend to continue the treatment for several years [26].

The second modality of treatment is lung transplantation. It is considered when drug therapy fails. The 1-year survival is 68–93% [27, 28]. Absence of GERD may play a great role in improving survival [27].

Last treatment modality is hematopoietic stem cell transplantation. It is still an experimental therapy. However, great improvement in FVC within 2 years occurred when using this method. Furthermore, it shows superiority to IV cyclophosphamide [29].

Aspiration Pneumonitis

A strong association between the degree of gastroesophageal reflux (GER) and the severity of ILD, which may raise the flag of micro-aspirations. However, it is still not clear whether the treatment of GER will improve or even prevent ILD [30, 31].

7.6.1.2 Vascular Diseases

SSc-associated pulmonary arterial hypertension (SSc-PAH).

Introduction

Pulmonary hypertension (PH) defined as mean pulmonary artery pressure (PAP) equals to or > 25 mmHg at rest. It can occur as a complication of SSc itself, which is SSc-PAH, or as a complication of ILD caused by SSc. Here, SSc-PAH is discussed.

It presents in 12–38% of SSc patients. Risk factors are increased number of telangiectases, lcSSc with anti-centromere antibody, dcSSc with ANA (dcSSc alone is less commonly associated with PAH), progressive decline in DLCO, and exercise-induced PAH on right heart catheterization.

Presentation

Patients usually present with exertional dyspnea, lethargy, and fatigue, which are the most common symptoms, and, less frequently, could be exertional angina, exertional syncope, symptoms of right ventricular failure (RVF) (due to Cor pulmonale), cough, hemoptysis, and Ortner's syndrome (horsiness due left recurrent laryngeal nerve palsy caused by pulmonary artery compression or other cardiac cause). On physical examination, if there is no right ventricular hypertrophy (RVH), loud pulmonary component of second heart sound is heard. However, If right ventricular hypertrophy present, then, parasternal heave, forth heart sound, prominent A wave in jugular venous pressure (JVP) could be noticed. Moreover, ascites and lower limb edema may be present. Recent studies showed that combination therapy with phosphodiesterase type 5 inhibitors or combination between (ERA/PDE5I) is superior than endothelin receptor antagonist alone by decreasing deterioration time, recent European guidelines recommend combination initial therapy, But it still has not established yet in American guidelines [32].

Screening

In regard to screening for SSc-PAH, physicians could use the same screening method as any patient newly diagnosed with SSc (Fig. 7.1). Also, other indications for earlier echocardiography screening are when symptoms, signs, and PFT findings are suggestive of PAH are present, such as DLCO <70% predicted or FVC/DLCO >1.6 and echocardiography with Doppler study findings are suggestive of PAH such as RVH, right ventricular enlargement (the chamber itself), right atrial enlargement, tricuspid regurge (TR), mid-systolic notch on the pulmonary artery Doppler flow tracing and shifting of the interventricular septum toward the left ventricle, pulmonary artery systolic pressure (PASP) >50 and the maximum tricuspid regurgitant jet velocity (TVR) >3.4.

Diagnosis

The SSc-PAH diagnosis is confirmed by right heart catheterization when mean pulmonary arterial pressure equals to or > 25 mmHg at rest and mean pulmonary capillary wedge pressure (PCWP) <15 mmHg after excluding other causes of PH such as having normal ventilation/perfusion scan (V/Q scan) (to rule out chronic thromboembolic disease), negative HIV and hepatitis serology, normal or mild ILD findings on

HRCT (to rule out significant ILD), and normal sleep study in the appropriate clinical context.

Prognosis

Although the advancement of treatment during the past decade has improved the survival, it's still worse than that in idiopathic PAH (IPAH) [33]. The 3-year survival is estimated to be 64% [33]. Moreover, early detection has a good impact in survival [34]. On the other hand, SSc-PAH associated with ILD has worse prognosis than that of SSc-PAH alone. The 3-year survival for SSc-PAH with ILD is 47% [35].

Treatment

In general, therapy is usually directed to the underlying cause of PAH and to the PAH itself if it persisted. However, since there is no specific treatment for SSc, the therapy will be directed to PAH itself. Nevertheless, many issues are involved in the treatment of SSc-PAH such as the decision of initiation of treatment, treatment modalities, duration of treatment, and follow-up of therapy.

The decision of initiation of treatment is all symptomatic patients defined by the World Health Organization (WHO) functional classes of II or more (i.e., at minimum to have dyspnea when doing ordinary activity). This category should receive treatment.

Treatment modalities are PAH specific drug therapy, supportive therapy, and lung transplantation. To start with, for the PAH specific drug therapy, there is no single drug that has shown superiority for treatment in SSc or other CTDs in general.

However, the drug classes that have shown effect in CTD-PAH are endothelin-1 receptor antagonists (ERA), phosphodiesterase type 5 (PDE5) inhibitors, and prostanoids (PGI-2). All of them improved the 6-min walk test (6MWT) [36]. Clinicians should, most of the time, start with monotherapy then step up for a combination if no improvement is observed. Furthermore, the choice for PAH-specific drug therapy depends on physician expertise, patient preference, and cost-effectiveness.

Also, supportive therapy should be considered for most patients. It consists of supplemental oxygen for patients with hypoxemia, to keep oxygen saturation > 90%. In addition, diuretics could be given for patients with fluid overload. Moreover, anticoagulation might be considered for all patients based on non-randomized trials, especially those who receive IV prostaglandins (due to the risk of catheter related thrombosis) but also one should weigh risk of bleeding against benefits [37]. Furthermore, warfarin is the drug of choice to reach a therapeutic INR of 1.5–2.5 [37]. On top of that, exercise, with a special training program (bicycle ergometer at lower and higher workload for 15–30 min/day, dumbbell training [0.5–1 kg], and respiratory training) could be advised. However, heart rate should be monitored not to reach above 120 beat/min and the oxygen saturation not to fall <90% (if a supplemental oxygen is given). These exercises has been tested and showed improvement in 6-min walk test (6MWT) [38, 39]. Lastly, digoxin is not usually used in PAH because there are no enough data to support its effectiveness [37]. Nevertheless, it is usually used in patients with COPD and biventricular failure [40].

As a last resort, when drug therapy fails, lung transplantation should be considered, specially, in patients with severe symptoms. The 2-year survival reaches 71% [27].

7.6.1.3 Airway Disease

Bronchiectasis

It is a common finding on HRCT, but usually not clinically manifested, reaching 59% of SSc patients, and this may be attributed to the high number of GERD and aspirations [41]. Clinicians should pay attention to bronchiectasis when intended to start immunosuppressive therapy due to the risk of sever lower respiratory tract infections [42].

Pleural Involvement

Pleural Effusion

Occurs in about 7% of SSc patients. Usually asymptomatic and occasionally associated with pericardial effusion. It resolves spontaneously.

Spontaneous Pneumothorax

It's a rare complication of SSc. Patients present with shortness of breath and/or pleuritic chest pain. The management depends on cardiopulmonary status and pneumothorax size on CXR. Supplemental oxygen and air drainage by needle aspiration or chest tube insertion should be considered depending on the clinical context.

Respiratory Muscle Weakness

This could lead to respiratory failure with or without hypercapnia [43, 44].

7.6.1.4 Systemic Lupus Erythematosus (SLE)

Background

SLE is a multisystem autoimmune disease and affects mostly women in childbearing age. Pulmonary involvement, manifested clinically or radiologically, occurs in around 25% of all SLE patients. They usually happen later in the course of the disease. Furthermore, most common pulmonary diseases are pleuritis (78%) followed by bacterial infections (58%), alveolar hemorrhage (26%), distal airway alterations (21%), opportunistic infections (14%), and, lastly, acute or chronic pulmonary thromboembolism (8%).

Pulmonary Manifestations

Pleural Diseases

Pleuritis

- Presents as pleuritic chest pain, shortness of breath, and fever. On physical examination, pleuritic friction rub may be heard. It is a clinical diagnosis. However, pleural biopsy could be done but rarely needed. If so, it shows peculiar immunofluorescent pattern characterized by staining of nuclei with anti-IgG, anti-IgM, and anti-C3 [45]. Treatment usually consists of NSAIDS for mild cases and steroid for severe cases.

Pleural Effusion

Presentation

It tends to be bilateral and small to moderate in size; however, large effusion may occur. It usually presents with shortness of breath, cough, and/or chest pain. Nevertheless, sometimes, it could be asymptomatic. Physical examination may show dullness on percussion, decrease tactile fremitus, decrease intensity of breath sound, and decrease vocal resonance.

Diagnosis

Although the following investigations could lead to the diagnosis of pleural effusion to be secondary to SLE, physicians should always rule out other common/serious causes of pleural effusion such as heart failure, parapneumonic effusion, and pulmonary embolism if suspected.

Chest radiograph shows blunting of costophrenic angle. Furthermore, pleural fluid analysis is shown in Table 7.4.

Treatment

Small asymptomatic pleural effusion needs no treatment. It resolves spontaneously. On the other hand, mild symptomatic effusion usually responds to NSAIDs [46], while severe symptomatic effusion is treated with steroids. Also, if patient is currently on steroids, increasing the dose may be required [46]. In refractory cases, tetracycline or talc pleurodesis might be an alternative option [47–49].

7.6.1.5 Parenchymal Lung Disease

Acute Lupus Pneumonitis (ALP)

Introduction

It's an uncommon but serious complication of SLE, which occurs in 2–8% of patients. It affects younger and newly diagnosed SLE patients and also could manifest as a fulminant pattern in pregnant women.

Presentation

Acute-onset fever, cough, shortness of breath, pleuritic chest pain, and, occasionally, hemoptysis. Physical examination shows signs of hypoxia and bibasilar crackles.

Diagnosis

It's a diagnosis of exclusion (Fig. 7.5). However, BAL, with or without transbronchial biopsy, must be done to rule out infection. Blood tests may show high levels of anti-Ro (anti-SS-A), which are associated with more likelihood of ALP. Chest radiograph may show bilateral alveolar infiltrates with predominance in lower lung fields. Also, pleural effusion may occur in half of the cases. Rarely, chest radiograph could be normal or showing nodules. Chest CT may show diffuse ground glass opacities. BAL, when done, the sample should be sent for cell count and differential, bacterial, fungal, and viral cultures, cytology, pneumocystis pneumonia (PCP) stain, and acid-fast bacilli (AFB) smear, and culture in the appropriate clinical context. Transbronchial biopsy, when done, shows non-specific diffuse alveolar damage (DAD) with or without alveolar hemorrhage and capillaritis. Less common pathologic features are alveolar edema, hyaline membrane formation, and immunoglobulin and complement deposition.

Treatment

Usually starts with empiric broad-spectrum antibiotics for 3 days. If no response, then, pulse steroids (1 g methylprednisolone daily for 3 days) should be started. Furthermore, adding another immunosuppressive agents like cyclophosphamide (CYC) could be considered [50]. In refractory cases, intravenous immunoglobulin (IVIG), plasma exchange, or rituximab may help [51–53].

Prognosis

It has poor prognosis with mortality reaching 50% [54]. BAL showing eosinophilia and neutrophilia have worse prognosis than lymphocytosis.

7.6.1.6 Diffuse Alveolar Hemorrhage (DAH)

Introduction

The prevalence ranges from <2% to 5.4% and it tends to recur. Furthermore, it occurs more frequently in lupus nephritis patients and with high levels of serum anti-DNA antibody.

Presentation

Usually presents with acute shortness of breath, cough, fever, and hemoptysis, although absence of hemoptysis dose not rule out DAH. The mean duration from onset of DAH to resolution of radiographic finding is 7.8 days. Physical examination reveals signs of respiratory distress and hypoxia.

Diagnosis

Blood tests may show acute drop in hemoglobin and low complement level. Chest radiograph may show bilateral alveolar infiltrates. But also could happen unilaterally in 18% of patients. Chest CT scan could show new bilateral ground glass opacities and consolidation. Moreover, magnetic resonance imaging (MRI) can suggest presence of blood. PFT show elevated DLCO (>130% predicted) due to excess hemoglobin in alveolar space. BAL is essential to rule out infection. Furthermore, bloody sample under microscope suggests DAH if hemosiderin-laden macrophages are present. Transbronchial biopsy could be done in stable patients. This may reveal bland hemorrhage (72%) or capillaritis (14%). Both of them are associated with intra-alveolar hemorrhage and hemosiderin-laden macrophages. Also, immunoglobulin G (IgG), complement 3 (C3), or immune complex deposition occurs in 50% of the cases. Thoracoscopic lung biopsy is rarely needed.

Treatment

Supportive therapy (i.e., mechanical ventilation) plays a major rule since most patients are admitted to the intensive care unit (ICU) [55, 56]. However, if infection is ruled out or BAL suggest hemorrhage, physician should start pulse intravenous steroids (methylprednisolone 1 g/day for 3 days) followed by 60 mg/day of oral prednisone plus intravenous CYC every 4 weeks (the CYC could be started after discharge from hospital) [55, 56]. In refractory cases, plasmapheresis is an effective alternative, which improves survival. Also, rituximab has shown promising results [56–58].

Prognosis
DAH has a very poor outcome with mortality ranges between 50% and 90% [55, 58].

7.6.1.7 Chronic ILD

Introduction
Occurs in around 9% of SLE patients [59, 60]. Moreover, the most common ILD patterns are NSIP, UIP, and lymphocytic interstitial pneumonia (LIP).

Presentation
The initial presentation could be a dry cough. Other symptoms are shortness of breath and decreased exercise intolerance. Physical examination could reveal fine bibasilar crackles; however finger clubbing is rare.

Diagnosis
It is made by symptoms, signs, PFT, and HRCT collectively. Lung biopsy is not usually required unless such diagnosis is doubted. Chest radiograph may be normal at the beginning but then progresses to irregular linear opacities and marked interstitial markings. HRCT may show GGO without honeycombing in NSIP. On the other hand, reticular pattern with basilar honeycombing occurs in UIP with/without traction bronchiectasis. Moreover, 30% of asymptomatic patients could have abnormal HRCT findings. PFT may show restrictive pattern with low DLCO. Also, it does not correlate with the severity of ILD in HRCT. BAL is helpful in rolling out infection. While biopsy needed to confirm the subtype of ILD when HRCT is controversial.

Treatment
In mild cases, systemic corticosteroid (prednisone 60 mg/day for at least 4 weeks) could be used [56]. However, for moderate to severe cases, a combination therapy of oral glucocorticoids and AZA is a choice [60]. Furthermore, in severe cases, a combination of oral glucocorticoids and CYC could be considered [60].

Prognosis
ILD associated with SLE has better prognosis compared to the idiopathic forms [61].

7.6.1.8 Pulmonary Vascular Diseases

Thromboembolic Disease

Introduction
Venous thromboembolic (VTE) events are well-known manifestations of SLE specially when antiphospholipid (aPL) antibodies are present. This, in turn, will establish the diagnosis of antiphospholipid syndrome. Patients diagnosed with antiphospholipid syndrome are at risk of recurrent DVT, PE, chronic thromboembolic pulmonary hypertension (CTEPH), abortions, DAH, and acute respiratory distress syndrome (ARDS). Furthermore, when small vessel occlusion occurs in three or more organs, the condition is known as catastrophic antiphospholipid syndrome (CAPS). SLE patients are at risk of VTE events with a prevalence of 9%. This percent would become as high as 42% if SLE patients had aPL. Moreover, aPL present in up to two thirds of SLE patients [62].

Presentation
Patients could present with deep vein thrombosis (DVT) or pulmonary embolism (PE). DVT presents with calf pain (usually unilateral), swelling, and redness. On the other hand, pulmonary embolism (PE) presents with shortness of breath, pleuritic chest pain, cough, and/or hemoptysis. Furthermore, CTEPH manifested as progressive shortness of breath and exercise intolerance.

Diagnosis
DVT is diagnosed by Doppler ultrasound (US). PE is confirmed by chest CT angiogram. Moreover, CTEPH needs all diagnostic procedures needed to diagnose PAH.

Treatment
Long-term anticoagulation with warfarin is highly recommended with targeting INR of 2.0–3.0. High-intensity warfarin (targeting INR 3.0–

4.0) showed no superiority to moderate intensity [63]. Some clinicians use long-term low-dose aspirin as a primary prevention [64].

CAPS is usually treated by systemic glucocorticoids, immunosuppressants, plasmapheresis, and/or IVIg in addition to anticoagulation [56].

Prognosis

For CAPS, the mortality reaches 50% [65].

7.6.1.9 SLE-Associated Pulmonary Arterial Hypertension (SLE-PAH)

Background

For definition of PAH, please see SSc-PAH.

The duration of SLE, since diagnosis, does not correlate with the risk of development SLE-PAH. Its prevalence varies between 0.5% and 15% in SLE patients. Risk factors are Raynaud's phenomenon, which occurs in 75% of SLE-PAH [54]; antiphospholipid antibodies (aPL), which present in 83% of SLE-PAH; and anti-U1 ribonuclear protein (RNP), which presents in >25% of SLE-PAH.

Presentation

Please see SSc-PAH.

Screening

Due to the rarity of PAH in SLE, annual echocardiogram screening should be directed to women in childbearing age, pregnant ladies, patients with Reynaud's phenomenon, anticardiolipin antibody, and anti-U1 RNP antibody [66].

Treatment

All patients should receive supportive therapy as needed (See SSc-PAH). On the other hand, mild PAH patients should receive immunosuppressive therapy alone, while moderate to severe PAH patients should receive PAH-specific therapy with or without immunosuppressive therapy [56].

PAH-specific therapies are effective in SLE-associated PAH specially epoprostenol, bosentan, sildenafil, ambrisentan, and tadalafil. They improved the 6MWT and functional class [67–70]. Adding immunosuppressive therapy (e.g., IV CYC with or without oral glucocorticoids) showed improvement in 6MWT and lowered PAP [71–74].

Acute Reversible Hypoxia

It's a rare complication of lupus, and patients usually present with acute and unexplained hypoxia and hypercapnia. Blood investigation may show high C3 levels. Chest radiograph could be normal. V/Q scan should show no evidence of PE. Lastly, arterial blood gases (ABG) shows increase alveolar-arterial (A-a) PO2 gradient. Furthermore, it responds quickly to high-dose systemic corticosteroids [75, 76].

7.6.1.10 Airway Disease

Upper Airway Involvement

Introduction

It occurs in around 30% of SLE patients. Also, it involves laryngeal mucosal inflammation or ulceration, cricoarytenoiditis, vocal cord paralysis, necrotizing vasculitis, and angioedema.

Presentation

Patients usually present with hoarseness and/or dyspnea. Moreover, they could develop angioedema symptoms such as lip and mouth swelling, dysphagia, odynophagia, and breathing difficulty.

Diagnosis

Chest radiograph and CT scan are usually normal. PFT may show flattening of the inspiratory or expiratory loop or both depending on the location of the obstruction. Furthermore, 3-D reconstructive images are needed to locate the site of obstruction. Fibro-optic laryngoscopy or bronchoscopy is needed for direct visualization of the vocal cord.

Treatment

Corticosteroids are of benefit in laryngeal mucosal inflammation or ulceration and vocal cord paralysis [77, 78]. However, in refractory cases, infectious causes should be considered (e.g., *Haemophilus influenzae* and *Streptococcus*.

Other rare pathogens are *Histoplasma*, *Coccidioides*, *Cryptococcus*, *Blastomycosis*, and *Candida*).

Lower Airway Involvement

Bronchiectasis

HRCT findings suggestive of bronchiectasis occur in around 21% of SLE patients. However, patients usually are asymptomatic [79].

Bronchiolitis Obliterans (BO)/Obliterative Bronchiolitis (OB)

It's a rare complication of SLE, which is characterized by severe airflow obstruction which is mostly irreversible. Patients usually present with progressive shortness of breath. Moreover, chest HRCT Shows mosaic attenuation pattern that gets accentuated in the expiratory images. PFT shows obstructive pattern. Biopsy is rarely required. Furthermore, anticholinergics were reported to have favorable outcome when compared to systemic steroids and immunosuppressive therapy [80, 81].

7.6.1.11 Muscle Involvement

Shrinking Lung Syndrome (SLS)

Introduction

It's an uncommon disorder, with a prevalence of 0.6–0.9% of SLE patients [80–82], characterized by unexplained dyspnea, decreased lung volumes, elevated diaphragm, and restrictive PFT pattern in the absence of parenchymal lung disease.

Presentation

Patients usually present with shortness of breath aggravated by being in supine position. Pleuritic chest pain is also reported. Physical examination reveals diminished breath sounds at the lung bases with or without crackles.

Diagnosis

Chest radiograph and HRCT show elevation of both diaphragms and basal atelectasis without evidence of parenchymal lung disease. PFT shows restrictive pattern with preservation of DLCO when corrected for alveolar volume (DL/VA). Also, respiratory muscle assessment could show reduced maximal inspiratory pressure (MIP) and stable maximal expiratory pressure (MEP).

Treatment

Oral glucocorticoids with or without other immunosuppressive therapy showed to be effective [83, 84]. Other options are AZA, methotrexate (MTX), CYC, and rituximab [82–87].

Prognosis

SLS has good prognosis when treated. Moreover, respiratory failure rarely occurs [64, 88].

7.6.1.12 Associated Lung Disorders

Adult Respiratory Distress Syndrome (ARDS)

It occurs in 4–15% of SLE patients. The most common cause of ARDS in SLE is sepsis. Other causes are ALP, DAH, and CAPS. Furthermore, it occurs more frequently in younger age group and is more progressive than in non-SLE patients. ARDS-related mortality contributes to 30% off all lupus deaths. Furthermore, mortality could reach up to 70%. The treatment is mainly supportive care.

Infectious Complications

Most of the SLE infectious complications happen in patients who are on immunosuppressive therapy. It accounts for 30–50% of all SLE deaths. Furthermore, bacterial infections are the most common (75%) followed by mycobacterial (12%) then fungal infections (7%) and lastly viruses (5%). It could mimic ALP or DAH, so, careful diagnostic approach is recommended. The diagnosis is usually conducted by chest radiograph and HRCT and also BAL to differentiate infectious from non-infectious causes (Fig. 7.5).

Pneumocystis Pneumonia (PCP) Prophylaxis

Since the incidence of PCP in SLE patients is very low (0.6%), it is not clear if all SLE patients on immunosuppressants should receive prophylaxis. But, at least patients at highest-risk of PCP infection (e.g., who receive biologic agents or immunosuppressants in addition to high dose daily steroid) should do so. The prophylactic drug of choice is trimethoprim-sulfamethoxazole (TMP-SMX) [89].

Lung Cancer

SLE patients are at increased risk of developing lung cancer. Furthermore, histologically, adenocarcinoma is the most common type (similar to the general population). However, there is a tendency for uncommon thoracic malignancies like carcinoids and bronchoalveolar carcinoma.

Drug Reactions

Please refer to Table 7.5.

7.7 Rheumatoid Arthritis (RA)

7.7.1 Introduction

RA is an autoimmune disorder characterized by joint involvement in a chronic and symmetrical fashion. Pulmonary involvement considered one of the most frequent extraarticular manifestations together with the cutaneous involvement. Furthermore, around 10–20% of RA deaths are attributed to pulmonary causes. The most common pulmonary involvements are ILD, airway disease, rheumatoid nodule, and pleural effusion.

1. Pulmonary manifestations.
2. Parenchymal involvement.
3. Interstitial lung disease (ILD).

7.7.1.1 Introduction

It's the most common pulmonary manifestation of RA with a prevalence of 20–63% radiographically by HRCT. And up to 9.4% of the patients have clinically significant symptoms. Usually happens in a well-established RA disease. However, in around 20%, it could precede it. The most common patterns are UIP followed by NSIP then desquamative interstitial pneumonia (DIP) and organizing pneumonia (OP). Also, risk factors for that are older age group, male gender, history of cigarette smoking, high titer of rheumatoid factor (RF), and anti-cyclic citrullinated peptides (anti-CCP) [90].

7.7.1.2 Presentation

Symptoms start to appear when lung function is greatly impaired. Moreover, pleuritic chest pain occasionally accompanied ILD symptoms. Please see SSc-ILD for more information.

7.7.1.3 Diagnosis

Chest radiograph might be normal in affected patients especially in early disease [91]. However, chest HRCT is the most important tool to diagnose early RA-ILD. UIP manifests as reticulation and honeycombing, while NSIP presents with GGO with/without bronchiectasis. The correlation between the radiographic and the histopathologic pattern is poor in NSIP [86]. Also, OP appears as diffuses patchy alveolar opacity and GGO. It's common to see different patterns simultaneously [90]. PFT may show restrictive pattern with declining of DLCO to be the earliest PFT sign [92, 93]. BAL might be utilized to rule out opportunistic infections, DAH, and/or drug reactions [86, 94, 95]. Biopsy is not recommended as a regular investigation unless the radiologic pattern is unclear and another treatment could make a difference [90].

7.7.1.4 Treatment

Patients with mildly progressive disease should receive high dose prednisone [96]. However, there are anecdotal reports of using daily oral CYC and corticosteroids in rapidly progressive extensive disease [97]. There is also another regimen of monthly IV CYC combined with corticosteroids. In refractory cases, physician could use rituximab, infliximab, or tocilizumab. The routine use of these agents has not been established yet due to the lack of strong evidence and the questionable safety, which is under investigation [98]. Of note, PCP prophylaxis should be given.

7.7.1.5 Prognosis

In general, RA-ILD has mild and slowly progressive nature. However, spontaneous resolution could happen [99].

When DLCO is <54%, it is suggestive of worse prognosis [99]. On the other hand, NSIP has better prognosis than UIP [100, 101].

7.7.2 Pleural Diseases

7.7.2.1 Pleural Effusion

Introduction

It's the second most common pulmonary involvement in RA (after ILD) with a prevalence ranges between 5% and 22%. It usually occurs unilaterally and small to moderate in size; however, large effusions may occur. Moreover, it is associated with RA flares. Risk factors are smoking, previous pleurisy, rupture of subpleural nodule, and high effusion protein levels (prevents resorption).

Presentation

Mostly asymptomatic, but if not, dyspnea, fever, and chest pain (if pleurisy) are the main manifestations [102].

Diagnosis

Chest radiograph shows blunting of costophrenic angles. Chest CT scan is more sensitive than chest radiograph. Furthermore, thoracentesis, if done, pleural fluid analysis could be diagnostic as following (Table 7.4). Pleural biopsy may be considered when TB or malignancy is suspected or when thoracentesis is not diagnostic. Also, the parietal pleura are the mainly involved part rather than the visceral one. When biopsy is done, it shows absence of the normal mesothelial cells covering the pleura, and they are replaced by pseudostratified layer of epithelioid cells with giant cells [103].

Treatment

If asymptomatic, mostly it will resolve spontaneously in up to 36 months. However, if symptomatic, for acute relief, a therapeutic thoracentesis could be done. If no need for acute treatment, then start with NSAIDs. After that, if failed, moderate dose of oral glucocorticoids (10–20 mg prednisolone daily), intrapleural corticosteroids, fibrinolytics, or immunosuppressive could be given. In refractory cases, pleurodesis (mechanical or chemical) is an option.

Complications

The following complications may develop if pleural effusion is not treated. First of all, pleural fibrosis and lung entrapment, which could be treated by decortications. Moreover, bronchopleural fistula could develop, which intervention with video-assisted thoracoscopy (VATS) did not show effectiveness in RA. An open approach with thoracotomy and direct closure may be helpful. Lastly, empyema which can be treated with antibiotics (Usually it's polymicrobial infection) and drainage through chest tube. Worth mentioning, that bronchopleural fistula has been reported in the vast majority of the empyema cases in RA.

7.7.3 Pulmonary Vascular Diseases

7.7.3.1 PAH

It has lower prevalence than in other CTDs [104]. For presentation, diagnosis and treatment (see PAH in SSc).

7.7.3.2 DAH

It's a very rare complication of RA [105]. "Risk factors are treatment with infliximab, leflunomide, and rituximab [106–108]. For presentation, diagnosis, and treatment, please see DAH in SLE.

7.7.4 Airway Diseases: Upper Airway Diseases

7.7.4.1 Cricoarytenoid Arthritis

Introduction

The cricoarytenoid joint function is to abduct and adduct the vocal cord when a person speaks. Good history taking could reveal upper airway symptoms in around two thirds of RA patients. The prevalence ranges between 26% and 55% with female predominance. Furthermore, joint abnormalities such as prominence, erosions, abnormal positioning of the vocal cord, and subluxation may occur [109].

Presentation

Patients usually presents with hoarseness of the voice (reaching 30%), dyspnea, sore throat, fullness sensation in the throat, shocking, stridor, dysphagia, and odynophagia.

Diagnosis

PFT shows fixed or variable upper airway obstruction. CT scan shows the abnormalities such as prominence, erosions, abnormal positioning of the vocal cord, and subluxation. Laryngoscopy may show vocal cord dysfunction.

Treatment

When patients presented with chronic symptoms, clinicians should start with medical treatment such as systemic or intra-articular steroid, which both have shown benefit. However, surgical options (e.g., tracheostomy, arytenoidectomy, arytenoidopexy) should be considered only if medical treatment failed [110].

On the other hand, patients may present with acute manifestations such as severe stridor and should get emergent tracheostomy [111].

Prognosis

Excellent results occur with aggressive therapy [112].

7.7.4.2 Vocal Cord Rheumatoid Nodule

Could mimic squamous cell carcinoma [111].

7.7.5 Airway Diseases: Lower Airway Diseases

7.7.5.1 Bronchiectasis

Prevalence ranges between 30% and 58% when elected by HRCT. However, only 1–5% of RA patients are symptomatic. Bronchiectasis usually is a late manifestation of RA, but it can precede the articular involvement. Furthermore, presentation and management is like any other bronchiectasis without rheumatoid arthritis.

7.7.6 Airway Obstruction and Bronchial Hyperreactivity

It occurs in about 60% of RA patients when documented by spirometry. Recurrent airway infections and smoking could precipitate airway disease in RA. Patients usually present with wheeze and productive cough. Furthermore, PFT may shows obstructive pattern. However, HRCT is more sensitive than PFT in detecting the obstruction. It shows air trapping, attenuation in lung heterogeneity, and bronchiectasis. The treatments are mainly inhaled corticosteroids and bronchodilators.

7.7.6.1 Bronchiolitis Obliterans (BO)

Introduction

It's a clinically progressive small airway disease, which is characterized by narrowing, ulceration, and scarring of the respiratory and terminal bronchioles. The prevalence varies between 8% and 65%. Also, risk factors are female gender, long-standing RA, D-penicillamine, gold salt, and methotrexate use [113, 114].

Presentation

Progressive dyspnea and dry cough are the most common presentations, while physical examination reveals inspiratory crackles and squeaks.

Diagnosis

PFT shows progressive irreversible airflow obstruction. However, HRCT is more sensitive than PFT in detecting the disease. It may show air trapping (mosaic pattern of regions of low attenuation which get accentuated on expiratory images). BAL is done to rule out infections if suspected, while biopsy shows airway narrowing, ulceration, scarring, and lymphoplasmacytic infiltrate.

Treatment
Physicians should stop offending agent and may start oral prednisone, some studies suggested the use of IV CYC as well [115, 116] or stop offending agent and start low dose oral macrolide (erythromycin 400–600 mg/day, clarithromycin 200–400 mg/day or azithromycin) for 6 months may be used as improvement was shown in the treatment of diffuse panbronchiolitis [117, 118].

Prognosis
Usually carries poor prognosis specially when using corticosteroids only. Thus, adding CYC or trying macrolides may be beneficial.

7.7.6.2 Follicular Bronchiolitis

Introduction
The bronchioles are invaded by lymphocytic, plasmacytic, and hyperplasic lymphoid follicles, and reactive germinal cells infiltrates. It has some overlap with COP and BO [114].

Presentation
Patients usually present with dyspnea and also may present with fever and cough.

Diagnosis
Chest radiograph may show reticular or reticulonodular opacities. Furthermore, HRCT shows bilateral centrilobular and peribronchial nodules associated with areas of GGO.

Also, PFT may show obstructive, restrictive, or both patterns. DLCO is usually decreased. BAL is done to rule out infections. Biopsy shows bronchioles, which are invaded by lymphocytic, plasmacytic, hyperplasic lymphoid follicles, and reactive germinal cells infiltrates.

Treatment
May start with corticosteroid then after tapering starts oral macrolides (erythromycin, clarithromycin, or azithromycin) for up to 1 year [119].

Prognosis
Follicular bronchiolitis has relatively good prognosis when treated.

7.7.7 Rheumatoid Nodule and its Complications: (Necrobiotic Nodule)

7.7.7.1 Rheumatoid Nodule

Introduction
Up to 32% of rheumatoid nodule occurs in the lungs. Also, because the most common site in the respiratory system is subpleural or interlobular, it could present by many different ways such as pneumothorax, cavities, pleural effusion, empyema, and bronchopleural fistula. Furthermore, it could be solitary or multiple nodules. On the other hand, radiologically, it could mimic non-small cell lung cancer. So, physicians should be meticulous when approaching such patients specially when there is history of smoking. Also, histologically, it has a great overlap with granulomatous diseases. For that, biopsy should be interpreted very carefully [120]. Risk factors for rheumatoid nodule are with male gender, positive rheumatoid factor (RF), long-standing disease (but may precede the diagnosis of RA), and smoking.

Presentation
Mostly asymptomatic. However, if symptomatic, it depends on the complication, e.g., cavities present with hemoptysis, pneumothorax presents with dyspnea and chest pain, pleural effusion presents with dyspnea, empyema presents with dyspnea and fever, and bronchopleural fistula presents with productive cough, dyspnea, and fever occasionally.

Diagnosis
Chest radiograph may show nodule but always should compare with previous chest radiographs to notice any changes in size or shape. Also, HRCT will give better details and physician should look for size, shape, lymph nodes, and effusions. It could be solid or as a cavity.

Treatment
If no complications, spontaneous resolution is the usual natural history. Moreover, rituximab has shown effectiveness in its resolution.

However, if complicated, treat accordingly (e.g., if secondary pneumothorax happened, it's better to perform surgical intervention to prevent recurrence).

Rheumatoid Nodulosis

It is multiple rheumatoid nodules in different places. Risk factors are methotrexate, etanercept, and leflunomide use. Actually, it could lead to the same presentations the rheumatoid nodule does. Furthermore, the treatment is usually to stop the offending drug and start hydroxychloroquine, D-penicillamine, colchicine, or sulfasalazine.

7.7.7.2 Caplan Syndrome (Rheumatoid Pneumoconiosis)

Introduction

It occurs in RA patients who get exposed to coal, silica, asbestos, and ceramics industry and roof tiles products. Furthermore, it characterized by rapid-onset lung nodules and could mimic TB or neoplasm. It occurs more commonly in Europe than in the United States. Also, it's more common in positive RF patients and in male.

Presentation

Most of the time patients are asymptomatic unless complicated by pneumothorax, pleural effusion, or progressive massive fibrosis, which is uncommon; they would present with dyspnea and/or chest pain. Also, rarely, patients may present with hemoptysis or *Aspergillus* colonization.

Diagnosis

Chest radiograph shows well-defined nodules starting from 0.5 cm in diameter and larger. Also, it could cavitate or calcify. Usually present in lung periphery [121]. HRCT may have a role in following up and detection of changes. Biopsy, since it could mimic TB or neoplasm, it is often done specially when there is high index of suspicion.

Treatment

There is no specific treatment, although some studies showed improvement when using corticosteroids when the lesions are compressive or rapidly progressive [122]. However, if complicated, treat accordingly.

Prognosis

It takes few weeks or months until nodules reach the final size. Usually, they remain at the final size for many years or may heal but leave behind an asteroid scar. Only 10% of the cavitations and the calcifications emerge.

7.7.8 Infections

7.7.8.1 Background

It's clear that lung infections is increased in RA patients since pneumonia is twice more common than in general population. However, it's very difficult to make sure if the risk of infection is due to RA itself or the immunosuppressive agents used to treat RA.

Immunosuppressive agents and risk of infection:

- **Corticosteroids**: It increases the risk of pneumonia by dose-depending mechanism. For most of patients, a dose of more than 10 mg/day is sufficient to cause it [123–126].
- **MTX**: With or without corticosteroids, it makes patients at risk of developing opportunistic infections, e.g., PCP and disseminated histoplasmosis [124, 127]. Usually occurs in the first 2 years of initiation the MTX [124].
- **Anti-tumor necrosis factor-alpha (TNF-a)**: Exposes patients to risk of many opportunistic infections, most importantly *Mycobacterium tuberculosis* (TB). Others like coccidioidomycosis, histoplasmosis, listeria, aspergillus, and norcodia have been reported [128].

7.7.8.2 Latent Tuberculosis Infection (LTBI) Screening [129]

Before initiating the treatment with any of the following biologic agents (adalimumab, certolizumab pegol, etanercept, infliximab, golimumab, abatacept, rituximab, or tocilizumab) a TB skin testing or interferon gamma release assay (IGRA) should be done to screen for latent TB infection (LTBI) regardless of the presence or absence of

TB risk factors. If negative results without presence of risk factors, then starting the treatment with the biologic agent is permissible. If negative results with the presence of TB risk factors, the physician should repeat the test in 1–3 weeks. If results are positive, CXR should be done. If negative CXR for TB signs, this is latent TB infection (LTBI), and referral to an infectious disease (ID) specialist should be undertaken. In this situation, the physician can initiate the treatment with the biologic agent after 1 month of starting the treatment of the LTBI. If positive CXR, then do sputum stain and culture for TB. If negative, it is LTBI. But if the sputum tested positive for TB, refer the patient to an ID specialist to start the treatment for active TB infection [129]. Of note, if patient is already on glucocorticoids, induration of 5 mm is considered positive [90].

For further reading, please see Infectious Disease Chap. 11.

7.7.8.3 Cancer

RA patients are at increased risk for developing lung cancer and lymphoma. The reason is not clear. But, a proposed theory could be due to RA itself, smoking, immunosuppressive therapy, or because RA is a middle age disease, which equals to the age at which cancers usually detected. Once mediastinal lymph node is detected, biopsy has to be undertaken as soon as possible.

7.7.8.4 Myopathy and Muscle Weakness

Introduction

Usually happens due to medication toxicity, rheumatoid vasculitis, and rheumatoid myositis. Physicians should suspect it when patients have progressive dyspnea with unclear cause and no improvement with treatment. Risk factors are the use of D-penicillamine and hydroxychloroquine.

Diagnosis

Blood tests show creatine-kinase (CK) within the normal limits. PFT show restrictive pattern. Also, FVC and VC in supine position is reduced by more than 10% than in upright. Furthermore, maximal inspiratory pressure (MIP) and maximal expiratory pressure (MEP) are reduced. DLCO is normal unless another pathology present. Biopsy may be needed to confirm the diagnosis.

7.7.8.5 Fibrobullous Disease

It's a rare complication of rheumatoid arthritis and usually occurs in the apical part of the lung. It could be a complication of a rheumatoid nodule even in the absence of a radiological evidence.

7.7.8.6 Amyloidosis

Secondary amyloidosis, which involves lungs, has been reported. It could present as nodules, ILD, or tracheobronchomalacia.

7.8 Sjogren Syndrome (SS)

7.8.1 Background

It's an autoimmune disease characterized by involvement of exocrine glands through infiltration of lymphocytes. A clinically significant pulmonary manifestation occurs in around 9–24% of SS patients. Also, pulmonary involvements in asymptomatic SS patients who were detected by PFT, CT scan, or BAL reach 75% of patients. Also, pulmonary manifestations usually occur late in the disease course. Furthermore, if they were clinically significant, it could increase the risk of mortality by fourfold [130]. Risk factors for pulmonary involvement are positive rheumatoid factor, hypergammaglobulinemia, positive anti-Ro and anti-La, and decreased FVC and FVC1, smoking, elderly patients, and male sex. Overall, rituximab is a promising drug to treat SS and its extra-glandular manifestations (because it targets B lymphocytes), unlike anti-TNF drugs.

- Pulmonary manifestations.
- *Airway involvement.*
- Upper airway.
- Nasal crusting.

  Around 18.5% of SS patients complain of nasal crusting. It is found in 50% during physical exam. The treatment usually consists of the use of room humidifiers and saline nasal spray as needed.

7.8.2 Epistaxis

It occurs in around 31.8% of patients with SS. The treatment is the same as for any patient with epistaxis.

7.8.3 Hoarseness of the Voice

This occurs in about 1/3 of SS patients. The diagnosis is done by laryngoscopy, which shows most commonly dryness or thick mucus covering the vocal cords. However, rarely, the presence of Bamboo node, which is a transverse yellow or white submucosal lesion, occurs in the vocal folds. Also, granulomatous and non-granulomatous nodules have been reported.

7.8.4 Xerotrachea and Xerobronchitis

Usually developed due to structural of functional disability of the mucociliary cells to clear the thickened secretions. It occurs in around 17% of SS patients. Those usually presents almost always with dry cough. Chest radiograph, HRCT, and PFT are normal. On the other hand, recurrent bronchitis, bronchopneumonia, atelectasis, and peribronchial and peribronchiolar scarring and narrowing might occur as complications.

7.8.5 Lower Airway Disease

7.8.5.1 Follicular Bronchiolitis (FB)

Introduction

It's a benign lymphoproliferative disorder, characterized by hyperplasic lymphoid follicles distributed along the bronchioles and the peribronchiolar interstituim unlike the LIP, which involves the whole parenchyma. It is a histopathological diagnosis; however, it could be suspected by history, CT scan, and PFT results. It's a common manifestation of SS. Usually, patients present with cough, dyspnea, and sometimes fever.

Investigation

CT scan shows bilateral peribronchial and centrilobular nodules with size range between 1 and 3 mm but could reach up to 12 mm. Other findings are reticular opacities, GGO, and intrathoracic lymphadenopathy. Furthermore, PFT usually shows restrictive pattern but also could be obstructive pattern or both. Biopsy shows hyperplasic lymphoid follicles distributed along the bronchioles and the peribronchiolar interstitium.

Treatment

Primary treatment of SS could be enough. However, systemic corticosteroid is shown to be effective [131].

Prognosis

Has good prognosis when treated with corticosteroid.

7.8.6 Chronic Obstructive Pulmonary Disease (COPD)

It is found to be more prevalent in SS patients through their disease course, especially smokers, who have 5 times higher chance compared to non-smokers to develop COPD [132].

7.8.7 Lung Parenchyma

7.8.7.1 ILD

Introduction

It's the most common pulmonary manifestations of SS. Furthermore, the most common subtype are NSIP followed by lymphcytic interstitial pneumonia (LIP) then UIP and lastly OP. It is more common when patients have anti-Ro antibodies.

Subtypes

NSIP

It occurs in about 28–61%. Presentation is usually chronic dyspnea. Chest radiograph may show bilateral interstitial infiltrates. PFT shows restrictive pattern with decreased DLCO. HRCT shows GGO (with subpleural and basilar predominance). Furthermore, reticular abnormalities with or without traction bronchiectasis could be found. Honeycombing happened with advanced disease. BAL is done to rule out infection when suspected. Biopsy shows uniform or homogenous pattern of cellular inflammation and/or fibrosis of the alveolar walls. Moreover, no need for treatment if patients are asymptomatic. However, if symptomatic with worsening symptoms, physician could give steroids (prednisone 1 mg/kg/day) [133]. Also, if refractory, immunosuppressive therapy (commonly AZA. Rarely CYC or cyclosporines) could be used [134–137]. The prognosis depends on the extent of fibrosis. The less fibrosis, the better prognosis [132].

Lymphocytic interstitial pneumonia (LIP)

It's one of the most common pulmonary manifestations of SS. It has potentials to progress into lymphoma. Thus, biopsy should always be considered if there is no response to standard therapy. The prevalence is 17% among SS patients who develop ILD [133] with female predominance [138]. Patients usually present with dyspnea and cough and, also, less commonly fever, weight loss and night sweat. Blood tests show polyclonal hypergammaglobulinemia (80% of cases). Chest radiograph may show bilateral reticular or reticulonodular opacities, more commonly in the lower zones. HRCT shows diffuse GGO and walled cysts (in 50% of cases). Also, interlobular septal thickening, centrilobular nodules, and bronchovascular bundle could be seen. PFT show restrictive pattern with low DLCO. BAL is done to rule out infection if suspected. Again, since it could progress to lymphoma, biopsy should always be considered if there is no response to standard therapy. Histopathology reveals infiltration of the interstitial septa and, sometimes, filling of the alveolar space by lymphocyte (B&T cells), plasma cells, and histiocytes. Patients usually treated with corticosteroids (start with prednisone 0.75–1.0 mg/kg/day then taper slowly for the following 3–6 months) [139–141]. Furthermore, initially, it responds well to corticosteroids. However, up to 1/3 of patients die due to progression of disease or due to the infectious complications resulted from the intensive immunosuppression therapy [142]. Rarely it could resolve spontaneously.

7.8.8 Pleural Involvement

7.8.8.1 Pleural Effusion

It's a very rare manifestation of SS. Therefore, when present, one should think of a secondary cause (i.e., in the setting of secondary SS), e.g., RA or SLE. Usually occurs bilaterally, but a unilateral presentation could happen. Pleural fluid analysis should be done for diagnosis (Table 7.4).

7.8.9 Pulmonary Vascular Disease

7.8.9.1 PAH

Introduction

It's a rare complication and usually occurs due to pulmonary artery vasculitis. Also, occasionally, it co-exists with Raynaud's phenomenon. Risk factors are Raynaud's phenomenon, ILD, skin vasculitis, hypergammaglobulinemia, positive anti-Ro, positive RF, and positive antiribonucleoprotein (anti-RNP) antibodies. Moreover, for presentation and diagnosis (see PAH in SSc). The mainstay of treatment is the use of PAH specific treatment (endothelin receptor antagonists, phosphodiesterase type 5 inhibitors, or prostanoids) with/without immunosuppressive therapy [143].

7.8.10 Cancer

7.8.10.1 Lymphoma

Introduction

The risk of SS patients to develop lymphoma in general, not only pulmonary lymphoma, is 44 times compared with healthy population [144], while pulmonary lymphoma prevalence is 1–2% among SS patients [145]. Furthermore, SS patients could develop benign lymphocytic infiltration, like in LIP, and this in turn could progress to lymphoma [145]. This benign lymphocytic infiltration is characterized by polyclonal B and T lymphocytes proliferation. Moreover, the most common type of lymphoma in SS patients is non-Hodgkin's lymphoma with a subtype of mucosa-associated lymphoid tissue (MALT) [145], while the most common pulmonary lymphoma is the low-grade extranodal marginal B-cell lymphoma of MALT type [145]. Risk factors are hypocomplementemia, cryoglobulinemia, vasculitis (palpable purpura), and severe exocrine involvement at time of diagnosis of SS [145].

Presentation

80% are asymptomatic at time of lymphoma diagnosis due to the incidental finding in radiological studies. If symptomatic: dyspnea, cough, weight loss, fatigue and sweat.

Diagnosis

Chest CT scan manifests as nodules (solitary or multiple), bilateral diffuse infiltrate, interstitial infiltration with slight lower zone predominance, mediastinal lymphadenopathy, and pleural effusion (usually do not occur alone rather happen with the parenchymal involvement). Furthermore, biopsy shows most commonly a non-Hodgkin's low-grade extranodal marginal B-cell lymphoma of MALT type [145]. Also, it has good prognosis with 5-year survival of more than 80% [146]. Of note, progression to high-grade lymphoma occasionally happens [145].

Pseudolymphoma

It's a rare and benign entity, also called pulmonary nodular lymphoid hyperplasia or bronchus-associated lymphoid tissue (BALT). It is characterized by infiltration of polyclonal lymphocyte and plasma cells. Usually it's asymptomatic but could present with dyspnea and cough. CT scan typically shows solitary nodule. However, less frequently, multiple nodules, which involve blood vessels, consolidation, mediastinal lymph node and/or pleural effusion, could be seen. Biopsy usually reveals bronchus-associated lymphoid tissue (BALT). Furthermore, corticosteroids or immunosuppressive therapy could be given [147]. It has good prognosis when treated [147]. However, rarely transforms into lymphoma.

Amyloidosis

Its prevalence is around 0.6%, and patients' presentation depends on the location such as larynx, trachea, bronchi, interstitium, and/or mediastinum. CT scan shows micronodular lesions (could be calcified or cavitary) predominantly in the subpleural area and in the lower lobes, while biopsy shows positive amyloid staining. The prognosis is usually good [148, 149].

7.9 Mixed Connective Tissue Disease (MCTD)

7.9.1 Introduction

It was first described in 1972 and defined as a combination of SSc, SLE, and polymyositis/dermatomyositis (PM/DM) with positive anti-ribonucleoprotein (Anti-RNP). Yet, it's not clear if it's a separate entity of disease or not. Furthermore, pulmonary manifestations occur in up to 65% of MCTD patients. Worth mentioning, that patients with MCTD could present with any pulmonary manifestations related to SLE, SSc, or PM/DM [150].

7.9.2 Pulmonary Manifestations

7.9.2.1 Lung Parenchyma

Interstitial Lung Disease (ILD)

Introduction

It occurs in around 50–65% of MCTD patients [150]. Also, esophageal dilatation is a risk factor for developing ILD [151].

Presentations

Please see ILD in SSc.

Diagnosis

In early stages, PFT shows reduction in DLCO only. Then, in late stages, it shows restrictive pattern with low DLCO. HRCT shows septal thickening, GGO, and non-septal linear opacities with predominance in the periphery or within the lower lobe. Also, in fact, no study encountered pathological findings, but thought to be NSIP and UIP.

Treatment
Physician should start corticosteroid (methylprednisolone 2 mg/kg/day) for 4–6 weeks then assess, if no improvement add CYC oral or IV to complete 6 months [152].

Prognosis
Good prognosis (in terms of preventing further progression of the disease) if treated during the acute inflammatory phase (GGO). Once signs of fibrosis on HRCT present, the response will be poor.

Alveolar Hemorrhage
It's an uncommon manifestation. Also, for presentation, diagnosis, and treatment refer to SLE-associated DAH.

Pulmonary Vascular Disease

PAH
Prevalence ranges between 3.4% and 27%. Furthermore, for presentation, diagnosis, screening and treatment, see SSc-PAH.

Pleural Diseases

Pleural Effusion
It's a common manifestation of MCTD with prevalence about 50% [153]. Pleural fluid analysis is usually exudative and with lymphocytic predominance. Moreover, it usually resolves spontaneously. However, if it persists, then a trial of corticosteroid could be effective.

7.10 Polymyositis (PM)/ Dermatomyositis (DM)

7.10.1 Introduction

Pulmonary manifestations play big role in the mortality and morbidity of PM/DM patients. Moreover, the main pulmonary complications are ILD, aspiration pneumonia, and hypoventilation due to muscle weakness.

7.10.2 Pulmonary Manifestations

7.10.2.1 Parenchymal Lung Disease

Interstitial Lung Disease (ILD)

Introduction
It's the most common pulmonary complication, which reaches up to 65% when screened by CXR, HRCT, or PFT. Furthermore, it can present as an acute, chronic, or asymptomatic with radiological findings only. When it is symptomatic, more than 60% of patients present with cough and dyspnea and normal radiograph, HRCT, or PFT. Also, it is more common in DM than in PM. However, recently, a new subtype of DM has been reported, the clinically amyopathic dermatomyositis (CADM), which is DM without muscle involvement. This subset, when associated with anti-CADM-140 antibodies, associated with higher prevalence of rapidly progressive ILD. Risk factors are positive antihistidyl tRNA synthetase antibody (anti-Jo-1), Krebs Von den Lungen-6 (KL-6), serum surfactant protein D, serum cytokeratin 19 fragment (CK-19), and anti-CADM-140 antibody (which associated with rapidly progressive ILD). All of them aren't present in every center as a routine test.

Presentations
Patients usually present with dyspnea and cough.

Diagnosis
PFT shows restrictive pattern with low DLCO. While HRCT could shows NSIP, UIP, OP, or DAD pattern. BAL to rule out infection or drug-induced pneumonitis. Biopsy is rarely needed because the HRCT findings correlate well with histopathology. Although transbronchial lung biopsy is inferior to open lung biopsy, it is a good choice if opportunistic infection or neoplasms are suspected because open lung biopsy associated with high mortality rate.

Treatment

Most commonly, corticosteroids with (CYC, AZA, cyclosporines) are given [154–161]. However, IVIG alone or with corticosteroids has shown good results in progressive disease [162, 163]. Also, tacrolimus and rituximab, individually, are promising drugs [164–166]. Anti-tumor necrosis factor-alpha (Anti-TNF-a) and MTX are less likely to be effective. In fact, they may induce irreversible lung fibrosis [167].

Prognosis

ILD in PM/DM increases mortality. A 5-year survival ranges between 60% and 86% [168, 169]. Also, worse prognosis is expected with DM compared to PM. Furthermore, when corticosteroids combined with other immunosuppressive therapy, approximately 1/3 of the patients will improve, 1/3 will remain the same, and 1/3 will deteriorate [154]. Moreover, rapidly progressive ILD has fatal outcome with 3-year survival of around 24% [170].

7.10.2.2 Aspiration Pneumonia

It occurs in around 17% [171] of PM/DM patients and is related to the dysfunction happens to the pharynx and esophagus muscles which lead to abnormal swallowing and frequent regurgitation. Risk factors are severe muscle disease [172]. Furthermore, investigations and treatment are like any other case of aspiration pneumonia.

7.10.2.3 Pulmonary Vascular Disease

PAH

Occasionally happens. For, presentation, diagnosis, and treatment, see SSc-PAH.

7.10.3 Pneumothorax (PNX) and Pneumomediastinum and Subcutaneous Emphysema

7.10.3.1 Introduction

They occur in two different clinical scenarios. The first one is vasculopathy with or without mild ILD (vasculopathy such as skin ulcers or bronchial wall necrosis). The second one is severe ILD with or without vasculopathy. Whenever one of these complications (PNX, pneumomediastinum, or subcutaneous emphysema) happens, one should suspect pulmonary vasculitis. Diagnosis is made by chest radiograph and chest CT scan. Moreover, physicians should start corticosteroid and immunosuppressive therapy together at the beginning then taper the steroid gradually [173].

7.10.4 Respiratory Failure and Hypoventilation

7.10.4.1 Introduction

This happens due to severe respiratory muscle weakness with prevalence around 21.8% [171].

7.10.4.2 Diagnosis

PFT shows restrictive pattern. Furthermore, FVC and VC in supine position are reduced by more than 10% than in upright. Also, maximal inspiratory pressure (MIP) and maximal expiratory pressure (MEP) are reduced. DLCO is normal unless another pathology is present. Chest radiograph may show decreased lung volumes, elevated diaphragms, and basal atelectasis.

7.10.4.3 Complications

Atelectasis and recurrent pneumonia may develop due to mucus plugging because of reduced cough reflex secondary to respiratory muscle weakness.

7.10.4.4 Treatment

Physicians should start immunosuppressive therapy. However, if failed, home mechanical ventilation could be used which could saves life and improves the quality of life.

7.10.4.5 Lung Cancer

There may be an association between lung cancer and myositis, especially DM.

Acknowledgments The Authors would like to thank Amr A. Telmesani, MD, for his contributions to this chapter in the previous edition.

References

1. McNearney TA, Reveille JD, Fischbach M, et al. Pulmonary involvement in systemic sclerosis: associations with genetic, serologic, sociodemographic, and behavioral factors. Arthritis Rheum. 2007;57(2):318–26.
2. Steen VD, Medsger TA. Changes in causes of death in systemic sclerosis, 1972-2002. Ann Rheum Dis. 2007;66(7):940–4.
3. Steen VD, Lanz JK Jr, Conte C, Owens GR, Medsger TA Jr. Therapy for severe interstitial lung disease in systemic sclerosis. A retrospective study. Arthritis Rheum. 1994;37(9):1290–6.
4. Le Pavec J, Launay D, Mathai SC, Hassoun PM, Humbert M. Scleroderma lung disease. Clin Rev Allergy Immunol. 2011;40(2):104–16.
5. Berezne A, Ranque B, Valeyre D, et al. Therapeutic strategy combining intravenous cyclophosphamide followed by oral azathioprine to treat worsening interstitial lung disease associated with systemic sclerosis: a retrospective multicenter open-label study. J Rheumatol. 2008;35(6):1064–72.
6. Tzelepis GE, Plastiras SC, Karadimitrakis SP, Vlachoyiannopoulos PG. Determinants of pulmonary function improvement in patients with scleroderma and interstitial lung disease. Clin Exp Rheumatol. 2007;25(5):734–9.
7. Airo P, Danieli E, Parrinello G, et al. Intravenous cyclophosphamide therapy for systemic sclerosis. A single-center experience and review of the literature with pooled analysis of lung function test results. Clin Exp Rheumatol. 2004;22(5):573–8.
8. Giacomelli R, Valentini G, Salsano F, et al. Cyclophosphamide pulse regimen in the treatment of alveolitis in systemic sclerosis. J Rheumatol. 2002;29(4):731–6.
9. Varai G, Earle L, Jimenez SA, Steiner RM, Varga J. A pilot study of intermittent intravenous cyclophosphamide for the treatment of systemic sclerosis associated lung disease. J Rheumatol. 1998;25(7):1325–9.
10. Tashkin DP, Elashoff R, Clements PJ, et al. Cyclophosphamide versus placebo in scleroderma lung disease. N Engl J Med. 2006;354(25):2655–66.
11. Hoyles RK, Ellis RW, Wellsbury J, et al. A multicenter, prospective, randomized, double-blind, placebo-controlled trial of corticosteroids and intravenous cyclophosphamide followed by oral azathioprine for the treatment of pulmonary fibrosis in scleroderma. Arthritis Rheum. 2006;54(12):3962–70.
12. Nadashkevich O, Davis P, Fritzler M, Kovalenko W. A randomized unblinded trial of cyclophosphamide versus azathioprine in the treatment of systemic sclerosis. Clin Rheumatol. 2006;25(2):205–12.
13. Dheda K, Lalloo UG, Cassim B, Mody GM. Experience with azathioprine in systemic sclerosis associated with interstitial lung disease. Clin Rheumatol. 2004;23(4):306–9.
14. Koutroumpas A, Ziogas A, Alexiou I, Barouta G, Sakkas LI. Mycophenolate mofetil in systemic sclerosis-associated interstitial lung disease. Clin Rheumatol. 2010;29(10):1167–8.
15. Liossis SN, Bounas A, Andonopoulos AP. Mycophenolate mofetil as first-line treatment improves clinically evident early scleroderma lung disease. Rheumatology. 2006;45(8):1005–8.
16. Mendoza FA, Nagle SJ, Lee JB, Jimenez SA. A prospective observational study of mycophenolate mofetil treatment in progressive diffuse cutaneous systemic sclerosis of recent onset. J Rheumatol. 2012;39(6):1241–7.
17. Saketkoo LA, Espinoza LR. Experience of mycophenolate mofetil in 10 patients with autoimmune-related interstitial lung disease demonstrates promising effects. Am J Med Sci. 2009;337(5):329–35.
18. Simeon-Aznar CP, Fonollosa-Pla V, Tolosa-Vilella C, Selva-O'Callaghan A, Solans-Laque R, Vilardell-Tarres M. Effect of mycophenolate sodium in scleroderma-related interstitial lung disease. Clin Rheumatol. 2011;30(11):1393–8.
19. Stratton RJ, Wilson H, Black CM. Pilot study of anti-thymocyte globulin plus mycophenolate mofetil in recent-onset diffuse scleroderma. Rheumatology. 2001;40(1):84–8.
20. Swigris JJ, Olson AL, Fischer A, et al. Mycophenolate mofetil is safe, well tolerated, and preserves lung function in patients with connective tissue disease-related interstitial lung disease. Chest. 2006;130(1):30–6.
21. Daoussis D, Liossis SN, Tsamandas AC, et al. Experience with rituximab in scleroderma: results from a 1-year, proof-of-principle study. Rheumatology. 2010;49(2):271–80.
22. Lafyatis R, Kissin E, York M, et al. B cell depletion with rituximab in patients with diffuse cutaneous systemic sclerosis. Arthritis Rheum. 2009;60(2):578–83.
23. Distler JH, Jungel A, Huber LC, et al. Imatinib mesylate reduces production of extracellular matrix and prevents development of experimental dermal fibrosis. Arthritis Rheum. 2007;56(1):311–22.
24. van Daele PL, Dik WA, Thio HB, et al. Is imatinib mesylate a promising drug in systemic sclerosis? Arthritis Rheum. 2008;58(8):2549–52.
25. Meyer KC, Decker C, Baughman R. Toxicity and monitoring of immunosuppressive therapy used in systemic autoimmune diseases. Clin Chest Med. 2010;31(3):565–88.
26. Tashkin DP, et al. Mycophenolate mofetil versus oral cyclophosphamide in scleroderma-related interstitial lung disease (SLS II): a randomised controlled, double-blind, parallel group trial. Lancet Respir Med. 2016;4(9):708–19.
27. Saggar R, Khanna D, Furst DE, et al. Systemic sclerosis and bilateral lung transplantation: a single centre experience. Eur Respir J. 2010;36(4):893–900.

28. Massad MG, Powell CR, Kpodonu J, et al. Outcomes of lung transplantation in patients with scleroderma. World J Surg. 2005;29(11):1510–5.
29. Burt RK, Shah SJ, Dill K, et al. Autologous non-myeloablative haemopoietic stem-cell transplantation compared with pulse cyclophosphamide once per month for systemic sclerosis (ASSIST): an open-label, randomised phase 2 trial. Lancet. 2011;378(9790):498–506.
30. Savarino E, Bazzica M, Zentilin P, et al. Gastroesophageal reflux and pulmonary fibrosis in scleroderma: a study using pH-impedance monitoring. Am J Respir Crit Care Med. 2009;179(5):408–13.
31. Johnson DA, Drane WE, Curran J, et al. Pulmonary disease in progressive systemic sclerosis. A complication of gastroesophageal reflux and occult aspiration? Arch Intern Med. 1989;149(3):589–93.
32. Mejía CCR, Alcolea BS, Ríos BJJ. Update in pulmonary arterial hypertension. Revista Clinica Espanola. 2016;216(8):436–44.
33. Fisher MR, Mathai SC, Champion HC, et al. Clinical differences between idiopathic and scleroderma-related pulmonary hypertension. Arthritis Rheum. 2006;54(9):3043–50.
34. Humbert M, Yaici A, de Groote P, et al. Screening for pulmonary arterial hypertension in patients with systemic sclerosis: clinical characteristics at diagnosis and long-term survival. Arthritis Rheum. 2011;63(11):3522–30.
35. Launay D, Humbert M, Berezne A, et al. Clinical characteristics and survival in systemic sclerosis-related pulmonary hypertension associated with interstitial lung disease. Chest. 2011;140(4):1016–24.
36. Kuwana M, Watanabe H, Matsuoka N, Sugiyama N. Pulmonary arterial hypertension associated with connective tissue disease: meta-analysis of clinical trials. BMJ Open. 2013;3(8):e003113.
37. Barst RJ, Gibbs JS, Ghofrani HA, et al. Updated evidence-based treatment algorithm in pulmonary arterial hypertension. J Am Coll Cardiol. 2009;54(1 Suppl):S78–84.
38. Grunig E, Lichtblau M, Ehlken N, et al. Safety and efficacy of exercise training in various forms of pulmonary hypertension. Eur Respir J. 2012;40(1):84–92.
39. Mereles D, Ehlken N, Kreuscher S, et al. Exercise and respiratory training improve exercise capacity and quality of life in patients with severe chronic pulmonary hypertension. Circulation. 2006;114(14):1482–9.
40. Mathur PN, Powles P, Pugsley SO, McEwan MP, Campbell EJ. Effect of digoxin on right ventricular function in severe chronic airflow obstruction. A controlled clinical trial. Ann Intern Med. 1981;95(3):283–8.
41. Solomon JJ, Olson AL, Fischer A, Bull T, Brown KK, Raghu G. Scleroderma lung disease. Eur Respir Rev. 2013;22(127):6–19.
42. Lavie F, Rozenberg S, Coutaux A, Koeger AC, Bourgeois P, Fautrel B. Bronchiectasis in a patient with CREST syndrome. Joint Bone Spine. 2002;69(5):515–8.
43. Chausow AM, Kane T, Levinson D, Szidon JP. Reversible hypercapnic respiratory insufficiency in scleroderma caused by respiratory muscle weakness. Am Rev Respir Dis. 1984;130(1):142–4.
44. Pugazhenthi M, Cooper D, Ratnakant BS, Postlethwaite A, Carbone L. Hypercapnic respiratory failure in systemic sclerosis. J Clin Rheumatol. 2003;9(1):43–6.
45. Pertschuk LP, Moccia LF, Rosen Y, et al. Acute pulmonary complications in systemic lupus erythematosus. Immunofluorescence and light microscopic study. Am J Clin Pathol. 1977;68(5):553–7.
46. Orens JB, Martinez FJ, Lynch JP 3rd. Pleuropulmonary manifestations of systemic lupus erythematosus. Rheum Dis Clin N Am. 1994;20(1):159–93.
47. Keane MP, Lynch JP 3rd. Pleuropulmonary manifestations of systemic lupus erythematosus. Thorax. 2000;55(2):159–66.
48. McKnight KM, Adair NE, Agudelo CA. Successful use of tetracycline pleurodesis to treat massive pleural effusion secondary to systemic lupus erythematosus. Arthritis Rheum. 1991;34(11):1483–4.
49. Gilleece MH, Evans CC, Bucknall RC. Steroid resistant pleural effusion in systemic lupus erythematosus treated with tetracycline pleurodesis. Ann Rheum Dis. 1988;47(12):1031–2.
50. Kamen DL, Strange C. Pulmonary manifestations of systemic lupus erythematosus. Clin Chest Med. 2010;31(3):479–88.
51. Pego-Reigosa JM, Medeiros DA, Isenberg DA. Respiratory manifestations of systemic lupus erythematosus: old and new concepts. Best Pract Res Clin Rheumatol. 2009;23(4):469–80.
52. Lim SW, Gillis D, Smith W, Hissaria P, Greville H, Peh CA. Rituximab use in systemic lupus erythematosus pneumonitis and a review of current reports. Intern Med J. 2006;36(4):260–2.
53. Eiser AR, Shanies HM. Treatment of lupus interstitial lung disease with intravenous cyclophosphamide. Arthritis Rheum. 1994;37(3):428–31.
54. Matthay RA, Schwarz MI, Petty TL, et al. Pulmonary manifestations of systemic lupus erythematosus: review of twelve cases of acute lupus pneumonitis. Medicine. 1975;54(5):397–409.
55. Schwab EP, Schumacher HR Jr, Freundlich B, Callegari PE. Pulmonary alveolar hemorrhage in systemic lupus erythematosus. Semin Arthritis Rheum. 1993;23(1):8–15.
56. Swigris JJ, Fischer A, Gillis J, Meehan RT, Brown KK. Pulmonary and thrombotic manifestations of systemic lupus erythematosus. Chest. 2008;133(1):271–80.
57. Santos-Ocampo AS, Mandell BF, Fessler BJ. Alveolar hemorrhage in systemic lupus erythematosus: presentation and management. Chest. 2000;118(4):1083–90.

58. Erickson RW, Franklin WA, Emlen W. Treatment of hemorrhagic lupus pneumonitis with plasmapheresis. Semin Arthritis Rheum. 1994;24(2):114–23.
59. Wiedemann HP, Matthay RA. Pulmonary manifestations of systemic lupus erythematosus. J Thorac Imaging. 1992;7(2):1–18.
60. Weinrib L, Sharma OP, Quismorio FP Jr. A long-term study of interstitial lung disease in systemic lupus erythematosus. Semin Arthritis Rheum. 1990;20(1):48–56.
61. Renzoni E, Rottoli P, Coviello G, Perari MG, Galeazzi M, Vagliasindi M. Clinical, laboratory and radiological findings in pulmonary fibrosis with and without connective tissue disease. Clin Rheumatol. 1997;16(6):570–7.
62. Ruiz-Irastorza G, Egurbide MV, Ugalde J, Aguirre C. High impact of antiphospholipid syndrome on irreversible organ damage and survival of patients with systemic lupus erythematosus. Arch Intern Med. 2004;164(1):77–82.
63. Crowther MA, Ginsberg JS, Julian J, et al. A comparison of two intensities of warfarin for the prevention of recurrent thrombosis in patients with the antiphospholipid antibody syndrome. N Engl J Med. 2003;349(12):1133–8.
64. Martens J, Demedts M, Vanmeenen MT, Dequeker J. Respiratory muscle dysfunction in systemic lupus erythematosus. Chest. 1983;84(2):170–5.
65. Asherson RA, Cervera R, Merrill JT, Erkan D. Antiphospholipid antibodies and the antiphospholipid syndrome: clinical significance and treatment. Semin Thromb Hemost. 2008;34(3):256–66.
66. Dhala A. Pulmonary arterial hypertension in systemic lupus erythematosus: current status and future direction. Clin Dev Immunol. 2012;2012:854941.
67. Barst RJ, Rubin LJ, Long WA, et al. A comparison of continuous intravenous epoprostenol (prostacyclin) with conventional therapy for primary pulmonary hypertension. N Engl J Med. 1996;334(5):296–301.
68. Galie N, Brundage BH, Ghofrani HA, et al. Tadalafil therapy for pulmonary arterial hypertension. Circulation. 2009;119(22):2894–903.
69. Galie N, Ghofrani HA, Torbicki A, et al. Sildenafil citrate therapy for pulmonary arterial hypertension. N Engl J Med. 2005;353(20):2148–57.
70. Galie N, Olschewski H, Oudiz RJ, et al. Ambrisentan for the treatment of pulmonary arterial hypertension: results of the ambrisentan in pulmonary arterial hypertension, randomized, double-blind, placebo-controlled, multicenter, efficacy (ARIES) study 1 and 2. Circulation. 2008;117(23):3010–9.
71. Gonzalez-Lopez L, Cardona-Munoz EG, Celis A, et al. Therapy with intermittent pulse cyclophosphamide for pulmonary hypertension associated with systemic lupus erythematosus. Lupus. 2004;13(2):105–12.
72. Jais X, Launay D, Yaici A, et al. Immunosuppressive therapy in lupus- and mixed connective tissue disease-associated pulmonary arterial hypertension: a retrospective analysis of twenty-three cases. Arthritis Rheum. 2008;58(2):521–31.
73. Sanchez O, Sitbon O, Jais X, Simonneau G, Humbert M. Immunosuppressive therapy in connective tissue diseases-associated pulmonary arterial hypertension. Chest. 2006;130(1):182–9.
74. Tanaka E, Harigai M, Tanaka M, Kawaguchi Y, Hara M, Kamatani N. Pulmonary hypertension in systemic lupus erythematosus: evaluation of clinical characteristics and response to immunosuppressive treatment. J Rheumatol. 2002;29(2):282–7.
75. Abramson SB, Dobro J, Eberle MA, et al. Acute reversible hypoxemia in systemic lupus erythematosus. Ann Intern Med. 1991;114(11):941–7.
76. Martinez-Taboada VM, Blanco R, Armona J, Fernandez-Sueiro JL, Rodriguez-Valverde V. Acute reversible hypoxemia in systemic lupus erythematosus: a new syndrome or an index of disease activity? Lupus. 1995;4(4):259–62.
77. Smith GA, Ward PH, Berci G. Laryngeal involvement by systemic lupus erythematosus. Trans Sect Otolaryngol Am Acad Ophthalmol Otolaryngol. 1977;84(1):124–8.
78. Teitel AD, MacKenzie CR, Stern R, Paget SA. Laryngeal involvement in systemic lupus erythematosus. Semin Arthritis Rheum. 1992;22(3):203–14.
79. Fenlon HM, Doran M, Sant SM, Breatnach E. High-resolution chest CT in systemic lupus erythematosus. AJR Am J Roentgenol. 1996;166(2):301–7.
80. Beylot-Barry M, Doutre MS, Bletry O, Beylot C. Lupus bronchiolitis obliterans: diagnostic difficulties. La Revue de medecine interne/fondee par la Societe nationale francaise de medecine interne. 1994;15(5):332–5.
81. Kawahata K, Yamaguchi M, Kanda H, et al. Severe airflow limitation in two patients with systemic lupus erythematosus: effect of inhalation of anticholinergics. Mod Rheumatol. 2008;18(1):52–6.
82. Toya SP, Tzelepis GE. Association of the shrinking lung syndrome in systemic lupus erythematosus with pleurisy: a systematic review. Semin Arthritis Rheum. 2009;39(1):30–7.
83. Soubrier M, Dubost JJ, Piette JC, et al. Shrinking lung syndrome in systemic lupus erythematosus. A report of three cases. Rev Rhum. 1995;62(5):395–8.
84. Walz-Leblanc BA, Urowitz MB, Gladman DD, Hanly PJ. The "shrinking lungs syndrome" in systemic lupus erythematosus—improvement with corticosteroid therapy. J Rheumatol. 1992;19(12):1970–2.
85. Benham H, Garske L, Vecchio P, Eckert BW. Successful treatment of shrinking lung syndrome with rituximab in a patient with systemic lupus erythematosus. J Clinical Rheumatol. 2010;16(2):68–70.
86. Costabel U, Guzman J, Bonella F, Oshimo S. Bronchoalveolar lavage in other interstitial lung diseases. Semin Respir Crit Care Med. 2007;28(5):514–24.

87. Van Veen S, Peeters AJ, Sterk PJ, Breedveld FC. The "shrinking lung syndrome" in SLE, treatment with theophylline. Clin Rheumatol. 1993;12(4):462–5.
88. Ernest D, Leung A. Ventilatory failure in shrinking lung syndrome is associated with reduced chest compliance. Intern Med J. 2010;40(1):66–8.
89. Weng CT, Liu MF, Weng MY, et al. Pneumocystis jirovecii pneumonia in systemic lupus erythematosus from southern Taiwan. J Clin Rheumatol. 2013;19(5):252–8.
90. Antin-Ozerkis D, Evans J, Rubinowitz A, Homer RJ, Matthay RA. Pulmonary manifestations of rheumatoid arthritis. Clin Chest Med. 2010;31(3):451–78.
91. Stack BH, Grant IW. Rheumatoid interstitial lung disease. Br J Dis Chest. 1965;59(4):202–11.
92. Frank ST, Weg JG, Harkleroad LE, Fitch RF. Pulmonary dysfunction in rheumatoid disease. Chest. 1973;63(1):27–34.
93. Popper MS, Bogdonoff ML, Hughes RL. Interstitial rheumatoid lung disease. A reassessment and review of the literature. Chest. 1972;62(3):243–50.
94. Ramirez P, Valencia M, Torres A. Bronchoalveolar lavage to diagnose respiratory infections. Semin Respir Crit Care Med. 2007;28(5):525–33.
95. Schnabel A, Richter C, Bauerfeind S, Gross WL. Bronchoalveolar lavage cell profile in methotrexate induced pneumonitis. Thorax. 1997;52(4):377–9.
96. Antoniou KM, Margaritopoulos G, Economidou F, Siafakas NM. Pivotal clinical dilemmas in collagen vascular diseases associated with interstitial lung involvement. Eur Respir J. 2009;33(4):882–96.
97. Kelly C, Saravanan V. Treatment strategies for a rheumatoid arthritis patient with interstitial lung disease. Expert Opin Pharmacother. 2008;9(18):3221–30.
98. Vij R, Strek ME. Diagnosis and treatment of connective tissue disease-associated interstitial lung disease. Chest. 2013;143(3):814–24.
99. Dawson JK, Fewins HE, Desmond J, Lynch MP, Graham DR. Predictors of progression of HRCT diagnosed fibrosing alveolitis in patients with rheumatoid arthritis. Ann Rheum Dis. 2002;61(6):517–21.
100. Flaherty KR, Toews GB, Travis WD, et al. Clinical significance of histological classification of idiopathic interstitial pneumonia. Eur Respir J. 2002;19(2):275–83.
101. Riha RL, Duhig EE, Clarke BE, Steele RH, Slaughter RE, Zimmerman PV. Survival of patients with biopsy-proven usual interstitial pneumonia and nonspecific interstitial pneumonia. Eur Respir J. 2002;19(6):1114–8.
102. Walker WC, Wright V. Pulmonary lesions and rheumatoid arthritis. Medicine. 1968;47(6):501–20.
103. Faurschou P, Francis D, Faarup P. Thoracoscopic, histological, and clinical findings in nine case of rheumatoid pleural effusion. Thorax. 1985;40(5):371–5.
104. Hassoun PM. Pulmonary arterial hypertension complicating connective tissue diseases. Semin Respir Crit Care Med. 2009;30(4):429–39.
105. Schwarz MI, Zamora MR, Hodges TN, Chan ED, Bowler RP, Tuder RM. Isolated pulmonary capillaritis and diffuse alveolar hemorrhage in rheumatoid arthritis and mixed connective tissue disease. Chest. 1998;113(6):1609–15.
106. Carloni A, Piciucchi S, Giannakakis K, Nori G, Zobel BB, Poletti V. Diffuse alveolar hemorrhage after leflunomide therapy in a patient with rheumatoid arthritis. J Thorac Imaging. 2008;23(1):57–9.
107. Heresi GA, Farver CF, Stoller JK. Interstitial pneumonitis and alveolar hemorrhage complicating use of rituximab: case report and review of the literature. Respiration. 2008;76(4):449–53.
108. Panagi S, Palka W, Korelitz BI, Taskin M, Lessnau KD. Diffuse alveolar hemorrhage after infliximab treatment of Crohn's disease. Inflamm Bowel Dis. 2004;10(3):274–7.
109. Brazeau-Lamontagne L, Charlin B, Levesque RY, Lussier A. Cricoarytenoiditis: CT assessment in rheumatoid arthritis. Radiology. 1986;158(2):463–6.
110. Dockery KM, Sismanis A, Abedi E. Rheumatoid arthritis of the larynx: the importance of early diagnosis and corticosteroid therapy. South Med J. 1991;84(1):95–6.
111. Chen JJ, Branstetter BF, Myers EN. Cricoarytenoid rheumatoid arthritis: an important consideration in aggressive lesions of the larynx. AJNR Am J Neuroradiol. 2005;26(4):970–2.
112. Chen, Joseph J., Barton F. Branstetter, Eugene N. Myers. Cricoarytenoid rheumatoid arthritis: an important consideration in aggressive lesions of the larynx. American Journal of Neuroradiology. 2005;26(4):970–72.
113. Mountz JD, Turner RA, Collins RL, Gallup KR Jr, Semble EL. Rheumatoid arthritis and small airways function. Effects of disease activity, smoking, and alpha 1-antitrypsin deficiency. Arthritis Rheum. 1984;27(7):728–36.
114. White ES, Tazelaar HD, Lynch JP 3rd. Bronchiolar complications of connective tissue diseases. Semin Respir Crit Care Med. 2003;24(5):543–66.
115. Penny WJ, Knight RK, Rees AM, Thomas AL, Smith AP. Obliterative bronchiolitis in rheumatoid arthritis. Ann Rheum Dis. 1982;41(5):469–72.
116. van de Laar MA, Westermann CJ, Wagenaar SS, Dinant HJ. Beneficial effect of intravenous cyclophosphamide and oral prednisone on D-penicillamine-associated bronchiolitis obliterans. Arthritis Rheum. 1985;28(1):93–7.
117. Azuma A, Kudoh S. Diffuse panbronchiolitis in East Asia. Respirology. 2006;11(3):249–61.
118. Kudoh S, Azuma A, Yamamoto M, Izumi T, Ando M. Improvement of survival in patients with diffuse panbronchiolitis treated with low-dose erythromycin. Am J Respir Crit Care Med. 1998;157(6 Pt 1):1829–32.
119. Hayakawa H, Sato A, Imokawa S, Toyoshima M, Chida K, Iwata M. Bronchiolar disease in rheumatoid arthritis. Am J Respir Crit Care Med. 1996;154(5):1531–6.

120. Leslie KO, Trahan S, Gruden J. Pulmonary pathology of the rheumatic diseases. Semin Respir Crit Care Med. 2007;28(4):369–78.
121. Caplan A. Certain unusual radiological appearances in the chest of coal-miners suffering from rheumatoid arthritis. Thorax. 1953;8(1):29–37.
122. Lakos G, Soos L, Fekete A, et al. Anti-cyclic citrullinated peptide antibody isotypes in rheumatoid arthritis: association with disease duration, rheumatoid factor production and the presence of shared epitope. Clin Exp Rheumatol. 2008;26(2): 253–60.
123. Doran MF, Crowson CS, Pond GR, O'Fallon WM, Gabriel SE. Frequency of infection in patients with rheumatoid arthritis compared with controls: a population-based study. Arthritis Rheum. 2002;46(9):2287–93.
124. Boerbooms AM, Kerstens PJ, van Loenhout JW, Mulder J, van de Putte LB. Infections during low-dose methotrexate treatment in rheumatoid arthritis. Semin Arthritis Rheum. 1995;24(6):411–21.
125. Saag KG, Koehnke R, Caldwell JR, et al. Low dose long-term corticosteroid therapy in rheumatoid arthritis: an analysis of serious adverse events. Am J Med. 1994;96(2):115–23.
126. Wolfe F, Caplan L, Michaud K. Treatment for rheumatoid arthritis and the risk of hospitalization for pneumonia: associations with prednisone, disease-modifying antirheumatic drugs, and anti-tumor necrosis factor therapy. Arthritis Rheum. 2006;54(2):628–34.
127. LeMense GP, Sahn SA. Opportunistic infection during treatment with low dose methotrexate. Am J Respir Crit Care Med. 1994;150(1):258–60.
128. Khraishi M. Comparative overview of safety of the biologics in rheumatoid arthritis. J Rheumatol Suppl. 2009;82:25–32.
129. Singh JA, Furst DE, Bharat A, et al. 2012 update of the 2008 American College of Rheumatology recommendations for the use of disease-modifying antirheumatic drugs and biologic agents in the treatment of rheumatoid arthritis. Arthritis Care Res. 2012;64(5):625–39.
130. Palm O, Garen T, Berge Enger T, et al. Clinical pulmonary involvement in primary Sjogren's syndrome: prevalence, quality of life and mortality—a retrospective study based on registry data. Rheumatology. 2013;52(1):173–9.
131. Wells AU, du Bois RM. Bronchiolitis in association with connective tissue disorders. Clin Chest Med. 1993;14(4):655–66.
132. Stojan G, Baer AN, Danoff SK. Pulmonary manifestations of Sjogren's syndrome. Curr Allergy Asthma Rep. 2013;13(4):354–60.
133. Parambil JG, Myers JL, Lindell RM, Matteson EL, Ryu JH. Interstitial lung disease in primary Sjogren syndrome. Chest. 2006;130(5):1489–95.
134. Deheinzelin D, Capelozzi VL, Kairalla RA, Barbas Filho JV, Saldiva PH, de Carvalho CR. Interstitial lung disease in primary Sjogren's syndrome. Clinical-pathological evaluation and response to treatment. Am J Respir Crit Care Med. 1996;154(3 Pt 1):794–9.
135. Deheinzelin D, de Carvalho CR, Tomazini ME, Barbas Filho JV, Saldiva PH. Association of Sjogren's syndrome and sarcoidosis. Report of a case. Sarcoidosis. 1988;5(1):68–70.
136. Hansen LA, Prakash UB, Colby TV. Pulmonary lymphoma in Sjogren's syndrome. Mayo Clin Proc. 1989;64(8):920–31.
137. Shi JH, Liu HR, Xu WB, et al. Pulmonary manifestations of Sjogren's syndrome. Respiration. 2009;78(4):377–86.
138. Cha SI, Fessler MB, Cool CD, Schwarz MI, Brown KK. Lymphoid interstitial pneumonia: clinical features, associations and prognosis. Eur Respir J. 2006;28(2):364–9.
139. Koss MN, Hochholzer L, Langloss JM, Wehunt WD, Lazarus AA. Lymphoid interstitial pneumonia: clinicopathological and immunopathological findings in 18 cases. Pathology. 1987;19(2):178–85.
140. Swigris JJ, Berry GJ, Raffin TA, Kuschner WG. Lymphoid interstitial pneumonia: a narrative review. Chest. 2002;122(6):2150–64.
141. Teirstein AS, Rosen MJ. Lymphocytic interstitial pneumonia. Clin Chest Med. 1988;9(3):467–71.
142. Ramos-Casals M, Tzioufas AG, Stone JH, Siso A, Bosch X. Treatment of primary Sjogren syndrome: a systematic review. JAMA. 2010;304(4):452–60.
143. Launay D, Hachulla E, Hatron PY, Jais X, Simonneau G, Humbert M. Pulmonary arterial hypertension: a rare complication of primary Sjogren syndrome: report of 9 new cases and review of the literature. Medicine. 2007;86(5):299–315.
144. Isaksen K, Jonsson R, Omdal R. Anti-CD20 treatment in primary Sjogren's syndrome. Scand J Immunol. 2008;68(6):554–64.
145. Kokosi M, Riemer EC, Highland KB. Pulmonary involvement in Sjogren syndrome. Clin Chest Med. 2010;31(3):489–500.
146. Thieblemont C, de la Fouchardiere A, Coiffier B. Nongastric mucosa-associated lymphoid tissue lymphomas. Clin Lymphoma. 2003;3(4):212–24.
147. Song MK, Seol YM, Park YE, et al. Pulmonary nodular lymphoid hyperplasia associated with Sjogren's syndrome. Korean J Intern Med. 2007;22(3):192–6.
148. Himmelfarb E, Wells S, Rabinowitz JG. The radiologic spectrum of cardiopulmonary amyloidosis. Chest. 1977;72(3):327–32.
149. Rubinow A, Celli BR, Cohen AS, Rigden BG, Brody JS. Localized amyloidosis of the lower respiratory tract. Am Rev Respir Dis. 1978;118(3):603–11.
150. Prakash UB. Respiratory complications in mixed connective tissue disease. Clin Chest Med. 1998;19(4):733–46. ix
151. Fagundes MN, Caleiro MT, Navarro-Rodriguez T, et al. Esophageal involvement and interstitial lung disease in mixed connective tissue disease. Respir Med. 2009;103(6):854–60.

152. Bodolay E, Szekanecz Z, Devenyi K, et al. Evaluation of interstitial lung disease in mixed connective tissue disease (MCTD). Rheumatology. 2005;44(5):656–61.
153. Bull TM, Fagan KA, Badesch DB. Pulmonary vascular manifestations of mixed connective tissue disease. Rheum Dis Clin N Am. 2005;31(3):451–64. vi
154. Fathi M, Vikgren J, Boijsen M, et al. Interstitial lung disease in polymyositis and dermatomyositis: longitudinal evaluation by pulmonary function and radiology. Arthritis Rheum. 2008;59(5):677–85.
155. Ideura G, Hanaoka M, Koizumi T, et al. Interstitial lung disease associated with amyopathic dermatomyositis: review of 18 cases. Respir Med. 2007;101(7):1406–11.
156. Jankowska M, Butto B, Debska-Slizien A, Rutkowski B. Beneficial effect of treatment with cyclosporin a in a case of refractory antisynthetase syndrome. Rheumatol Int. 2007;27(8):775–80.
157. Kawasaki M, Kaneda K, Kaneko H, Sekigawa I, Takasaki Y, Ogawa H. Two cases of dermatomyositis associated with interstitial pneumonia: a comprehensive study of gene expression. Clin Exp Rheumatol. 2008;26(2):379–80.
158. Kotani T, Makino S, Takeuchi T, et al. Early intervention with corticosteroids and cyclosporin A and 2-hour postdose blood concentration monitoring improves the prognosis of acute/subacute interstitial pneumonia in dermatomyositis. J Rheumatol. 2008;35(2):254–9.
159. Mielnik P, Wiesik-Szewczyk E, Olesinska M, Chwalinska-Sadowska H, Zabek J. Clinical features and prognosis of patients with idiopathic inflammatory myopathies and anti-Jo-1 antibodies. Autoimmunity. 2006;39(3):243–7.
160. Suda T, Fujisawa T, Enomoto N, et al. Interstitial lung diseases associated with amyopathic dermatomyositis. Eur Respir J. 2006;28(5):1005–12.
161. Yamasaki Y, Yamada H, Yamasaki M, et al. Intravenous cyclophosphamide therapy for progressive interstitial pneumonia in patients with polymyositis/dermatomyositis. Rheumatology. 2007;46(1):124–30.
162. Danieli MG, Malcangi G, Palmieri C, et al. Cyclosporin A and intravenous immunoglobulin treatment in polymyositis/dermatomyositis. Ann Rheum Dis. 2002;61(1):37–41.
163. Murota H, Muroi E, Yamaoka T, Hamasaki Y, Katayama I. Successful treatment with regimen of intravenous gamma globulin and cyclophosphamide for dermatomyositis accompanied by interstitial pneumonia, opportunistic infection and steroid psychosis. Allergol Int. 2006;55(2):199–202.
164. Guglielmi S, Merz TM, Gugger M, Suter C, Nicod LP. Acute respiratory distress syndrome secondary to antisynthetase syndrome is reversible with tacrolimus. Eur Respir J. 2008;31(1):213–7.
165. Levine TD. Rituximab in the treatment of dermatomyositis: an open-label pilot study. Arthritis Rheum. 2005;52(2):601–7.
166. Selva-O'Callaghan A, Labrador-Horrillo M, Munoz-Gall X, et al. Polymyositis/dermatomyositis-associated lung disease: analysis of a series of 81 patients. Lupus. 2005;14(7):534–42.
167. Hengstman GJ, De Bleecker JL, Feist E, et al. Open-label trial of anti-TNF-alpha in dermato- and polymyositis treated concomitantly with methotrexate. Eur Neurol. 2008;59(3–4):159–63.
168. Marie I, Hachulla E, Cherin P, et al. Interstitial lung disease in polymyositis and dermatomyositis. Arthritis Rheum. 2002;47(6):614–22.
169. Douglas WW, Tazelaar HD, Hartman TE, et al. Polymyositis-dermatomyositis-associated interstitial lung disease. Am J Respir Crit Care Med. 2001;164(7):1182–5.
170. Won Huh J, Soon Kim D, Keun Lee C, et al. Two distinct clinical types of interstitial lung disease associated with polymyositis-dermatomyositis. Respir Med. 2007;101(8):1761–9.
171. Marie I, Hachulla E, Cherin P, et al. Opportunistic infections in polymyositis and dermatomyositis. Arthritis Rheum. 2005;53(2):155–65.
172. Medsger TA Jr, Robinson H, Masi AT. Factors affecting survivorship in polymyositis. A life-table study of 124 patients. Arthritis Rheum. 1971;14(2):249–58.
173. Terao M, Ozawa K, Inui S, Murota H, Yokomi A, Itami S. A case of dermatomyositis complicated with pneumomediastinum. Mod Rheumatol. 2007;17(2):156–9.

8

Rheumatic Disorders and the Nervous System

Emad Alkohtani and Amal Alkhotani

8.1 Introduction

The nervous system can be affected by many rheumatologic disorders. The involvements are different in various diseases. Some rheumatologic diseases have prominent nervous system features, e.g. SLE, while in others these are minor (Table 8.1).

Patients with rheumatologic disorders can have nervous system involvement secondary to medications including immunosuppressive therapy or related to associated comorbidities. It also can be related or a sequel of the disease process itself.

The objective of this chapter is to provide a systemic approach to patients with various rheumatic conditions presenting with neurological syndromes.

8.1.1 Specific Objectives

By the end of the chapter, the reader should be able to:

1. Recognize different neurological manifestations associated with SLE.
2. Compose a diagnostic approach to SLE patients presenting with acute headache.
3. Compose a diagnostic approach to SLE patients presenting with chronic headache.
4. Manage SLE patients presenting with acute stroke.
5. Recall the different causes of stroke in SLE patients.
6. Recall the differential diagnosis of generalized seizure in SLE patients.
7. Recall the differential diagnosis of focal seizure in SLE patients.
8. Use appropriate investigation for SLE patients presenting with seizure.
9. Recognize SLE patients with seizure who will require long-term antiepileptic medications.
10. Compose a diagnostic approach and manage SLE patients presenting with spinal cord dysfunction.
11. Recognize neurological manifestations of rheumatoid arthritis (RA).
12. Recognize RA patients at high risk of cervical spine disease.
13. Manage RA patients with suspected cervical spine disease.
14. Recognize causes of neuropathy in RA patients.
15. Compose a diagnostic approach to RA patients presenting with neuropathy.
16. Compose a diagnostic approach to patients with neuropathy and skin rash.

E. Alkohtani
King Abdullah Medical City, Makkah, Saudi Arabia
e-mail: Emad.alkhotani@gmail.com

A. Alkhotani (✉)
Umm Al-Qura University, Makkah, Saudi Arabia
e-mail: amkhotani@uqu.edu.sa

Table 8.1 Neurological involvement in rheumatic diseases

Condition	Neurological syndromes
Antiphospholipid syndrome	Transverse myelopathy, stroke, migraine, memory loss, demyelination, movement disorders
Temporal arteritis/ giant cell arteritis and Takayasu's arteritis	Headache, visual loss, papilloedema, amaurosis fugax, stroke
Systemic vasculitis	Peripheral neuropathy, mononeuritis multiplex, stroke, polymyositis, meningoencephalitis
Eosinophilic granulomatosis with polyangiitis	Peripheral or cranial neuropathy, mononeuritis multiplex, encephalopathy
Dermatomyositis—Polymyositis	Proximal myopathy
Mixed connective tissue disease	Proximal myopathy
Rheumatoid arthritis	Rheumatoid vasculitis causing stroke and/or neuropathy, atlantoaxial subluxation, polymyositis; mononeuritis multiplex, peripheral neuropathy
Systemic lupus erythematosus	Aseptic meningitis, demyelinating syndrome, chorea, myelopathy, seizures, anxiety/mood disorders; psychosis, Guillain-Barre´ syndrome, plexopathy; cranial and/or peripheral neuropathy, myasthenia gravis, autonomic disorder, stroke, migraine, headache
Behçet's disease	Meningitis, encephalitis, seizure, stroke, headache
Scleroderma	Proximal myopathy, plexopathy, intracerebral inflammation
Ankylosing spondylitis	Spinal stenosis
Granulomatosis with polyangiitis and polyarteritis nodosa	Peripheral or cranial neuropathy, mononeuritis multiplex, ocular disorders
Sjogren's syndrome	Myelopathy, polyneuropathy, motor neurone syndromes, cognitive Dysfunction

Table 8.2 Neuropsychiatric syndromes associated with systemic lupus erythematosus

NPSLE associated with the central nervous system	NPSLE associated with the peripheral nervous system
– Aseptic meningitis – Cerebrovascular disease – Demyelinating syndromes – Headaches – Movement disorders (chorea) – Myelopathy – Seizure disorders – Acute confusional state – Anxiety disorders – Cognitive dysfunction – Mood disorders – Psychosis	– Acute inflammatory demyelinating syndromes (Guillain-Barre´ syndrome) – Autonomic neuropathy – Mononeuropathy, single or multiplex – Myasthenia gravis – Cranial neuropathy – Plexopathy – polyneuropathy

8.2 Systemic Lupus Erythematosus (SLE)

In 1999, the American College of Rheumatology (ACR) established 19 different neuropsychiatric SLE syndromes (NPSLE) (Table 8.2).

In this chapter, the diagnostic approach to patients with SLE presenting with different neurological complaints will be presented. In general, obtaining good and detailed history and examination will assist to narrow the differential diagnosis and help with obtaining specific diagnostic tests (Table 8.3).

8.2.1 Headache

The prevalence of headache in patients with SLE is reported around 47.1–57% [1–3]. The differential diagnosis and approach to headache in SLE patients is different for acute versus chronic headache (Figs. 8.1 and 8.2). Patients with SLE can present with headache as primary disorders or can be secondary to other causes. The objective is to rule out serious causes before attributing it to primary headache disorder.

Table 8.3 Summary of NPSLE syndromes and differential diagnosis

<table>
<tr><th>NPSLE manifestations</th><th>Diseases to exclude</th><th>Notes</th></tr>
<tr><td>Headache</td><td>Aseptic meningitis, CNS infections, venous sinus thrombosis</td><td rowspan="8">1. Diagnosis of NPSLE is by exclusion of other important causes by ordering routine tests:
a. Laboratory: CBC, electrolyte, renal, and liver function tests
b. CSF: WBC, protein, glucose, gram stain and culture, viral PCR
c. Imaging: Either CT brain or MRI brain and spinal cord according to the case
d. EEG, EMG, NCV
2. Treatment is by glucocorticoids and immunosuppressive drugs and anticoagulant in certain conditions
– In refractory cases, you can add one or all of the following:
a. Plasmapharesis
b. Intravenous immunoglobulin
c. rituximab</td></tr>
<tr><td>Cognitive dysfunction</td><td>Drug side effects, depression, endocrine disorders like adrenal disease, stroke</td></tr>
<tr><td>Stroke</td><td>Thromboembolic causes, cerebral vasculitis</td></tr>
<tr><td>Seizure</td><td>Infection, electrolyte abnormalities, uraemia, hypertension, medication side effects, hypoxia or rarely brain tumour</td></tr>
<tr><td>Acute confusional state</td><td>Metabolic causes like renal or liver failure, CNS infections, medication side effects, seizure, structural lesion, e.g. tumour</td></tr>
<tr><td>Myelopathy</td><td>Infectious myelitis, neuromyelitis optica</td></tr>
<tr><td>Movement disorders</td><td>Hereditary causes like Huntington's, Wilson, metabolic causes, structural like brain tumour</td></tr>
<tr><td>Peripheral neuropathy</td><td>Metabolic causes like diabetes, infectious causes, vitamin deficiency, etc.</td></tr>
</table>

8.2.1.1 Approach

Obtain a careful history of the headache: onset, duration, types, and precipitating, aggravating, and relieving factors. Headache that increases with coughing or sneezing and also that is worse with lying down raises the possibility of raised intracranial pressure. The presence of history of visual obscuration is also suggestive of increased intracranial pressure. Ask about any associated neurological symptoms that will make primary headache unlikely and necessitate neuroimaging. In female patients, ask about the relation of headache to the menstrual cycle. Headaches that worsen in relation to menstrual cycle likely will be migraine related.

In addition, a comprehensive evaluation of SLE itself (current active symptoms like joint pains, skin rashes, and urinary symptoms, duration, organ involvements, and prior NPSLE attacks).

Detailed drug history should be obtained as some may precipitate or worsen headaches, e.g. some nonsteroidal anti-inflammatory drugs (NSAIDs) like ibuprofen can cause aseptic meningitis.

On examination, look carefully for signs of meningitis and focal neurological deficits, and *do not forget* to look for papilledema.

Workup depends on your initial findings (Figs. 8.1 and 8.2).

Indications for neuroimaging:

1. New-onset headache or worsening of pre-existing headache.
2. Features suggestive of increased intracranial pressure from history or examination, e.g. papilledema.
3. Altered level of consciousness.
4. Focal neurological signs and symptoms.
5. Associated seizure.

   Treatment depends on the cause of the headache. Patients with venous sinus thrombosis will require treatment with anticoagulants. Meningitis should be treated with antibiotic therapy. If the headache is attributed to primary headache disorders, use abortive therapy as indicated. If primary headache is frequent, preventive therapy should be considered according to the headache type.

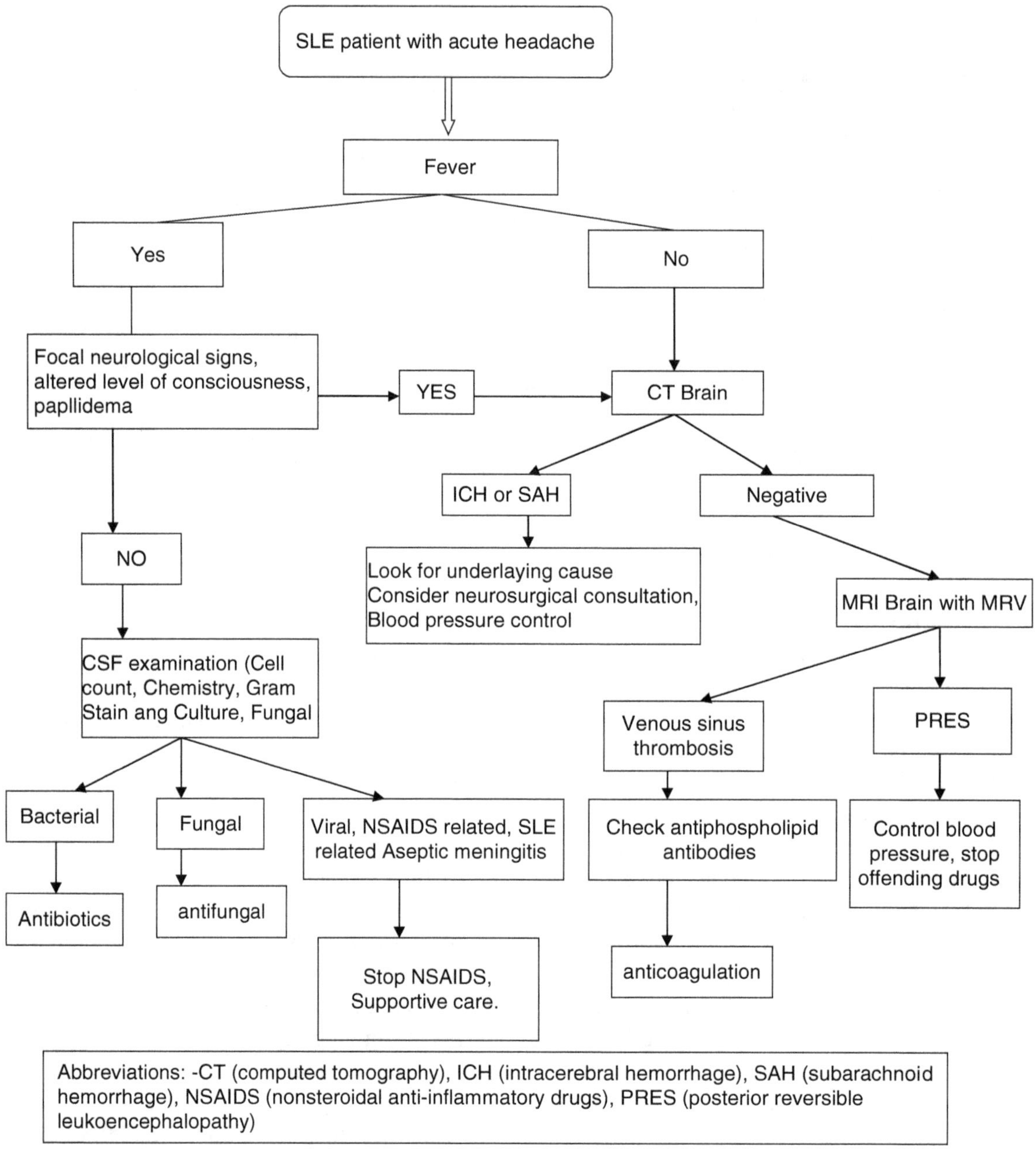

Fig. 8.1 Diagnostic approach to SLE patients with acute headache

8.2.2 Stroke

Cerebrovascular diseases account for around 2–17% [2–4] of all NPSLE events.

Approach to SLE patients with acute stroke is the same as in non-SLE patients (Fig. 8.3).

Keep in mind that in SLE patients, further consideration of the aetiology of the events should be considered. When patients with SLE present with acute neurological deficit within a 4.5-h window, immediate evaluation with brain CT scan is warranted to rule out presence of intracerebral haemorrhage. In absence of contraindication, thrombolytic therapy should be administered. Patient who arrived outside the thrombolytic window should have CT brain before starting antiplatelet therapy. The

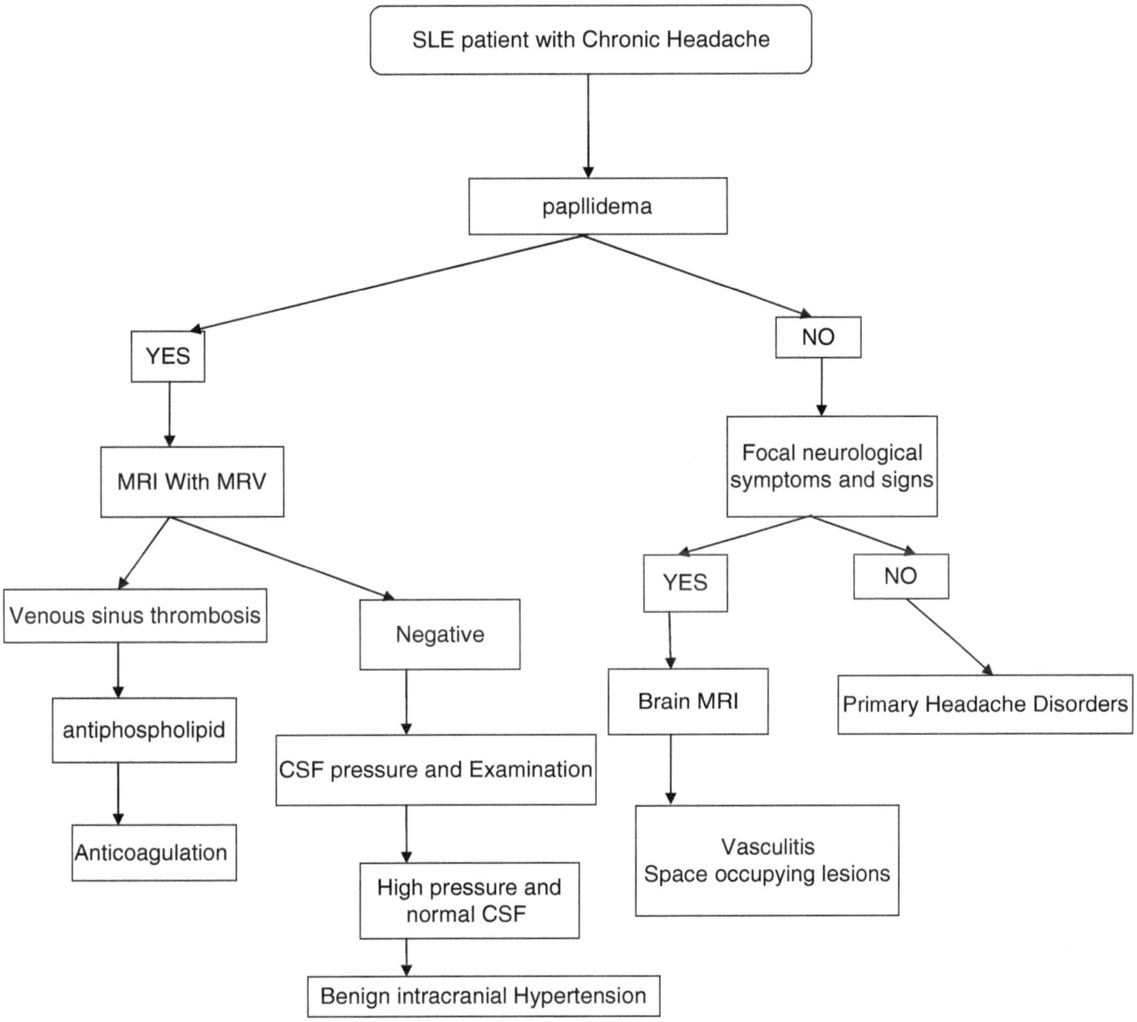

Fig. 8.2 Approach to SLE patient with chronic headache

initial workup for any SLE patient with stroke should include:

1. Fasting blood glucose.
2. Fasting lipid profile.
3. Carotid Doppler.
4. Holter monitoring.
5. Echocardiogram.
6. Antiphospholipid antibodies.

Disease activity should be determined (anti-dsDNA level, urinalysis, complement level (C3 and C4), creatinine). Specific treatment for active disease with immunosuppressive therapy should be considered. All patients should get cardiovascular risk factor modifications. In patients with negative antiphospholipid antibodies and with no indication for anticoagulation such as atrial fibrillation, antiplatelet therapy is the cornerstone for the prevention of further events. Patient with antiphospholipid antibodies should be anticoagulated with warfarin at an INR >3.0 or combined antiplatelet-anticoagulant (INR 2.0–3.0). There is no consensus agreement on this [5].

8.2.3 Seizure

Seizure is a transient neurological dysfunction that results from excessive abnormal discharges of cortical neurons. Seizure can be generalized or focal in onset. The differential diagnosis of generalized-onset seizure is different than focal-onset seizure (Table 8.4).

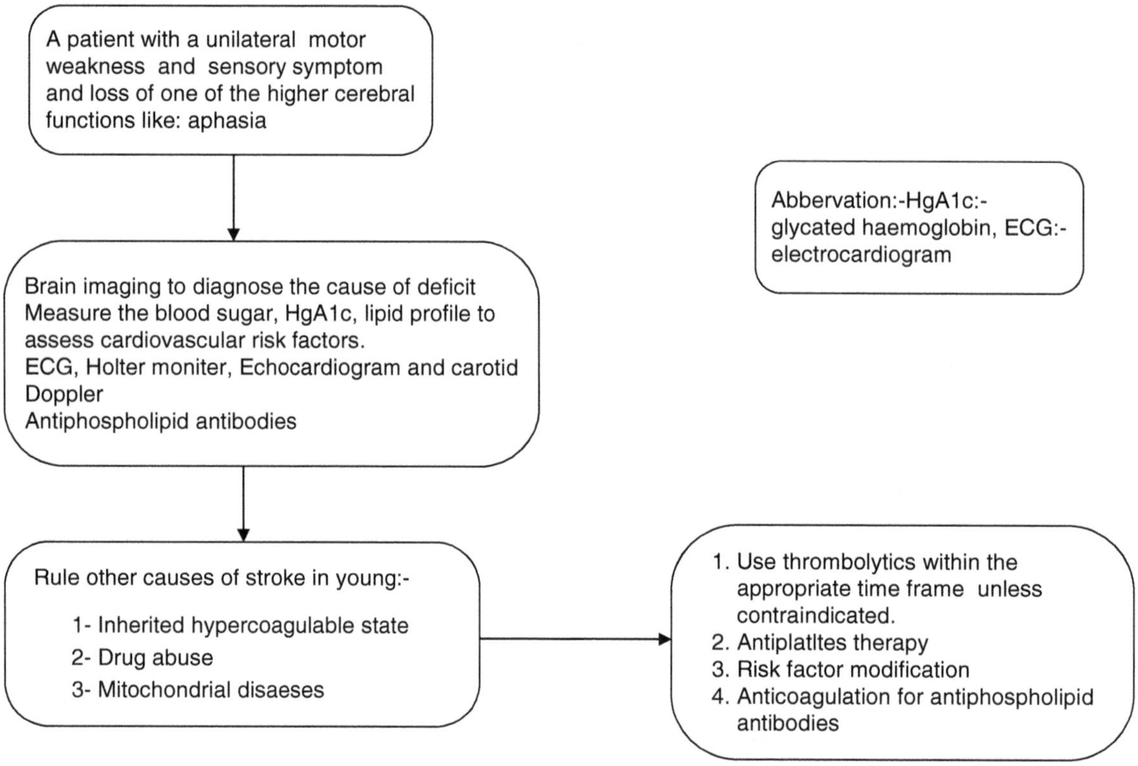

Fig. 8.3 Approach to SLE patients with acute stroke

Table 8.4 Cause of generalized versus partial onset seizure

Generalized seizure	Partial-onset seizure
Electrolyte imbalance	Venous sinus thrombosis
Medication side effect	Posterior reversible encephalopathy
Uraemia	Limbic encephalitis
Infection	Infection
NPSLE	Stroke

Different aetiological factors can cause seizure in SLE patients (Tables 8.5 and 8.6). The prognosis and the need for further treatment of seizure are dependent on the cause of seizure [6, 7].

Table 8.5 Causes of seizure in SLE patients

Electrolyte imbalance
Uraemia
Medication side effect
Posterior reversible encephalopathy
Infection (meningitis, encephalitis, cryptococcal meningitis)
Limbic encephalitis
Venous sinus thrombosis
NPSLE (single unprovoked seizure)

Table 8.6 workup of SLE patients present with single seizure

Electrolytes
Renal profile
Liver profile
CBC
Brain MRI and MRV
EEG

8.2.3.1 Tips in History

1. Disease activities.
2. Seizure onset, duration, and postictal events.
3. Determine the seizure type by asking if there was a preceding aura and by taking exact description of seizure from a witness.
4. History of fever.
5. Any associated other neurological symptoms or signs.
6. Medication history.
7. History of comorbidities, e.g. hypertension or renal failure.

8. Similar events in the past.
9. History of prior CNS insults, e.g. stroke.
10. Family history of epilepsy.

Treatment with an antiepileptic is not indicated for a single unprovoked seizure and for seizure secondary to metabolic causes. Use an antiepileptic in the presence of recurrent events, abnormal EEG, and abnormal neuroimaging which carry a higher risk of recurrence without treatment.

If seizure happens in a setting of high disease activities, treatment with immunosuppressive therapy is indicated.

8.2.4 Myelopathy

It is a condition that results from inflammation of the spinal cord. Although it is considered rarer than other NPSLE syndromes, its development carries poor functional outcome. The classical presentation is with symptoms of spinal cord dysfunction including motor weakness, sensory loss with sensory level, and loss of sphincter control. The presentation differs according to the specific localization of the cord inflammation (Table 8.7).

Patients with SLE can present with transverse myelitis and rarely can also present with longitudinal myelitis where more four segments of the cord are involved. The development of longitudinal myelitis carries a worse prognosis and mandates aggressive immunosuppressive therapy. In the presence of longitudinal myelitis, brain MRI should be done to rule out brain demyelination. Anti-NMO antibodies (neuromyelitis optica) should be sent for those patients.

Table 8.7 Symptoms and signs of myelopathy according to the spinal level

Cervical cord	Motor weakness affecting four limbs (lower motor neuron signs at the level with upper motor neuron signs below the level of the lesion in chronic stage) Sensory loss below the level with cervical sensory level Loss of sphincter control Respiratory compromise in high cervical lesion
Thoracic cord	Motor weakness below the lesion (usually upper limb preserved unless T1 involved) Sensory loss below the lesion with truncal sensory level Loss of sphincter control

When dealing with patients with symptoms of acute cord dysfunction, one should rule out surgical causes first as an early intervention will affect the outcome (Fig. 8.4). When surgical causes are excluded, patients should have CSF examination to rule out infectious causes of myelitis. Treatment with immunosuppressive therapy should be delayed. Combine it with antiviral therapy until negative culture is obtained.

Different immunosuppressive regimens have been used in patients with myelopathy including pulse steroid therapy with or without intravenous cyclophosphamide or plasmapheresis. Aggressive therapy with combined three modalities can be used for patients with more severe disease especially with longitudinal myelitis, although one case series did not show superior outcome with the combined three modalities [8]. That observation may be explained by the fact that patients who had combined therapy had severe disease at their presentation. In a subgroup of patients with antiphospholipid antibodies, the use of anticoagulation is recommended.

8.3 Rheumatoid Arthritis

Rheumatoid arthritis (RA) is the most common inflammatory destructive joint disease. Besides its articular manifestations, patients with RA exhibit multiple extra-articular manifestations. The nervous system can be involved at varying degrees in patients with RA [9]. Both central and peripheral nervous system can be involved (Fig. 8.5). Central nervous system involvements can happen in the form of necrotizing vasculitis or as a result from cervical spine involvements and the development of atlantoaxial subluxation. Peripheral nervous system involvement can be primary due vasculitis or secondary to the joint deformities or compression from rheumatoid nodules. Also the nervous system can be involved secondary to drug side effect.

The approach to patients with rheumatoid arthritis and atlantoaxial subluxation as well to patients presenting with neuropathy will be discussed (Fig. 8.6).

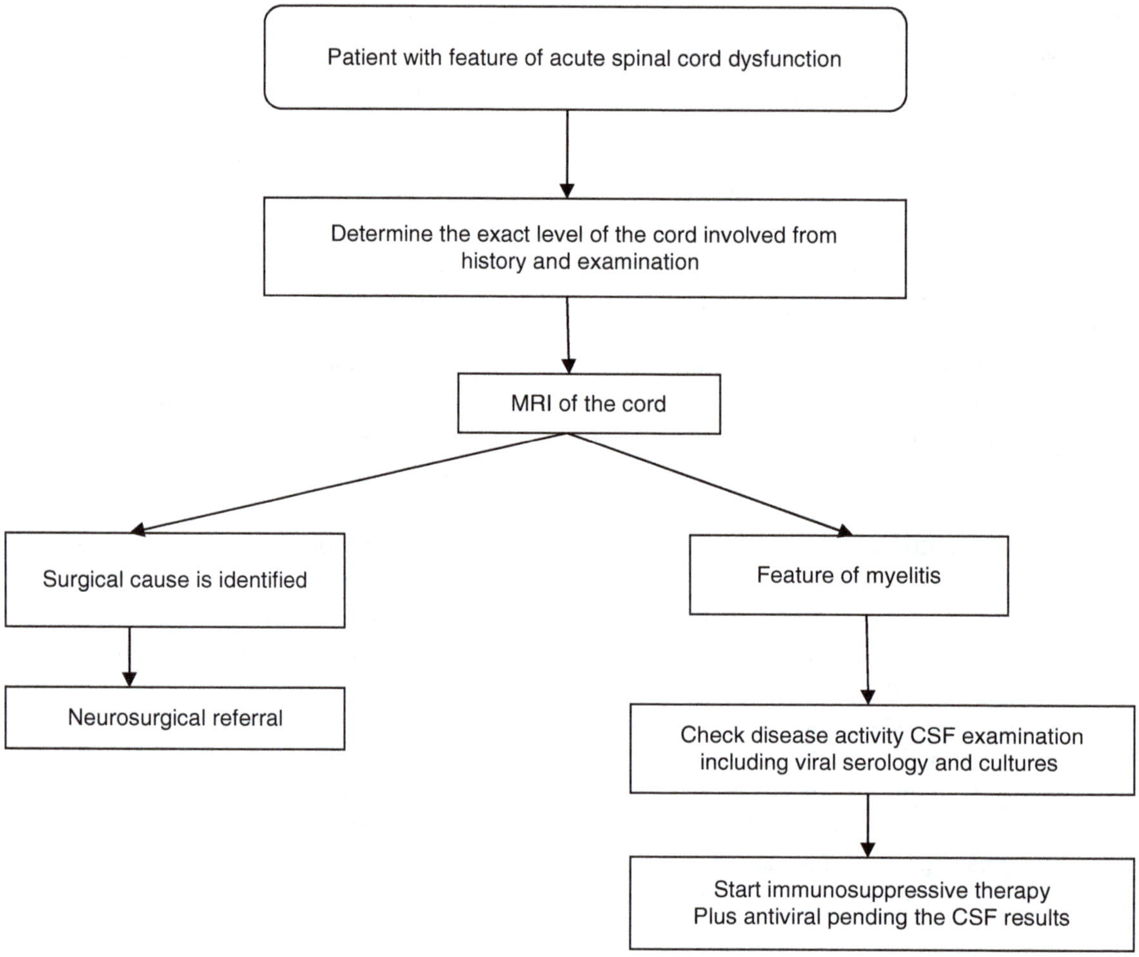

Fig. 8.4 Approach to patient with suspected myelopathy

Fig. 8.5 Causes of neurological manifestations of RA

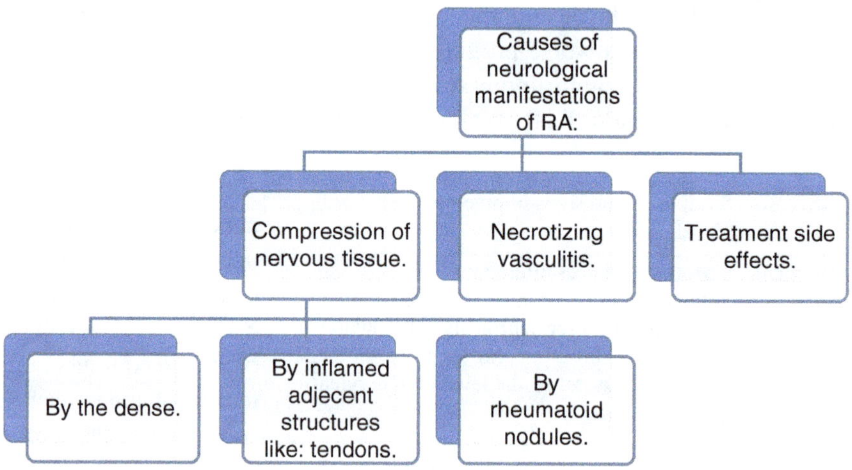

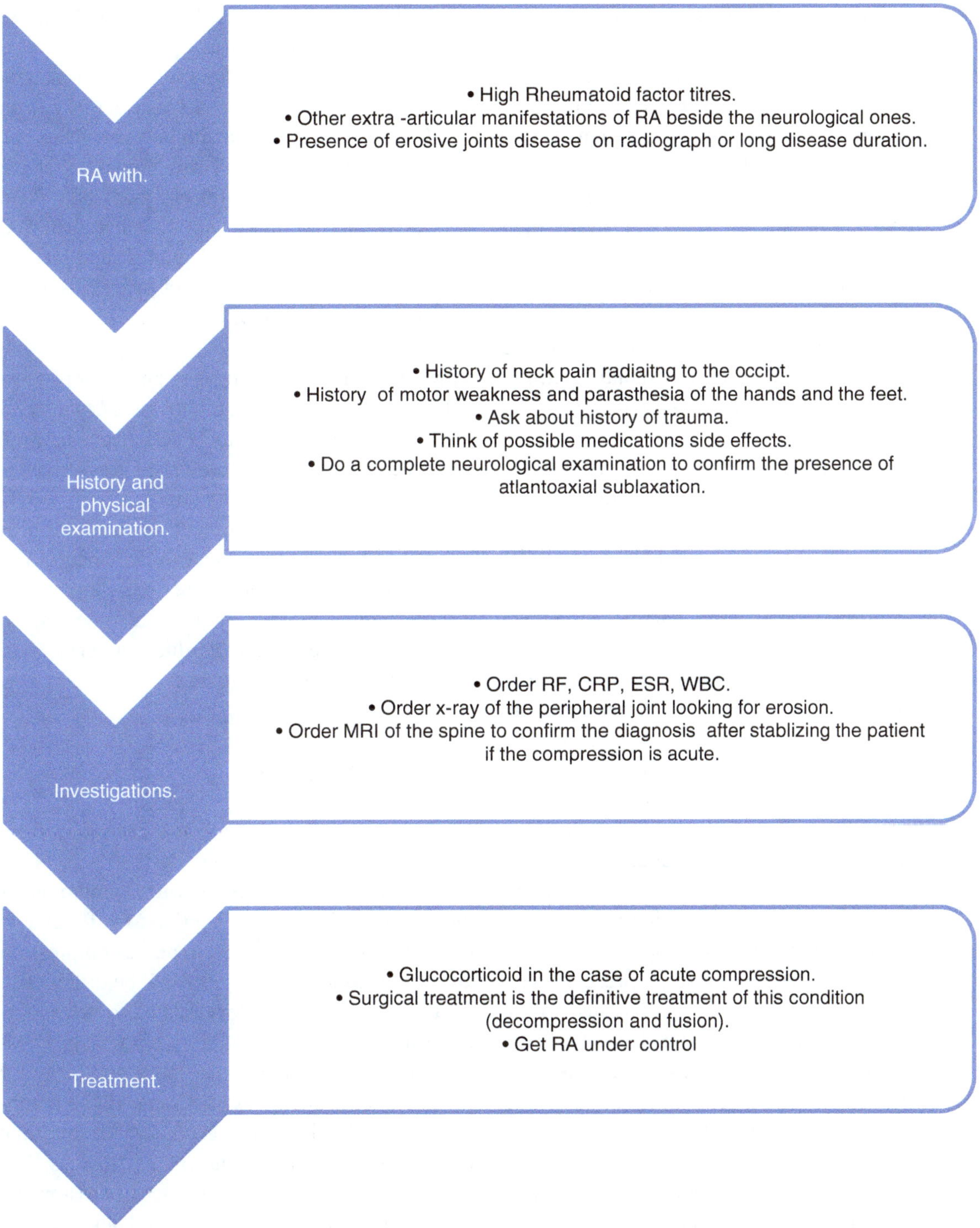

Fig. 8.6 Approach to RA patient with suspected atlantoaxial subluxation

8.3.1 Atlantoaxial Subluxation

1. RA is the most common inflammatory disorder affecting the cervical spine. The involvement of cervical spine is related to active erosive RA and early age of onset [10].
2. Craniocervical complications arise in 30–50% of patients with RA more than 7 years; however, the atlantoaxial subluxation with myelopathy develops in 2.5% of RA more than 14 years [11].
3. Cervical spine involvements by RA include atlantoaxial subluxation, cranial settling, subaxial subluxation, or combinations of the above.
4. Atlantoaxial subluxation is the most common type of cervical spine affection.
5. The subluxation can be anterior, posterior, or lateral, and the anterior subluxation is the most common type that results from laxity of the primary and secondary ligamentous structures.
6. It is very important to recognize this particular complication especially in neurologically normal patients, as early recognition and treatment will improve outcome.
7. Patients with atlantoaxial subluxation can be asymptomatic, or more commonly involve complaints of neck pain. Patients may present with occipital neuralgia, facial pain, ear pain, or pain in the suboccipital region.
8. In cases where cord compression already developed, patients would present with weakness, sensory symptoms related to the cord compression, as well as loss of sphincter control. *(When you deal with any RA patients presenting with any of the above symptoms, consider atlantoaxial subluxation).*
9. Detailed neurological examination is mandatory with careful evaluation for signs of myelopathy.
10. In order to prevent the development of neurological sequels, an evaluation for possible atlantoaxial subluxation radiologically is mandatory for any patient with RA at presentation and periodically thereafter and prior to any surgical procedures.
11. If atlantoaxial subluxation is suspected, besides assessing the disease activity with DAS-28 score, for example (see Chap. 1), and peripheral joint X-ray, the status of the cervical spine should be assessed. Plain X-ray that includes lateral, anteroposterior, open mouth odontoid views and lateral flexion-extension dynamics is necessary to assess joint stability.

More advanced imaging is required for patients with neurological symptoms to assess multilevel disease. MRI is better than CT scan to evaluate the neurological structures as well as to provide better look at the ligamentous structures.

The mainstay of treatment is early surgical intervention before the onset of severe neurological dysfunction, appropriate and aggressive disease-modifying therapy to control the disease activity, and adequate rehabilitation services to optimize neurological outcome.

8.3.2 Neuropathy

Neuropathy in patients with RA can result from nerve compression or secondary to vasculitis. When RA patients present with symptoms of mononeuropathy, it is essential to differentiate between neuropathy related to nerve compression and vasculitis as the treatment will be different.

Take appropriate history related to neurological complaints. The onset of symptoms, progression, and whether there is sensory and/or motor deficits should be checked. Check if the symptoms are all related to one nerve or multiple nerves (mononeuritis multiplex). Assess RA activity, severity with the presence of erosions on X-rays, functional decline, duration, and medications used for RA. On examination, try to identify the deficit and if you can which nerve is involved (Table 8.8). Examine all other peripheral nerves to assess whether it is a single or multiple processes. Examine the activity of RA and

Table 8.8 Things to look for in common nerve involvements

Nerve	Motor symptoms	Sensory symptoms	Notes
Radial nerve	Wrist drop due to weakness of extensors of the wrist and the fingers. Loss of elbow extension if the upper third of the nerve is affected	Loss of sensation over the anatomical snuff box	Flex the elbow, pronate the forearm, and extend the wrist and the fingers to demonstrate wrist drop if it is not clear
Median nerve	Loss or weakness of the thumb abduction mainly Loss of wrist flexors	Loss of sensation over the palmer aspect of the thumb, index, middle, and lateral half of the little finger and the corresponding part of the palm if it is affected above the wrist	Pen touching test for lesion at the wrist. Ochsner clasping for lesion in the cubital fossa
Ulnar nerve	Weakness of most of the small muscles of the hand which will lead clawing of the hand	Loss of sensation over the little finger the medial half of the ring finger	Froment's test can be used to demonstrate loss of thumb adduction in ulnar nerve affection
Femoral nerve	Weakness in knee extension	Loss of sensation over the medial aspect of the thigh and the leg	
Sciatic nerve	Weakness of all the muscles below the knee that results mainly in foot drop and weakness of the hip flexion	Loss of sensation over the posterior aspect of the thigh, all the aspects of the lower limb below the knee except for the medial aspect of the leg	It divides into the common peroneal nerve and the posterior tibial nerve at the level of the knee
Common peroneal nerve	Foot drop	Usually minimal sensory loss over the lateral aspect of the dorsum of the foot	Loss of eversion is another feature

assess deformity. Look for rheumatoid nodules. Nerve conduction studies (NCS) and electromyogram (EMG) will help to establish the diagnosis of nerve involvements. If it develops in a site of entrapment, e.g. carpal tunnel for median nerve and tarsal tunnel for posterior tibial nerve, the condition is most likely to be related to nerve compression rather than vasculitis and requires supportive care and may require surgical intervention. Neuropathy that develops in a non-compression site is related to vasculitis. Those patients may exhibit mononeuropathy or features of multiple nerve involvement (mononeuritis multiplex). Usually it happens in the setting of active erosive disease and with seropositive disease. Treatment with steroid should be initiated together with the use of disease-modifying therapy to achieve disease control. Patients with RA can also present with features of peripheral neuropathy that can be sensory, sensory-motor, or motor neuropathy. The approach to such patients will be discussed in the next part.

8.4 Neuropathy with Skin Rash

When neuropathy either mononeuropathy, mononeuritis multiplex, or peripheral neuropathy occurs in a setting of skin rash, vasculitis should be considered as an etiological factor. Vasculitis is a condition that results from inflammation of the blood vessels. It can be primary or secondary to other conditions, e.g. connective tissue disease, infection (hepatitis C), hypersensitivity reaction, and paraneoplastic condition. (See Chap. 19 for full details about vasculitis.)

Figure 8.7 shows the diagnostic approach to patient with neuropathy and rash.

8.4.1 Tips in History and Physical Examinations

1. Identify the nature of neuropathy (sensory, sensory-motor, motor, mono, multiple versus peripheral).

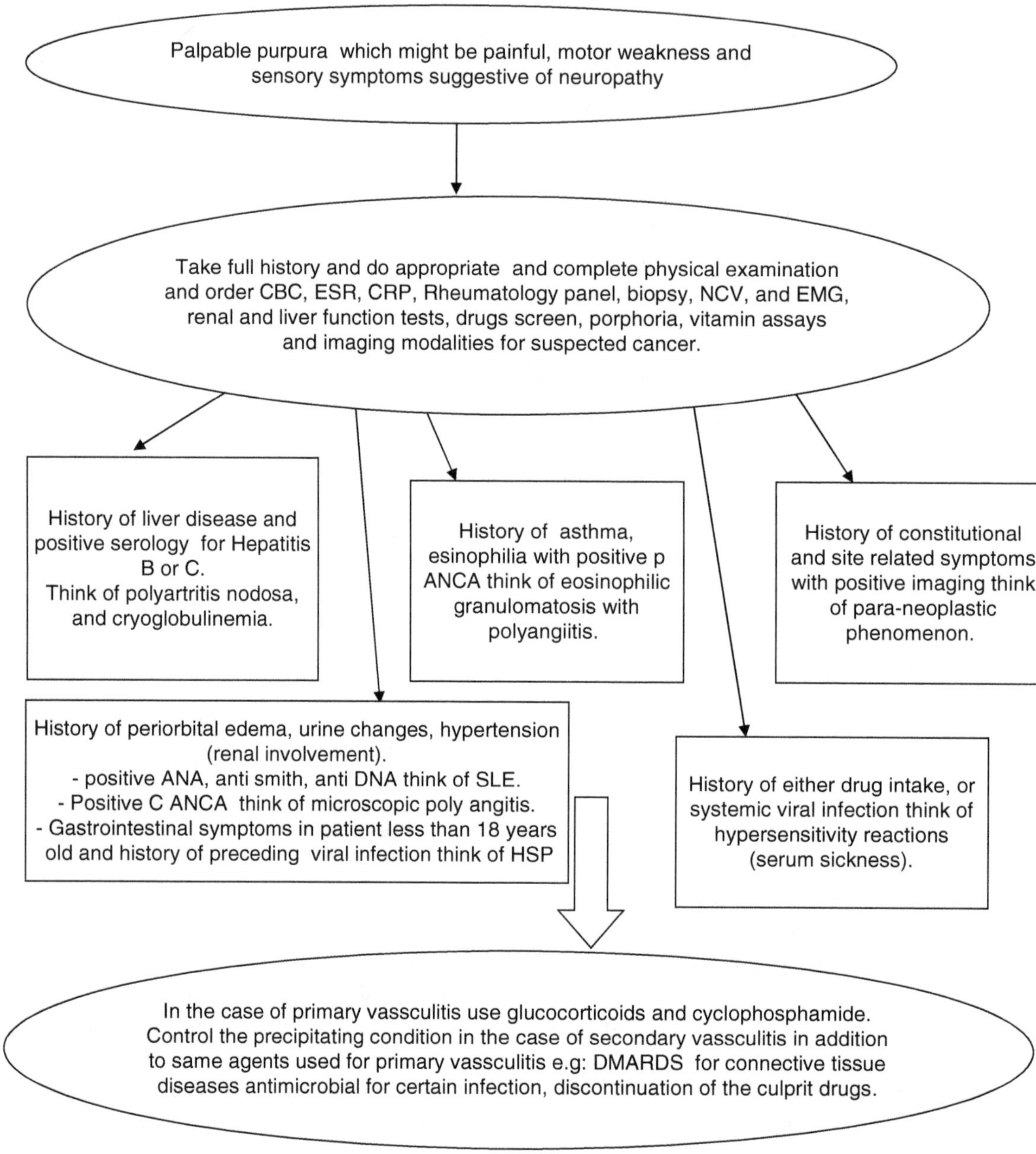

Fig. 8.7 Approach to patient with rash and neuropathy

2. Symptoms of asthma like shortness of breath may suggest Churg-Strauss syndrome, *eosinophilic granulomatosis with polyangiitis [EGPA]*, or *allergic granulomatosis*.
3. Symptoms of renal involvement like periorbital oedema and hypertension may suggest ANCA-associated vasculitis including microscopic polyangiitis and Henoch-Schonlein purpura (HSP).
4. The age of the patient may give a clue since HSP is rare in a patient who is older than 18.
5. Associated gastrointestinal symptoms are important findings in HSP.
6. Symptoms of liver involvement are essential to be established as hepatitis C is associated with cryoglobulinaemic vasculitis and hepatitis B is strong risk factor for polyarteritis nodosa.

7. History of recent use of drugs or recent systemic viral infection that can be associated with hypersensitivity reactions.
8. Symptoms of connective tissue diseases like SLE, RA, and Sjogren disease are suggestive for a secondary cause of vasculitis.
9. Constitutional symptoms can be associated with rheumatologic diseases or solid tumours like lung cancer or lymphoma in what is known as paraneoplastic phenomenon.
10. Family history of similar presentation as some genetically determined disease, e.g. porphyria can present with skin rash and neuropathy.
11. High risk factors, e.g. multiple sexual partner and IV drug abusers, may suggest infections like HIV and/or syphilis.
12. The patient's job is important to exclude exposure to certain toxins.
13. Pay attention to the patient's nutritional status as vitamin deficiencies can lead to neuropathy and rash that might be mistaken for vasculitis.
14. Thorough systemic examination is mandatory to help narrow your differential diagnosis.

8.4.2 Laboratory Investigations and Imaging Modalities

1. CBC, C-reactive protein, and ESR to assess the presence of inflammatory condition in the body like vasculitis and connective tissue disease.
2. NCS and EMG help to categorize the type of neuropathy [12].
3. Nerve biopsy is the ultimate gold standard to diagnose vasculitis as a cause of neuropathy [12].
4. Rheumatologic autoantibody profile like ANA, ANCA, RF, anti-DNA, anti-RO, anti-Jo, and anti-CCP will help identify if vasculitis were secondary to connective tissue disease (see for details in Chap. 4).
5. Assess the patient's liver, renal, thyroid, as well as glucose levels to help narrow the differential diagnosis.
6. Serology for hepatitis B and C, HIV, and cryoglobulin level and VDRL to exclude secondary syphilis.
7. Vitamin assays like B12, folate, and E to exclude vitamin deficiency as the cause of patient presentation.
8. Toxicology screen looking for drug toxicities.
9. Look for porphyrins according to which subtype you suspect in the patient.
10. Use the different imaging modalities to look for solid tumour or lymphoma if you think they are the culprit.

8.4.3 Treatment

1. Immunosuppressive therapy with glucocorticoids is the mainstay of treatment. Depending on disease severity, the addition of cyclophosphamide should be considered to minimize the risk of relapse, morbidity, and mortality [13].
2. Control the precipitating condition in the case of secondary vasculitis in addition to same agents used for primary vasculitis, e.g. DMARDs for connective tissue diseases, antimicrobial for certain infection, discontinuation of the culprit drugs, etc.

Acknowledgments The Authors would like to thank Fahd M. Almalki, MD, for his contributions to this chapter in the previous edition. The authors also would like to thank Dr. Waleed Hafiz for his assistance in the development of this chapter.

References

1. Hanly JG, Urowitz MB, Su L, Bae SC, Gordon C, Wallace DJ, et al. Prospective analysis of neuropsychiatric events in an international disease inception cohort of SLE patients. Ann Rheum Dis. 2010;69(3):529–35.
2. Ainiala H, Loukkola J, Peltola J, Korpela M, Hietaharju A. The prevalence of neuropsychiatric syndromes in systemic lupus erythematosus. Neurology. 2001;57(3):496–500.
3. Brey RL, Holliday SL, Saklad AR, Navarrete MG, Hermosillo-Romo D, Stallworth CL, et al. Neuropsychiatric syndromes in lupus: preva-

lence using standardized definitions. Neurology. 2002;58(8):1214–20.
4. Joseph FG, Lammie GA, Scolding NJ. CNS lupus: a study of 41 patients. Neurology. 2007;69(7):644–54.
5. Ruiz-Irastroza G, Cuadrado MJ, Ruiz-Arruza I, Brey R, Crowther M, Dreksen R, et al. Evidencebased recommendations for the prevention and long term management of thrombosis in antiphospholipid antibody positive patients. Report of a task force at the 13th international congress on Antiphospholipid antibodies. Lupus. 2011;20(2):206–18.
6. Bertsias GK, Ioannidis JP, Aringer M, Bolen E, Bombardieri S, Bruce IN, et al. EULAR recommendations for the management of systemic lupus erythematosus with neuropsychiatric manifestations: report of a task force of the EULAR standing committee for clinical affairs. Ann Rheum Dis. 2010;69(12):2074–82.
7. Alkhotani A. Neuropsychiatric lupus. SQUMJ. 2013;13(1):19–23.
8. Kovacs B, Lafferty TL, Brent LH, DeHoratius RJ. Transverse myelopathy in systemic lupus erythematosus: an analysis of 14 cases and review of the literature. Ann Rheum Dis. 2000;59(2):120–4. Review
9. Sofat N, Malik O, Higgens CS. Neurological involvements in patients with rheumatic disease. QJM. 2006;99(2):69–79.
10. Ahn JK, Hwang JW, Lee J, Lee YS, Jeon CH, Cha HS, Koh EM. Risk factors for development and progression of atlantoaxial subluxation in Korean patients with rheumatoid arthritis. Rheumatol Int. 2011;31(10):1363–8.
11. Wasserman BR, Moskovich R, Razi AE. Rheumatoid arthritis of the cervical spine clinical consideration. Bull NYU Hosp Jt Dis. 2011;69(2):136–48.
12. Seo JH, Ryan HF, Claussen GC, Thomas TD, OH SJ. Sensory neuropathy in vasculitis a clinical, pathologic, and electrophysiologic study. Neurology. 2004;63:874–8.
13. Mathew L, Talbot K, Love S, Puvanarajah S, Donaghy M. Treatment of vasculitic peripheral neuropathy: a retrospective analysis of outcome. QJM. 2007;100(1):41–51.

9

Proximal Myopathy: A Systematic Diagnostic Approach

Hani Almoallim, Hadiel Albar,
and Fahtima Mehdawi

9.1 Introduction

Patients with muscle disorders are a diagnostic challenge to physicians, because of the various ways of presentation. A comprehensive approach should be followed systematically in order to reach the correct diagnosis. Weakness is a common symptom among patients including those with central or peripheral nervous systems diseases and those with muscular and/or neuromuscular diseases. Muscle weakness is not only a regular finding in rheumatologic diseases, but in inflammatory myopathies as well. This chapter focuses on skills needed to approach any patient that presents with weakness, specifically proximal myopathy.

In addition to IIM and CTD, proximal myopathy has a wide range of differential diagnosis including drugs, alcohol, thyroid disease, hereditary myopathies, malignancy, and infections. Clinical assessment should aim to distinguish proximal myopathy from other conditions that present with weakness. Patients with proximal myopathy who need prompt attention, like those with cardiac, respiratory, or pharyngeal muscle involvement, should be identified early and quickly.

In this chapter, the aim is to provide a systematic diagnostic approach to adult patients presenting with proximal myopathy. This is an essential step to establish the correct diagnosis in order to conduct the appropriate management.

9.1.1 Objectives

By the end of this chapter, you will be able to:

1. Identify true muscular weakness by history and physical examination.
2. Construct diagnostic approach to proximal myopathy.
3. Manage a case of inflammatory myopathy.

9.2 Clinical Presentation of Proximal Myopathy

Myopathies are diseases that primarily affect the muscles and are usually characterized clinically by weakness, fatigue, or stiffness. Symmetrical proximal muscle weakness, wasting, normal sensation, and normal stretch reflexes are classical findings in patients with myopathies particularly in IIM and myopathies associated with

H. Almoallim
Medical College, Umm Al-Qura University (UQU), Makkah, Saudi Arabia

H. Albar
King Faisal Specialist Hospital & Research Center, Jeddah, Saudi Arabia

F. Mehdawi (✉)
Doctor Soliman Fakeeh Hospital, Jeddah, Saudi Arabia

CTD. Aching muscle cramps can also occur. Clinical presentations sometimes can be complex, hence the need to follow a comprehensive approach to weakness.

9.2.1 History

Weakness is a common complaint with different interpretations by patients. The aim of history taking is to try to define what the patient means by "weakness." The generalized feeling of tiredness and/or fatigability is usually associated with systemic diseases like congestive heart failure, cirrhosis, and anemia. In these patients there is usually a long-standing history of a chronic disease like ischemic heart disease and/or chronic liver disease. The activity in these patients is usually limited by dyspnea, chest pain, joint pain, fever, and/or depressed mood. Long-standing chronic diseases can lead to cachexia with severe muscle atrophy, wasting, and consequent generalized weakness. The sense of generalized tiredness and/or fatigability should be differentiated from the complaints of generalized body aches and pains in patients with fibromyalgia. The generalized body aches and pains have their own approach that is beyond the scope of this chapter.

Once it is established that the weakness is not a consequence of a non-muscular, generalized, systemic disease and there are no generalized body aches and pains, then it is essential to find out whether this weakness is localized to certain areas. Hemiparesis (weakness affecting upper and lower limbs on the same side of the body) should direct the history towards central nervous system diseases like stroke. Paraparesis (weakness of both lower limbs) and/or quadriparesis (weakness of the four body limbs) should limit the differential diagnosis to spinal cord and/or cerebral cortex and/or brain stem diseases. Monoparesis (weakness of one limb) is usually a disease of a peripheral nervous system including disc prolapse causing radiculopathy by compressing on a spinal nerve to peripheral nerve involvement in vasculitis. Figure 9.1 is a schematic that should be fol-

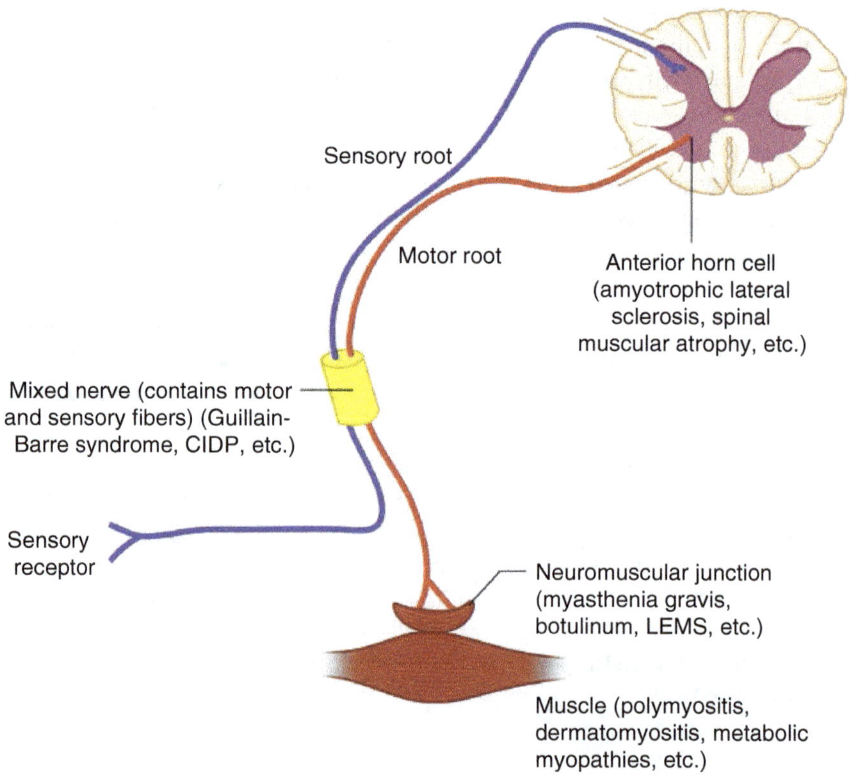

Fig. 9.1 The four anatomic stations underlying lower motor neuron weakness

lowed while obtaining history and examining patients with weakness.

Symmetrical weakness occurs in large number of diseases including inflammatory myositis, inherited muscle dystrophy, endocrine disorders, and neuromuscular junction diseases. In symmetrical and diffuse weakness, it is important to know if the weakness is proximal or distal. There are several clues in the history that point towards proximal myopathy (muscles of the trunk, shoulders, and thighs). The patient will have difficulty combing hair, difficulty climbing up the stairs, difficulty standing from a sitting position, and/or difficulty in getting up from bed. In distal myopathy, the patient will complain about difficulties while performing fine work like handling the objects by hands and driving. These patients may also present with wrist drop or foot drop. It must be noted that there are diseases affecting proximal muscles in an asymmetrical fashion like diabetic amyotrophy as well as diseases with both proximal and distal muscle weakness in symmetrical and/or asymmetrical fashion like in systemic lupus erythematosus (SLE) with myopathy and vasculitis, respectively. Inclusion body myositis, a rare IIM in elderly patients, presents with both proximal and distal myopathies simultaneously. The focus should be simply to identify the localization of the weakness, and then with comprehensive approach to history taking like what is described in Chap. 1, the differential diagnosis should be easier to obtain.

There are special characters for weakness that signify certain alerts to specific diagnoses. Ascending pattern of weakness should direct the attention towards demyelinating diseases like acute inflammatory demyelinating polyneuropathy (Guillain-Barre syndrome). Descending patterns that start centrally and proceed progressively to distal areas should direct the attention to infections like botulism. The weakness that is worsened by repetitive movement at the end of the day with double vision and drooping eyelids should direct the attention towards neuromuscular disorders like myasthenia gravis.

An extensive review of rheumatologic symptoms should follow; this was outlined thoroughly in Chap. 1. Detailed history of joint pain, skin rashes, fever, recent infections, bleeding tendencies, history suggestive of malignancies, and/or drug history (particularly statins and glucocorticoids) should all be obtained. Endocrine disorders should also be ruled out by reviewing common symptoms like neck swelling, diarrhea/constipation, and heat/cold intolerance. Further details are found below. Detailed family history should be obtained as there are several rare hereditary myopathies that run in families (see below). A family history may also be present in other causes of weakness including dermatomyositis, polymyositis, and potassium-related paralyses. A thorough neurological history is important. Sensory deficits, impaired level of consciousness, speech or visual defect, seizure, and sphincter control should be obtained from patients with weakness. In addition, social history will further help narrow the diagnosis; thus, history of smoking, alcohol, illicit drug use, and exposure to toxins like organic phosphorus should be obtained.

There are life-threatening symptoms associated with IIM like dysphagia and nasal regurgitation resulting from skeletal muscle involvement of the pharynx and upper third of the esophagus and/or chest pain and heart failure from cardiac muscle involvement. These should be identified promptly as they need urgent medical intervention. Breathlessness might suggest respiratory muscle involvement. Respiratory failure can occur in some diseases like Guillain-Barre syndrome, myasthenia gravis, and amyotrophic lateral sclerosis. Table 9.1 summarizes some of the common symptoms of diseases presenting with weakness.

9.2.2 Physical Examination

The physical examination is an objective confirmation of the distribution and the severity of the muscle weakness. The first step is to observe the patient doing certain activities like raising arms, standing up from a chair, or writing. This will determine if the weakness is proximal, distal, or combined. A comprehensive neurological examination should follow with higher function examination and examination of cranial nerves. You may find ptosis, ophthalmoplegia, and/or poor gag reflex in myasthenia gravis patients. The next

Table 9.1 Associated symptoms presented with muscle weakness

Disease	Symptoms
Dermatomyositis	Skin rash, e.g., upper eyelids (*heliotrope rash*), erythema of the knuckles (*Gottron rash*), anterior chest (*v sign*), or back (*shawl sign*) Weight loss, anorexia, bleeding tendency, abnormal vaginal bleeding, chronic cough (malignancy).
Inclusion body myositis	Frequent falls, dysphagia
Myasthenia gravis	Squint, dysphagia Compression symptoms of thymoma (cough, SOB)
Lambert-Eaton syndrome	Autonomic symptoms, e.g., dry mouth, impotence History of lung cancer
Mixed connective tissue disease and overlap syndrome	Other connective tissue disease's symptoms; arthritis, skin rash
Rhabdomyolysis	History of trauma, seizure, dark urine

step is performing detailed motor examination. This starts with inspection of the muscle bulk and determining whether if it is normal, atrophied, or hypertrophied. In addition to observation for any fasciculation that might suggest LMND, tone, power, reflexes, and gait should also be examined. Clear distinctions between signs of upper motor neuron disease (UMND) (hypertonia, hyperreflexia, and upgoing plantar response) and signs of LMND (for lesions from the anterior horn cell until muscles) (hypotonia, normal or low or absent reflexes, and equivocal or downgoing plantar response) should be made. Usually with signs of UMND, patients may present with hemiparesis, paraparesis, and quadriparesis or with variable locations in the central nervous system as in multiple sclerosis. Since weakness is a prominent sign present in both UMND and LMND, it is essential to assess the power and document the degree of weakness, as well as for proper future monitoring of this disease while on

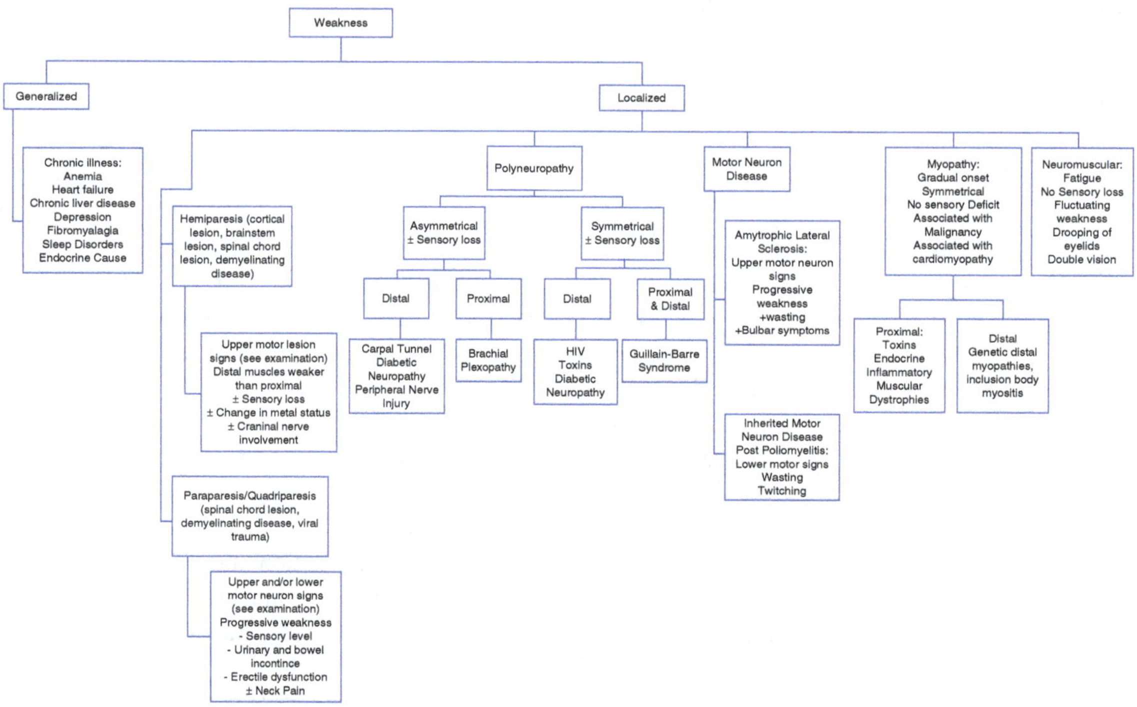

Fig. 9.2 Clinical approach to weakness

treatment. Clinical approach to weakness is illustrated in Fig. 9.2. Grades of power are shown in Table 9.2.

Reflexes are usually intact in proximal myopathy, and any signs of abnormal reflexes suggest neurological cause. The last step in the neurological examination is examining sensory level. For example, in peripheral neuropathy loss of sensation is parallel to the weakness. After comprehensive neurological examination, a search for extra-muscular signs should follow. The examination of the face, hands, lower limbs, chest, and abdomen is important, since any abnormality can help in the differential diagnosis. Few signs of common diseases presenting with myopathy are shown in Table 9.3.

There are certain associations essential to be recognized while performing the physical examination. These associations may easily reveal the diagnosis without spending efforts on unnecessary investigations. Changes in the mental status, for example, with muscle weakness may indicate electrolyte imbalance. Cardiovascular assessment may reveal signs of cardiomyopathy, which is associated with some inflammatory and hereditary myopathies. Pulmonary assessment may reveal crackles of interstitial lung disease associated with some inflammatory myopathies. Lymph node examination is essential as malignancies are associated with a significant number of IID including lymphoma. Small joint examination is essential as well to detect any tenderness and/or swelling suggestive of rheumatoid arthritis (RA) and/or systemic lupus erythematosus (SLE)-associated myopathies. Skin examination is helpful: signs like Gottron's papules in dermatomyositis, erythema nodosum in sarcoidosis, and skin bronzing in adrenal insufficiency (see Dermatology chapter). Also a search for any signs possibly related to underlying malignancy like finger clubbing, fecal occult blood, and hepatosplenomegaly should be made. Table 9.4 lists findings with their most likely definitive diagnosis. The vital signs should be measured to exclude any life-threatening problems. Postural hypotension can be seen in autonomic neuropathy, e.g., in diabetes mellitus and Lambert-Eaton syndrome. Also, body mass index (BMI) should be measured to assess if the patient is underweight suggestive of a malignant disease process.

Table 9.2 Grades of power

5	Normal muscle strength, full resistance
4	Reduced, but still against resistance
3	Further reduced, only against gravity
2	Only moves with gravity
1	Flicker of movement
0	No movement

9.3 Differential Diagnosis of Proximal Myopathy

Several conditions cause proximal myopathy. Myopathies can be classified into idiopathic or acquired. The clinical history and physical exam-

Table 9.3 Common signs with specific myopathies

	Head and neck	Hands	Chest and abdomen
Dermatomyositis	– Upper eyelids (heliotrope ash) – Lymphadenopathy or any mass (malignancy)	– Erythema of the knuckles (Gottron rash) – Clubbing (lung cancer)	– Erythema of anterior chest (v sign), or back (shawl sign) – Axillary lymphadenopathy, breast lump or abdominal mass
Overlap syndrome and MCTD	– Fish mouth, pinched nose (in scleroderma) – Malar rash, discoid lupus (in SLE)	Sclerodactyly, Raynaud's (in scleroderma). Arthritis (in SLE)	Signs of lung fibrosis and serositis
Lambert-Eaton syndrome	– Dry mouth and skin (autonomic neuropathy)	– Clubbing (lung cancer)	– Chest finding if there are complications for lung cancer e.g. pleural effusion, lymphadenopathy
Myasthenia gravis	SVC syndrome (thymoma)	–	–

Table 9.4 Correlation between findings and suggestive diagnoses of weakness

Findings	Suggestive diagnosis
Acute focal weakness decreased muscle power, hyperreflexia, hypertonia, positive Babinski sign, ± sensory deficit, ± loss of bladder/bowel control	Stroke, or spinal cord injury
Diffuse or localized peripheral weakness, muscle atrophy, fasciculations, hypotonia, loss of reflexes	Lower motor neuron disease
Asymmetrical distal weakness, muscle atrophy, hypotonia, loss of reflexes, sensory deficit "Glove and stocking" distribution	Peripheral neuropathy Diabetic neuropathy
Acute onset of combined weakness (ascending), fasciculations, loss of deep tendon reflexes, sensory deficit	Guillain-Barre syndrome
Facial weakness, fatigability, ptosis	Myasthenia gravis
Symmetrical weakness of proximal muscles, muscle wasting, with some types, muscle tenderness, normal reflexes, no sensory level	Proximal myopathies
Symmetrical distal weakness, with myotonic contractions	Myotonic dystrophy
Cardiomyopathy, and proximal muscle weakness	Inflammatory myopathies, hereditary myopathies
Mental status changes with proximal weakness	Myopathy-inducing electrolyte disorder (calcium or magnesium)

ination are essential in identifying the presence of a myopathy and narrowing down the differential diagnosis. In adults a major cause of myopathy is medication like statins [1]. Myopathy due to endocrine causes, for example, thyroid disease, Cushing disease, and adrenal diseases, should be diagnosed promptly because treating the primary condition will result in resolution of the myopathy [2]. Inflammatory diseases typically affect older adults including both proximal and steroid responsive disorders like polymyositis and dermatomyositis and distal and proximal myopathies with less response to steroid like inclusion body myositis. Rheumatologic disorders causing weakness, such as SLE and RA, can occur in young and elderly persons. Figure 9.3 summarizes the differential diagnosis of proximal myopathy. Further details about these disorders will be mentioned briefly in this section.

9.3.1 Toxins- and Drug-Induced Myopathy

Considering toxin and drug exposure in the differential diagnosis of every single patient presenting with proximal myopathy is essential. The timely diagnosis allows for optimum recovery. There are many drugs that cause proximal myopathy, such as lipid-lowering drugs, glucocorticoids, antimalarial drugs, antiretroviral drugs, alcohol, and cocaine [1]. There is an acute presentation in drug-induced myopathy. Statin therapy associated with muscle problems is seen in approximately 10–25% of patients treated in clinical practice. Statin-induced myopathy can present as myalgia and myositis or sometimes is severe enough to cause rhabdomyolysis. The average onset of statin-induced myopathy is weeks to months. The only treatment is discontinuation of statin which results in resolution of muscle symptoms [3]. Glucocorticoids are a common cause of muscle weakness. Long-term use of glucocorticoids results in an insidious onset of proximal myopathy. Muscle enzymes are usually normal. Relief of the weakness occurs with lowering the dose of glucocorticoids [4]. Alcohol-induced myopathy generally follows a history of long-standing alcohol intake and/or consumption of large amount of alcohol. Table 9.5 summarizes pertinent features of the common causes of toxin- and drugs-induced myopathy.

9.3.2 Endocrine Myopathy

Hormones play an essential role in body metabolism. Deficiency or excess in most hormones will affect muscle metabolism. In endocrine-related muscle diseases, the presentation is more likely to be fatigue than true muscle weakness. The

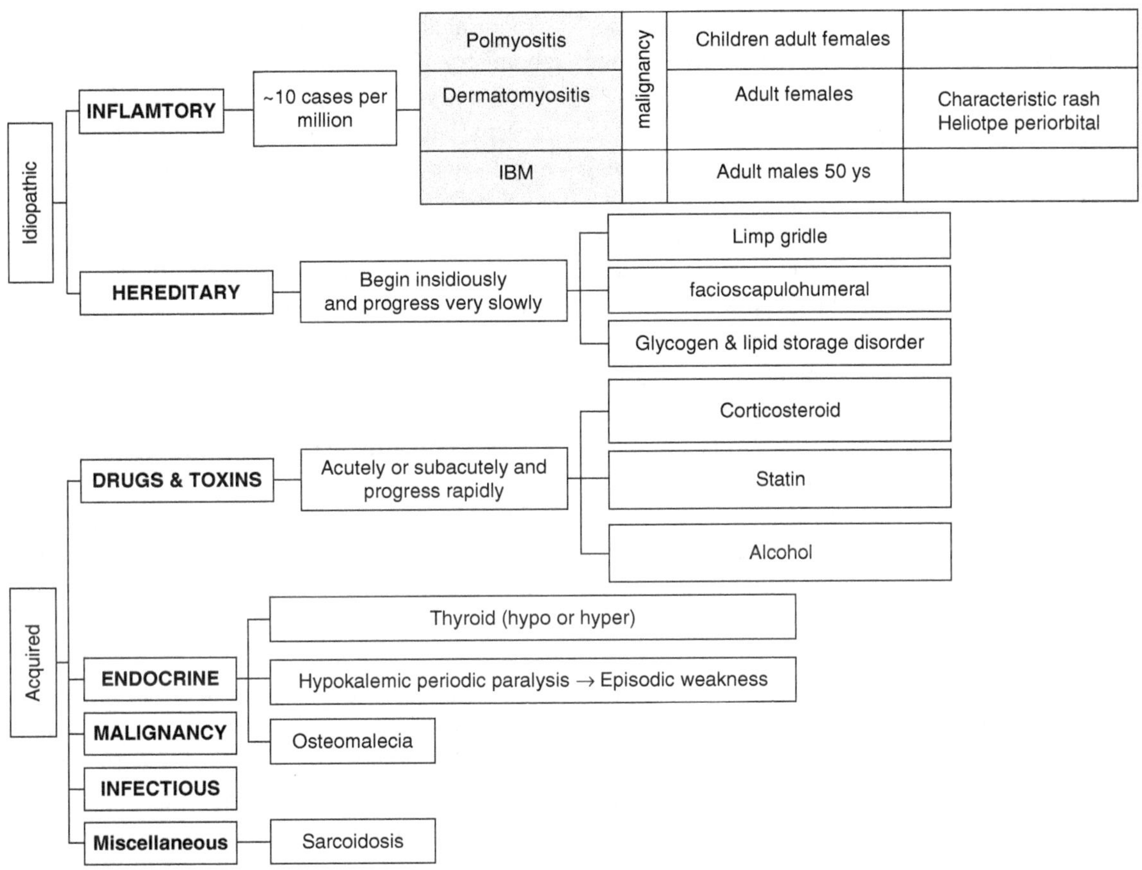

Fig. 9.3 Differential diagnosis of proximal myopathy

Table 9.5 Features of toxin- and drug-induced myopathy

Toxin/drug	Effect on muscle	Characteristics	Management
Alcohol	Large consumption of alcohol will cause direct muscle necrosis	Acute and chronic presentation Calf muscles Tenderness Swelling Generalized muscle cramps	Resolution with cessation of alcohol
Glucocorticoid	Direct catabolic effect Chronic use of prednisone at a daily dose of ≥30 mg/day Risk increases in elderly and malignancy	Proximal lower muscles Progressive Accompanied with atrophy No tenderness	Improved muscle strength within 3–4 weeks after lowering the dose
Statin	Varying degrees of muscle necrosis Severe complications such as rhabdomyolysis and myglobinuria Dose and duration dependent	Myalgia Malaise Muscle tenderness Muscle pain may be related to exercise	Muscle weakness will resolve with decreasing the dose or cessation of the statin

serum CK level is often normal (except in hypothyroidism). Nearly all endocrine myopathies respond to treatment [5].

Abnormalities in thyroid hormone can lead to a wide range of muscle diseases. For example, hypothyroid patients have frequent muscle complaints such as cramps, pain, and weakness. Almost one third of hypothyroid patients present with proximal myopathy. They present mainly with shoulder and hip muscle weakness. Treatment by thyroid replacement usually leads to resolution of symptoms and laboratory abnormalities [6]. Proximal myopathy is a very common presentation in hyperthyroid patients and may be the only symptom of the disease. Bulbar, respiratory, and even esophageal muscles may be affected, causing dysphagia and aspiration. Other neuromuscular disorders may occur in association with hyperthyroidism including hypokalemic periodic paralysis, myasthenia gravis, and a progressive ocular myopathy. Because proximal weakness is a presenting sign of hyperthyroidism and hypothyroidism, checking thyroid-stimulating hormone (TSH) is essential. Adrenal insufficiency causes muscle fatigue rather than true muscle weakness. Conn's syndrome can lead to proximal myopathy which is related to hypokalemia [7]. Pituitary disorders like acromegaly if long-standing can cause myopathy [8]. Neuromuscular complications of diabetes mellitus (DM) are mainly due to neuropathy which can be presented as asymmetrical proximal weakness. Ischemic infarction of the thigh muscles can present with severely uncontrolled diabetes [9] (see Chap. 21 (Diabetes and Rheumatology)). Table 9.6 summarizes pertinent findings of myopathies caused by endocrine disorders.

9.3.3 Dystrophic Myopathies

Dystrophic myopathies are a distinct group of inherited muscle disorders that generally present chronically. They are slowly progressive in nature resulting in muscle atrophy with exception of metabolic myopathies, where symptoms on occasion can be precipitated acutely. Each type of dystrophic myopathy has some characteristic structural abnormalities on muscle immunohistochemistry. Congenital myopathies present predominantly in the perinatal period. Some can present later in childhood, and these children may have a milder course of the disease. Multiple gene defects can give rise to similar clinical and ultrastructural phenotypes; thus, muscle immunohistochemistry should be tested to reach a final diagnosis. Table 9.7 shows the features of dystrophic myopathy [10].

9.3.4 Inflammatory Myopathies

Inflammatory myopathies are a group of complex diseases of unknown etiology. The most common types are dermatomyositis, polymyositis, and inclusion body myositis. Table 9.8 represents the current classification for IIM. The incidence of inflammatory myopathies is 5–10/million cases per year [11]. These diseases are characterized by progressive muscle weakness with extra-muscular organ involvement and high serum muscle enzymes. Generally there is a female predominance 2:1, but in inclusion body myositis, the opposite is seen as it is three times more common in males [12]. The main pathophysiology is related to autoimmunity, though recent studies show that the mechanism of muscle damage is multiple and complex [13].

The clinical features of inflammatory myopathy in general are muscle weakness occurring within weeks to months. The distribution of weakness is mainly proximal in dermatomyositis and polymyositis, but as the disease progresses, distal muscles may become affected. On the other hand, distal muscle weakness is the initial presentation of inclusion body myositis. The onset of polymyositis is usually after the second decade of life. Dermatomyositis has two peaks, the first peak at around 10–15 years of age and the second peak between 40 and 70 years. Inclusion body myositis occurs after the age of 50. Table 9.9 summarizes the pathological and clinical features of the most common IID.

Dermatomyositis is known for its cutaneous manifestations. The rashes can precede, follow, or occur simultaneously with the myopathy.

Table 9.6 Pathophysiology and characteristics of endocrine myopathies

Endocrine disease	Pathophysiology	Characteristics
Hypothyroidism	Exact mechanism is unknown T4 is essential for metabolism Decrease in T4 leads to decrease in glycogenolysis which leads to impaired muscle function	Proximal myopathy occurs in one third (shoulder and hip girdle muscles) Muscle cramps, stiffness, pain are common complaints More common in women Muscle hypertrophy is a rare sign (Hoffman's sign) Delayed deep tendon reflexes
Hyperthyroidism	Exact mechanism is unknown Impaired muscle function may be due to increased cellular metabolism and energy utilization, increased catabolism and protein degradation, and inefficient energy utilization	Muscle weakness ± tenderness and atrophy in 60–80% of patients Presentation may be acute or chronic Two-thirds of patients with hyperthyroid myopathy report proximal weakness, mainly hip flexors and quadriceps Cramps are less common Atrophy is usually absent Bulbar symptoms may be present Associated with other neuromuscular diseases: Myasthenia gravis Periodic paralysis Progressive ocular myopathy
Hyperparathyroidism		25% of patients will have insidious onset of proximal myopathy, legs more than arms Atrophy is a common feature Fatigue, muscle pain, and hyperreflexia are common
Adrenal insufficiency		100% of patients present with weakness, but usually there is no objective proximal myopathy
Primary hyperaldosteronism		Weakness is a common complaint Weakness and paralysis are usually due to the hypokalemia
Cushing syndrome (see Glucocorticoid myopathy)		

Gottron's papules and heliotrope rash are pathognomonic features of dermatomyositis [14]. Dermatomyositis and polymyositis are also known to cause manifestations related to the cardiovascular system, respiratory system, and gastrointestinal system.

Patients diagnosed with IID tend to have a higher risk of developing malignancies. Patients with dermatomyositis or polymyositis have an increased risk of developing malignancy. Those with dermatomyositis are three to six times more likely and those with polymyositis are two to four times more likely than the normal population to develop ovarian, gastric, pancreatic, and lung cancer and non-Hodgkin lymphoma. Thus screening for malignancies is highly recommended in this population [15].

9.3.5 Myopathy Due to Infectious Disease

Infectious diseases may cause an acute presentation of weakness with muscle cramps, myoglobinuria, and rhabdomyolysis. Among the infectious causes, viral infections are the most

Table 9.7 Features of dystrophic myopathy

Type of myopathy	Distribution	Characteristic	Mode of inheritance
Duchenne	Proximal	Age of onset 3–5 years Weakness starts in the trunk Spreads to arms and legs Gower's sign Calf hypertrophy Wheelchair by ages 9–10 Cardiomyopathy Scoliosis/respiratory problems Cognitive impairment	X-linked
Becker's	Proximal	Age of onset 3–20 years Less severe than Duchenne	X-linked
Limb-girdle	Proximal	Age of onset 3–20 years Shoulder and hip muscles Low back pain Sparing of the face Cardiac involvement Contractures No cognitive impairment	AR/AD
Facioscapulohumeral muscular dystrophy (FSHD)	Proximal	Age of onset is variable (average 10–20 years) Infant form wheelchair by 9 years Severe facial weakness Inability to close eyes Inability to smile Weakness can involve shoulder and hips Early onset: Hearing loss, seizures, cognitive impairment	AD
Myotonic dystrophy	Distal	Age of onset is variable Most common adult-onset muscular dystrophy Type 1, type 2 Affects facial muscle, arms, legs Multisystem: Cardiac, cataract, sexual organs, cognitive impairment Excessive daytime sleepiness	AD

Table 9.8 Classification of idiopathic inflammatory myopathies

1. Primary idiopathic dermatomyositis
2. Polymyositis or dermatomyositis with malignancy
3. Juvenile dermatomyositis (or polymyositis)
4. Inclusion body myositis
5. Rare forms of idiopathic myositis
   - Granulomatous myositis
   - Eosinophilic myositis
   - Focal myositis
   - Orbital myositis

common. Myalgia is the most common symptoms, but can last up to 2–3 weeks. Usually myopathy due to viral infections is self-limiting, but severe cases may cause myoglobinuria and renal impairment.

Human immunodeficiency virus (HIV) is an important differential when approaching myopathy; the condition is often referred to as HIV polymyositis. HIV polymyositis can be a presenting manifestation of HIV infection or can occur in later stages. Patients with HIV polymyositis may present with asymptomatic elevation of CK levels, or as severe muscle tenderness and muscle weakness. HIV-related myopathy appears to have a better prognosis than idiopathic inflammatory myopathies. See the treatment section for how to manage HIV polymyositis.

Table 9.9 The pathogenetic mechanisms and clinical features of the most common IID

Condition	Pathogenesis	Age/sex	Clinical features	
Dermatomyositis	Humeral mediated process CD4 cells and B lymphocytes attack the vascular endothelium; result in necrosis of capillary and ultimately muscle atrophy	10–15 years 40–70 years F: M—2:1	Symmetrical proximal muscle weakness Pathognomonic: Heliotrope (purple) Periorbital edema; violaceous papules (Gottron's papules) or macules (Gottron's sign)	Both dermatomyositis and polymyositis: • 10% have interstitial lung disease (may lead to respiratory failure and death) • Increase rate of malignancy • Dysphagia, nasal regurgitation, and/or aspiration with increased age • Cardiac involvement in the form of myocarditis, conduction defects, and arrhythmias • Constitutional symptoms
Polymyositis	Cellular mediated process CD8 cytotoxic cells recognize MHC-1 on the muscle fiber, and this is the initiation of the necrotic process	Second decade of life F: M—2:1	Diagnosis by exclusion No skin manifestation Associated with HIV Histopathology is considered the most effective way to establish the diagnosis of PM	
Inclusion body myositis	The mechanism is poorly understood, but histopathology shows inflammatory cells surrounding myofibers and rimmed vacuoles, and some myofibers are attacked by CD8 cytotoxic cells	>50 years 3 times more in men	Insidious onset and progressive asymmetric distal weakness with wrist and index finger flexors weaker than extensors. Associated with early atrophy and poor response to steroid	

9.4 Diagnostic Approach

A thorough history and physical examination is the cornerstone to reach the diagnosis. Investigations should be tailored to screen for reversible causes of a myopathy (Fig. 9.4).

When the cause of muscle weakness is unclear, appropriate testing should be performed, and it is recommended to start with blood tests including electrolytes (potassium, calcium, phosphate, and magnesium), thyroid-stimulating hormone (TSH) level, alkaline phosphatase and 25 (OH) vitamin D level, and HIV [16].

9.4.1 Muscle Enzyme

The measurement of serum levels of muscle enzymes is of critical value for the evaluation and monitoring of muscular disorders. Creatine kinase (CK), lactate dehydrogenase (LD), alanine aminotransferase (ALT), aspartate aminotransferase (AST), and aldolase are the serum muscle enzymes that are measured in clinical practice. In patients with suspected myopathy who do not demonstrate CK elevation, testing for aldolase can be helpful, but it is less sensitive and less specific [17].

Approach to high level of CK is demonstrated thoroughly in Table 9.10. It must be noted that CK elevation is, however, not specific to myopathy and further testing should be performed in a comprehensive approach. Table 9.11 shows the differential diagnosis to high CK level.

While diagnosing myocardial infarction, besides symptoms and abnormal ECG findings, there will be rise in CK-MB, the isoenzyme of CK, electrophoretically distinguished and high in concentration in the cardiac tissue. However, it is neither specific nor sensitive as troponins [18].

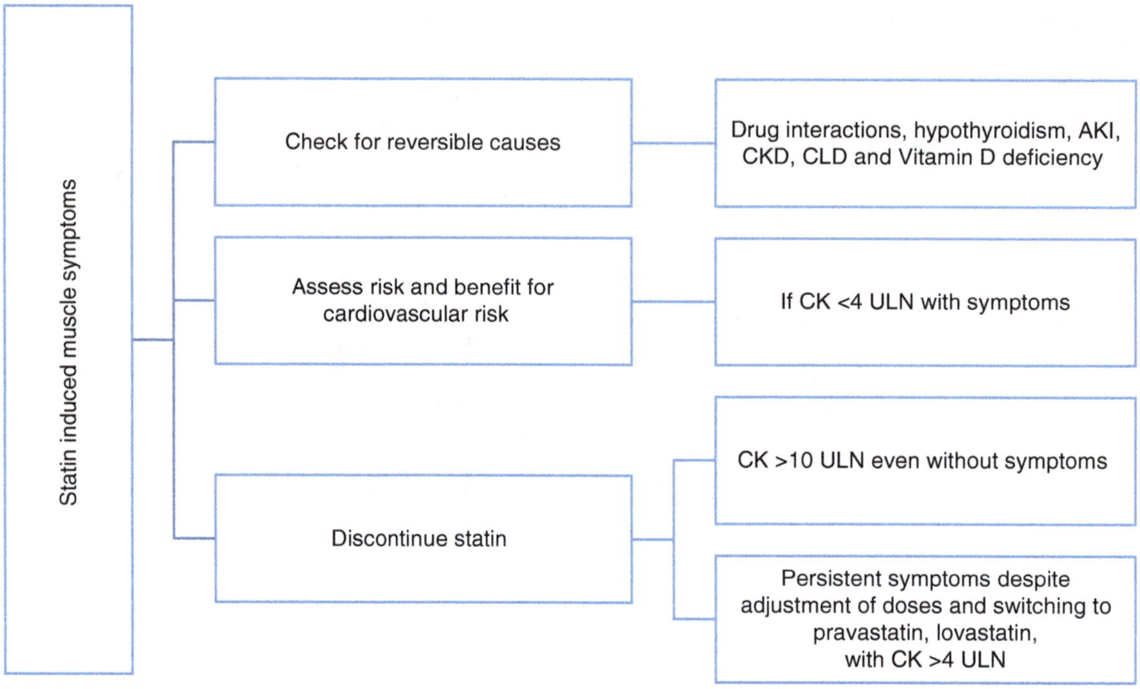

Fig. 9.4 Approach to statin-induced myopathy

CK might be falsely elevated secondary to ethnicity (can be high in Afro-Caribbean men), exercise (can remain elevated for up to 72 h), intramuscular injections, needle electromyography (EMG), medications, hypothyroidism, and motor neuron disease [16].

9.4.2 Rhabdomyolysis

Muscle injury due to vigorous exercise, medication, infection, and metabolic derangements can cause rhabdomyolysis. Severe myalgia, weakness, and red to brown urine due to myoglobinuria are classical initial presenting features. Rise of CK levels is typically seen after 2–12 h of injury and reaches its maximum within 24–72 h. A decline is usually seen within 3–5 days of cessation of muscle injury. Myoglobinuria is present in 50–75% of patients at the time of initial evaluation. Thus it is recommended to perform routine dipstick urine analysis in any patient with extremely elevated CK level and myopathy. There are serious metabolic derangements that complicate this massive muscle destruction in the body. Electrolyte imbalance and acute renal failure are serious examples.

9.4.3 Other Tests

In addition to CK, to diagnose rheumatologic myopathy, erythrocyte sedimentation rate (ESR) C-reactive protein (CRP), antinuclear antibody assay (ANA), rheumatoid factor, anti-double-stranded DNA, antiphospholipid antibodies, and anti-centromere antibodies should be ordered. In case of inflammatory myopathy, check for anti-Jo1 antibody, directed against histidyl-tRNA synthetase. Recognition of anti-Jo1 syndrome is important because such patients can develop extra-muscular features, such as interstitial lung disease, Raynaud's phenomenon, and arthritis [19].

Table 9.10 Approach to high CK level

Episodic Range from normal to rhabdomyolysis	Mild 3–four-fold ULN	High 100 fold ULN
Endocrine Hypothyroidism Hyperthyroidism Cushing's syndrome Acromegaly Electrolyte imbalance	*Drugs* Antimalarial, cholesterol-lowering drugs (statins), cocaine, alcohol, colchicine → 10- to 20-fold	*Rhabdomyolysis* Acute, massive muscle injury due to: Trauma, seizures, electrolyte imbalances, infections The degree of myoglobinuria might Correlate with the risk of acute renal failure CK levels decrease rapidly to normal after managing the cause
Metabolic myopathies Glycogen and lipid storage disease Carnitine palmitoyl transferase (CPT) Muscle phosphorylase deficiency	*Systemic vasculitis* Polyarteritis nodosa Wegener's Behçet's disease Sarcoidosis	
	Connective diseases Rheumatoid arthritis Systemic lupus erythematosus Sjögren's syndrome Scleroderma Specific autoantibodies anti-U1 RNP and anti-PM/Scl	*Infectious myopathies* Viral (EBV, HIV), bacterial, mycobacterium, fungal, parasitic
Periodic paralysis Primary hypokalemic periodic paralysis	*Inclusion body myositis* 80 percent of patients	*Polymyositis & dermatomyositis* Abnormal EMG and muscle biopsy findings correlation between the height of CK elevation at diagnosis and the severity of disease
	Dystrophic myopathies Limb-girdle dystrophies Facioscapulohumeral dystrophy, myotonic dystrophy CK levels peak by age 2 and then progressively fall, often to the normal range, as more and more muscle is replaced by fat and fibrosis	
	Motor neuron disease (amyotrophic lateral sclerosis)	

Table 9.11 Differential diagnosis to high CK level

• Differential diagnosis of CK with weakness	• Differential diagnosis of CK without weakness
– Inflammatory – Metabolic – Endocrine – Drug induced – Infectious (viral)	– Strenuous exercise – After EMG studies – Trauma – Post-surgery – Intramuscular injections – Metabolic and congenital myopathy – Medications – Race (African Americans)

9.4.4 Electromyography (EMG)

Electromyography (EMG) is a test that is used to record muscle electrical activity and assess the nerves that control the muscles. An abnormal electromyogram can indicate a neuropathy or neuromuscular disease. Characteristic EMG findings of myopathy include short duration and decreased amplitude of action potential unlike neuropathies that are characterized by increased duration and amplitude of action potential.

Although there are no pathognomonic features that distinguish different forms of myopathy, EMG can help distinguish inflammatory from non-inflammatory forms of myopathy. Normal EMG examination, however, would not exclude myopathy [18]. In case of polymyositis, the site of muscle biopsy should be opposite to where the EMG was conducted [16].

9.4.5 Muscle Magnetic Resonance Imaging (MRI)

MRI evaluates deep muscles not readily accessible by EMG and plays a role in the diagnostic process by identifying subclinical signs of muscle involvement. Fat-suppressed and short tau inversion recovery techniques differentiate between active myositis, pictured as edema, and chronic inactive myositis in patients with inflammatory myopathy, presented as fat [20]. A secondary role for muscle MRI is to provide information about the best site for muscle biopsy by showing which muscles are involved in the myopathic process.

9.4.6 Muscle Biopsy

Establishing the diagnosis of IID is essentially based on histopathological grounds. There are currently advanced therapies that can be used effectively in these patients. The justification of using these drugs or even steroids should be based on muscle biopsy. Open surgical biopsy is preferable to closed needle biopsy because of the patchy nature of inflammation in PM and so that adequate tissue could be obtained. However, in some circumstances, the biopsy is performed by expert radiologists. Muscle biopsy is a reliable instrument in the diagnosis of PM in 85% of the patients [18]. It is an outpatient procedure that may cause pain, bleeding, infection, or sensory loss. No special preparation is required other than that patients should discontinue using anticoagulants before the procedure [21].

The best muscles to biopsy are those moderately affected by the disease process but not atrophied. Previous sites of injections, EMG examination, or trauma should be avoided. The most common biopsy sites are the deltoid, quadriceps for proximal myopathy, and gastrocnemius for distal myopathies.

Technology using genetic markers is advancing rapidly. In inflammatory myopathies, immune staining for major histocompatibility classes I and II (MHC-I/II) is upregulated in myofibrils, whereas MHC-I immune staining alone is nonspecific [22].

9.4.7 Screening for Malignancy

Idiopathic inflammatory myopathies PM and DM have positive relation to malignancy; retrospective studies' results justify CT of the chest, abdomen, and pelvis in addition to age-appropriate screening tests such as colonoscopy and mammography for any patient newly diagnosed. This is shown in Southeast Asia where input of otolaryngologists is invaluable due to the higher incidence of nasopharyngeal carcinoma for DM patients. Recent advances in understanding of pathogenesis of idiopathic inflammatory myopathies have led to discovery of biomarkers like type 1 interferon and myeloid cell signatures to distinguish active disease from chronic injury [17].

9.4.8 Genetic Testing

Genetic testing is becoming increasingly useful in confirmation of patient with muscular dystrophies and heritable myopathies. These mutations can be identified through peripheral blood DNA analysis. Molecular testing often eliminates the need for muscle biopsy.

9.5 The Management of Myopathy

9.5.1 Inherited Myopathy

For most patients with congenital myopathy or muscular dystrophy, the treatment is mainly supportive. Physical therapy, occupational therapy, management of contractures, nutrition, and genetic counseling together play a role in managing congenital myopathies. In patients with Duchenne muscular dystrophy, treatment with prednisone has been shown to improve strength and muscle bulk and slow the rate of natural progression of the disease. Patients should also be monitored over time for complications related to kyphoscoliosis or involvement of cardiac, respiratory, or bulbar muscles. Finally, genetic counseling should be offered to all patients with inherited myopathy and their family members.

9.5.2 Acquired Myopathy

Management of proximal myopathy depends on underlying etiology. Treatable causes should be sought and treated accordingly. Discontinuation of offending drug is likely to improve symptoms in patients with drug-induced myopathy, e.g., statins [5]. Dose reduction should be considered for those patients in whom abrupt discontinuation of drug may not be possible, e.g., steroid myopathy [6]. In HIV-related myositis, treatment with the combination of highly active antiretroviral therapy (HAART) and steroids may be beneficial.

Treatment of IIM is largely empirical because of paucity of well-controlled trials. Current evidence is mostly based on retrospective or open prospective trials involving small numbers of patients. Corticosteroids are the cornerstone in the treatment of PM and DM [19, 20]. In the absence of placebo-controlled trials, the optimal initial dose and duration of therapy are uncertain, but patients are generally started on 0.75–1 mg/kg body weight/day of prednisolone. Intravenous pulse methylprednisolone is initially considered for those with cardiac, respiratory, or pharyngeal muscle involvement to obtain quicker response. Because maximal improvement may not be seen for several weeks, the usual practice is to start tapering the dose of prednisolone only after about 4–12 weeks, guided by clinical improvement. Many patients relapse when corticosteroids are discontinued, and therefore, a maintenance dose of 5–10 mg/day is often required for several years. About a third of patients with PM or DM, and those with IIM, might fail to show any response to prednisolone. Second-line immunosuppressive drugs are tried in patients who do not respond to corticosteroids alone and in those with progressive disease and internal organ involvement. Choice of drug is largely empirical and depends on disease severity, extra- muscular manifestations, and personal experience of treating physician, again because of paucity of well-conducted trials.

Azathioprine [23] or methotrexate is usually preferred. Intravenous immunoglobulin (Ig), the only agent for which there is positive evidence from randomized placebo-controlled trial [21, 24], is especially useful for patients with dysphagia and treatment-resistant DM. Intravenous Ig is, however, expensive and limited in availability. Cyclophosphamide, given as monthly intravenous pulses for 3–6 months, is also an option for patients with respiratory muscle weakness, interstitial lung disease, or cardiac involvement [25]. Plasmapheresis has also been studied, but was not found to be helpful in a double-blind placebo-controlled trial [26]. Rituximab, a CD20 monoclonal antibody that depletes B cells, has been reported to have a favorable effect in small open-label uncontrolled trials [27, 28]. A new double-blind, placebo-phase trial in refractory adult and pediatric myositis using rituximab revealed good results [29]. Tumor necrosis factor inhibitors such as infliximab, adalimumab, and etanercept are ineffective in treating IID and may cause deterioration or trigger the disease [30]. Other biological agents that may be considered as experimental treatments include alemtuzumab, which is reportedly effective in polymyositis [31], and anti-complement C3 (eculizumab), which may be effective for the treatment of dermatomyositis. Overall, the long-term outcome of inflammatory myopathies has substantially improved, with a 10-year survival rate of more than 90% . Table 9.12 shows a step-by-step approach in the management of IID [32].

Input of physiotherapist is also valuable because randomized controlled trials among patients with IIM have demonstrated that exercise therapy, adapted to the patient's condition, is

Table 9.12 Approach to treatment of inflammatory myopathies

Clinical situation	Treatment for IID
New-onset disease	Prednisone (0.75–1 mg / kg) for 4–12 weeks
Weakness is severe + cardiac, respiratory, pharyngeal involvement	Intravenous glucocorticoids (1000 mg/day) for 3–5 days and then switch to oral
If patient responds to glucocorticoids	Start a glucocorticoid-sparing agent • Azathioprine • Methotrexate
If response to glucocorticoids is insufficient	Intravenous immune globulin (2 g/kg in divided doses over 2–5 days)
If response to glucocorticoids and intravenous immunoglobulin is insufficient	Consider initiating treatment with rituximab

Dalakas, Marinos C. "Inflammatory muscle diseases." *New England Journal of Medicine* 372.18 (2015): 1734–1747

beneficial and safe [33]. Benefits of exercise not only include improved muscle endurance, strength, and functional abilities but also prevent muscle wasting and fibrotic contractures.

Acknowledgments The authors would like to thank Haytham Abbas, MD, for his contributions to this chapter in the previous edition.

References

1. Dalakas MC. Toxic and drug-induced myopathies. J Neurol Neurosurg Psychiatry. 2009;80:832–8.
2. Horak HA, Pourmand R. Neurol Clin. 2000;18(1):203–13.
3. Thompson PD, Clarkson P, Karas RH. Statin-associated myopathy. JAMA. 2003;289:1681.
4. Afifi AK, Bergman RA, Harvey JC. Steroid myopathy. Clinical, histologic and cytologic observations. Johns Hopkins Med J. 1968;123:158.
5. Horak HA, Pourmand R. Endocrine myopathies. Neurol Clin. 2000;18:203–13. https://doi.org/10.1016/S0733-8619(05)70186-9.
6. McKeran RO, Slavin G, Ward P, et al. Hypothyroid myopathy. A clinical and pathological study. J Pathol. 1980;132:35.
7. Cicala MV, Mantero F. Primary aldosteronism: what consensus for the diagnosis. Best Pract Res Clin Endocrinol Metab. 2010;24:915–21. https://doi.org/10.1016/j.beem.2010.10.007.
8. Del Porto LA, Liubinas SV, Kaye AH. Treatment of persistent and recurrent acromegaly. J Clin Neurosci. 2011;18:181–90. https://doi.org/10.1016/j.jocn.2010.10.003.
9. Yildirim Donmez F, Feldman F. Muscle compromise in diabetes. Acta Radiol. 2008;49:673–9. https://doi.org/10.1080/02841850802105269.
10. Emery AE. The muscular dystrophies. Lancet. 2002;359:687.
11. Briani C, Doria A, Sarzi-Puttini P, Dalakas MC. Update on idiopathic inflammatory myopathies. Autoimmunity. 2006;39:161e70.
12. Yazici Y, Kagen LJ. Clinical presentation of the idiopathic inflammatory myopathies. Rheum Dis Clin North Am. 2002;28:823–32.
13. Targoff IN. Immune manifestations of inflammatory muscle disease. Rheum Dis Clin N Am. 1994;20:857–80.
14. Kovacs SO, Kovacs SC. Dermatomyositis. J Am Acad Dermatol. 998(39):899–920.
15. Sigurgeirsson B, Lindelof B, Edna O, Allander E. Risk of cancer in patients with dermatomyositis or polymyositis. N Engl J Med. 1992;326:363–7.
16. Ghaoui R, Clarke N, Hollingworth P, Needham M. Muscle disorders: the latest investigations. Intern Med J. 2013;43(9):970–8.
17. Suresh E, Wimalaratna S. Proximal myopathy: diagnostic approach and initial management. Postgrad Med J. 2013;89(1054):470–7.
18. Weisberg LA, Strub RL, Garcia CA, Strub AC. Diseases of muscle and neuromuscular junction. In: Essentials of clinical neurology: University Park Press; 1983.
19. Inflammatory myopathies. Postgrad Med J. 2006;82:417–24. 59
20. Greenberg SA. Inflammatory myopathies: evaluation and management. Semin Neurol. 2008;28:241–9.
21. Dalakas MC, Illa I, Dambrosia JM, et al. A controlled trial of high-dose intravenous immune globulin infusions as treatment for dermatomyositis. N Engl J Med. 1993;329:1993–2000.
22. Chawla J. Stepwise approach to myopathy in systemic disease. Front Neurol. 2011;2:49.
23. Bunch TW. Article first published online: 23 Nov 2005. https://doi.org/10.1002/art.1780240107.
24. Wang DX, Shu XM, Tian XL, et al. Intravenous immunoglobulin therapy in adult patients with polymyositis/dermatomyositis: a systematic literature review. Clin Rheumatol. 2012;31:801–6.
25. Al-Janadi M, Smith CD, Karsh J. Cyclophosphamide treatment of interstitial pulmonary fibrosis in polymyositis/dermatomyositis. The Journal of Rheumatology, 1989;16(12):1592—6. http://europepmc.org/abstract/MED/2625692.

26. Miller FW, Leitman SF, Cronin ME, et al. Controlled trial of plasma exchange and leukapheresis in polymyositis and dermatomyositis. N Engl J Med. 1992;326:1380–4.
27. Levine TD. Rituximab in the treatment of dermatomyositis: an open-label pilot study. Arthritis Rheum. 2005;52:601–7.
28. Chung L, Genovese MC, Florentino DF. A pilot trial of rituximab in the treatment of patients with dermatomyositis. Arch Dermatol. 2007;143:763–7.
29. Rituximab in the treatment of refractory adult and juvenile dermatomyositis and adult polymyositis. Arthritis Rheum. 2013;65(2):314–24. https://doi.org/10.1002/art.37754.
30. Brunasso AMG, Aberer W, Massone C. New onset of dermatomyositis/polymyositis during anti-TNF-α therapies: A systematic literature review. The Scientific World Journal; 2014. https://doi.org/10.1155/2014/179180.
31. Thompson BEN, Corris P, Miller JAL, Cooper RG, Halsey JP, Isaacs JD, Rheumatologist C. Alemtuzumab (Campath-1H) for Treatment of Refractory Polymyositis. The Journal of Rheumatology. 2008;35(10):2080–2. http://www.jrheum.org/content/35/10/2080.abstract.
32. Yin G, Liang Y, Deng R, Wang Y, Xie QB, Zuo C. [Survival analysis and risk factors for survival in idiopathic inflammatory myopathies: a retrospective cohort study]. Sichuan Da Xue Xue Bao Yi Xue Ban. 2013;44(5):818–22. Chinese. PMID: 24325120.
33. Habers GE, Takken T. Safety and exercise training in patients with an idiopathic inflammatory myopathy: a systematic review. Rheumatology (Oxford). 2011;50:2113–24.

10

Rheumatic Diseases and Bone Issues

Altaf Abdulkhaliq

10.1 Introduction

Bone is a target tissue in many inflammatory diseases including rheumatic diseases such as rheumatoid arthritis (RA), ankylosing spondylitis (AS), systemic lupus erythematosus (SLE), and psoriatic arthritis.

A relationship between inflammation and bone disease has been established in a variety of clinical settings and animal models of inflammatory disease [1–4]. It has been established that the nature of the inflammatory disease can influence on the extent and type of bone disease and that even a small rise in the level of systemic inflammation can impact on bone remodeling and increase fracture risk [5].

The inflammatory joint disorders, namely, rheumatic diseases, are usually accompanied with extra-articular side effects, mainly bone loss, or osteoporosis that would result in an increased risk of fractures and deformities, which are in turn associated with increased morbidity and mortality [6]. Therefore, such types of musculoskeletal diseases are considered as one of the major causes of disability around the world and can explain the enormous cost of the musculoskeletal conditions to the community.

A. Abdulkhaliq (✉)
College of Medicine, Umm Al-Qura University, Makkah, Saudi Arabia
e-mail: aaabdulkhaliq@uqu.edu.sa

In order to easily understand the underlying pathology and mediators that affect bones in rheumatic conditions, a brief overview on bone structure, biology, physiology, and essential molecular mechanism and signaling pathways needs to be explained clearly.

10.2 Objectives

1. To explain the underlying bones pathology among patients with rheumatic diseases.
2. To identify the common bone lesions occur with rheumatic diseases.
3. To recognize the serious impact of developing secondary osteoporosis among patients with rheumatic diseases.
4. To provide an updated approach for prevention and treatment of glucocorticoid-induced osteoporosis (GIOP) and bone fractures among patients with rheumatic diseases receiving glucocorticoids.

10.3 Bone Structures

Bone is a dynamic and highly specialized form of connective tissue, in which the extracellular components are mineralized, thus giving the property of marked rigidity and strength while retaining some degree of elasticity. Bone represents a store of calcium and other inorganic ions

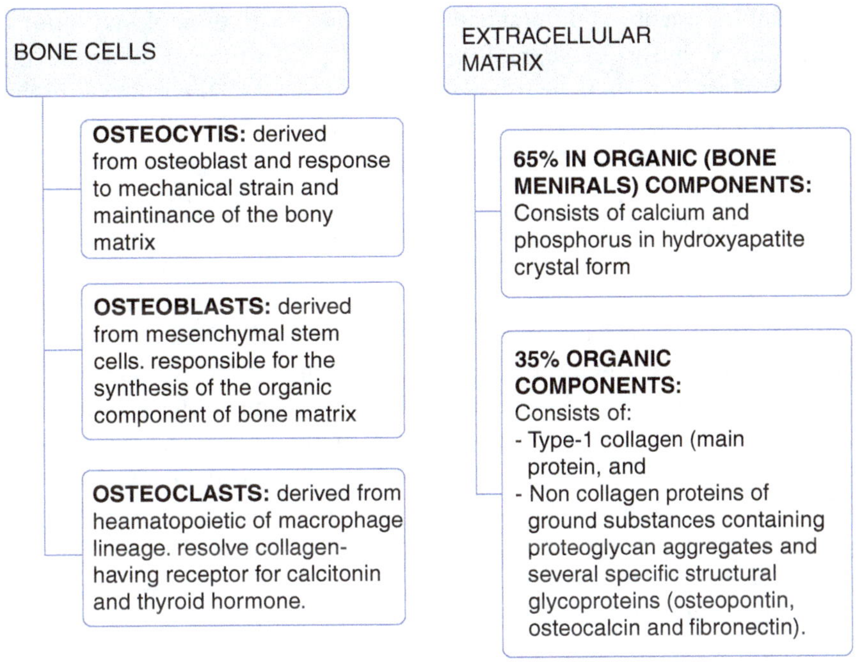

Fig. 10.1 Components of bone structure

and actively contributes to the maintenance of calcium homeostasis.

Two types of bone can be identified macroscopically: compact or cortical bone and cancellous or trabecular bone. Microscopically both types of bone have the same histological structure. Like other supporting connective tissues, bone is composed of cells and extracellular matrix that is made up of 35% of organic component and 65% inorganic component [7]. The inorganic part consists of calcium and phosphorus in hydroxyapatite crystal form, while the organic component consists of type 1 collagen and ground substance containing proteoglycan aggregates and several specific structural glycoproteins [8] (Fig. 10.1).

10.4 Bone Remodeling and Bone Cells

Bone remodeling is the lifelong process whereby old bone is removed by bone resorbing cells and subsequently replaced by new bone via the action of bone-forming cells to maintain the bone structure. Bone remodeling occurs normally in all individuals, and in adults about 25% of trabecular and 3% of cortical bone is replaced by such process each year [9]. Bone remodeling also helps to maintain mineral homeostasis via the liberation of calcium and phosphorus into the circulation. The remodeling process occurs at discrete sites on cortical and cancellous bone surfaces and involves the integrated and sequential actions of osteoclasts (bone resorbing cells) and osteoblasts (bone-forming cells), comprising anatomic structures known as basic multicellular units (BMUs).

10.4.1 Bone Cells

Mesenchymal stem cells have the potential to differentiate into various cell types including osteoblasts, chondrocytes, adipocytes, myoblasts, and fibroblasts. Determination of the final fate of the differentiation process is determined by and depending on the signaling transcription pathways that are activated during the initial phase of differentiation of mesenchymal progenitor cells [10, 11].

Among the important signaling pathways that are responsible to direct the differentiation into osteoblast lineage are the mitogen-activated protein kinase (MAPK) and protein kinase A (PKA)-dependent pathway [12] and Wnt-signaling pathway with its related β-catenin protein [13, 14]. Moreover, of the transcriptional factors, at least two are shown to be absolutely essential for osteoblast differentiation from mesenchymal precursors including Runx2 [15–17].

The plasma membrane of activated osteoblast is rich in alkaline phosphatase and exhibits receptors for parathyroid hormone (PTH) [18], whereas the nuclei have receptors for estrogens [19], vitamin D3 [20], and glucocorticoids [21], which all are involved in the regulation of osteoblast differentiation and activity.

Osteoblasts contribute in the synthesis and secretion of new organic part of bone matrix (but not yet mineralized), called osteoid, between the secreting osteoblast layer and in contact with older bone matrix of previously formed bone. This process is referred to as *bone apposition* and is completed by further mineralization of the newly formed bone matrix (*deposition of calcium* salts into matrix), a process regulated by osteoblast too. At the end of the secreting period of osteoblasts, those osteoblasts are embedded within the bone and differentiated into osteocytes.

Osteoclasts originate from hematopoietic stem cells (HSCs), precisely from cells of the colony-forming unit of macrophage (CFU-M) that differentiate to multinucleated, giant, motile cells on stimulation with macrophage colony-stimulating factor (M-CSF) and receptor activator of nuclear factor-kappa B "NF_kB" ligand (RANKL) (Fig. 10.2).

Firstly, the osteoclast progenitors proliferate and differentiate into mononuclear preosteoclasts and then fuse with each other to form multinucleated cells. The terminal differentiation in this lineage is characterized by acquisition of mature phenotypic markers, such as the calcitonin receptor, tartrate resistant acid phosphatase (TRAP), and integrin αvβ3 [22]. The mature and active osteoclasts are characterized by a moderate

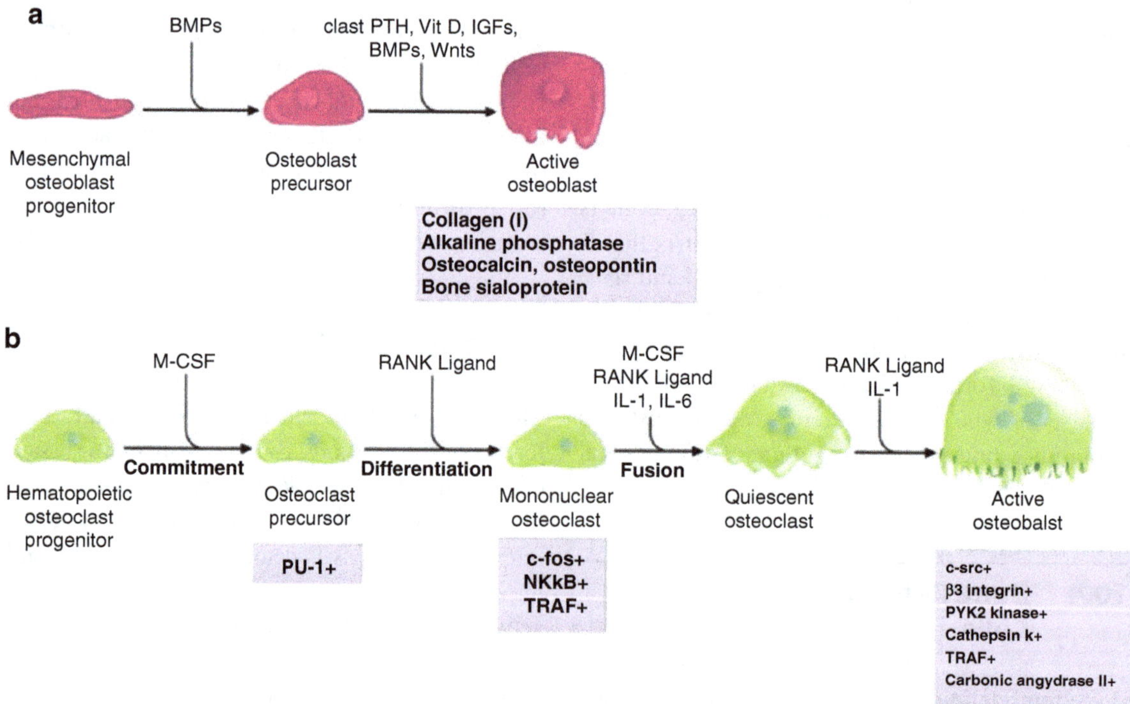

Fig. 10.2 Pathways regulating the development of (**a**) osteoblasts and (**b**) osteoclasts. Hormones, cytokines, and growth factors that control cell proliferation and differentiation are shown above the arrows. Transcription factors and other markers specific for various stages of development are depicted below the arrows. BMPs, bone morphogenetic proteins; Wnts, wingless-type mouse mammary tumor virus integration site; PTH, parathyroid hormone; Vit D, vitamin D; IGFs, insulin-like growth factors; Runx2, Runt-related transcription factor 2; M-CSF, macrophage colony-stimulating factor; PU-1, a monocyte- and B lymphocyte-specific ets family transcription factor; NFB, nuclear factor B; TRAF, tumor necrosis factor receptor-associated factors; RANK ligand, receptor activator of NFB ligand; IL-1, interleukin-1; IL-6, interleukin-6 [24]

rough endoplasmic reticulum, a well-developed Golgi apparatus, and abundant mitochondria, while the surface of their plasma membrane facing bone matrix is having ruffled border (clear or sealing zone), which is devoid of organelles but rich in actin microfilaments that form a ring of contractile protein serving to attach the cell to the bone surface via integrin receptors during the resorptive process [8]. *The clear zone* is a site of adhesion of the osteoclast to the bone matrix and creates a microenvironment where bone resorption takes place. From the ruffled border, osteoclasts secrete collagenase (and other proteolytic enzymes) and pump protons (low pH) into microenvironment and thus promoting the localized digestion of matrix and the dissolving of bone mineral (calcium salt crystal), respectively.

Several systemic and local factors have influenced osteoclasts and their bone resorption ability. In normal physiological conditions, the osteoclast activity is highly balanced by those factors. However, in pathological conditions, this balance becomes disturbed such as during excessive activation of the immune system, due to the secretion of additional pro-inflammatory cytokines, produced mainly by activated T cells [23].

10.4.2 The Remodeling Cycle

The remodeling cycle is comprised of four distinct phases including activation, resorption, reversal, and formation phase (Fig. 10.3). Bone remodeling starts with activation of the lining cells via increasing the surface expression of RANKL.

In the activation phase, RANKL interacts with its receptor RANK, thus triggering the recruitment of osteoclast progenitors to bone where they proliferate and differentiate into osteoclasts and attach tightly to the bone matrix.

Next is *the resorption phase*, when the activated osteoclasts possess ruffled borders under which the proteolytic enzymes are secreted and the *hydrogen ions are pumped* resulting in digestion of collagens and dissolving the mineralized

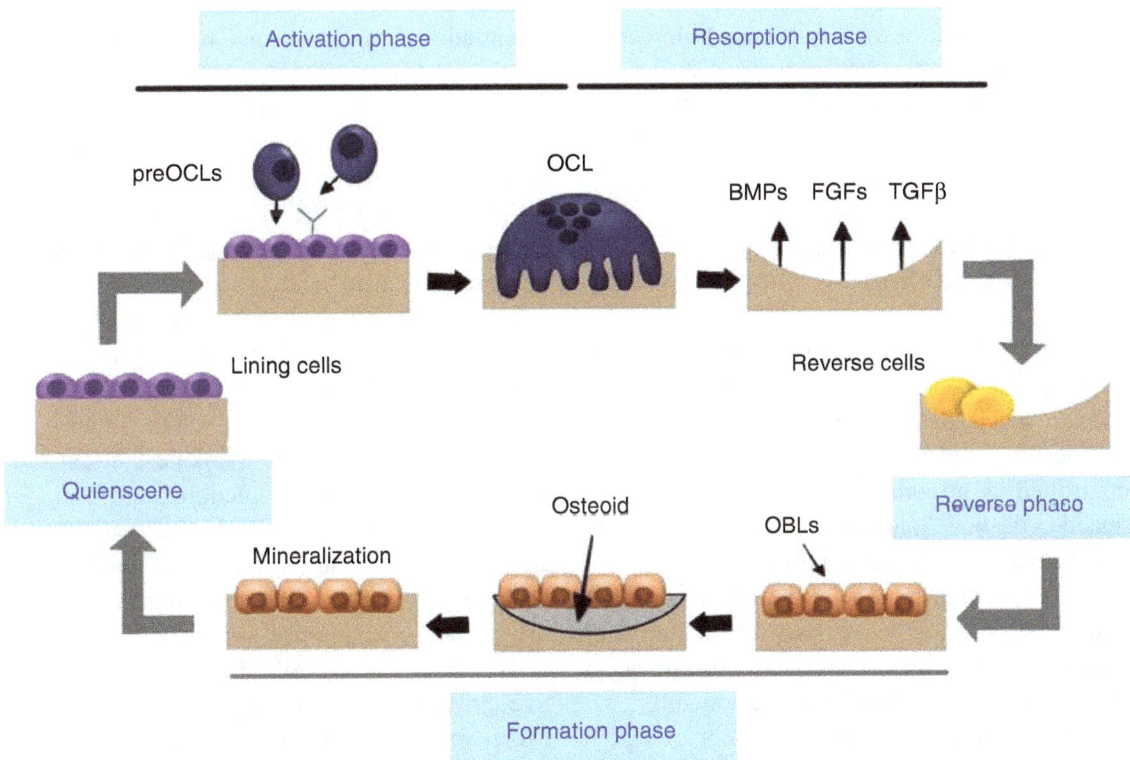

Fig. 10.3 Process and phases of normal bone remodeling [26]

matrix with the formation of a resorption cavity and allowing the release of several growth factors usually stored in the bone matrix. In addition, there is an accumulation of high concentration of calcium that directly controls osteoclasts activity resulting in cell retraction [25] and movement of osteoclasts across the bone surface to resorb a new area. At the end of this stage, osteoclasts undergo apoptosis after a life span of about 3 weeks, and thus the process of remodeling requires the continual production of osteoclast precursors.

In *the reversal phase*, the remnant debris of matrix degradation will be removed, while the released growth factors including bone morphogenetic proteins (BMPs), fibroblast growth factors (FGFs), and transforming growth factor-β (TGFβ) are likely to be responsible for recruitment of osteoblasts to cover the bottom of the resorption cavity, forming osteoid tissue until the cavity is filled.

In the final *formation phase* of bone remodeling, osteoblasts initially synthesize the organic matrix and then preside over its mineralization, thus completing the bone remodeling process. Toward the end of this process, some osteoblasts start to flatten and become quiescent lining cells; others become embedded in the matrix and differentiate into osteocytes, while the remaining of osteoblasts will undergo programmed cell death.

10.4.3 Factors Influencing Remodeling

The rate at which new osteoblasts and osteoclasts are supplied and the timing of apoptosis of these cells are crucial determinants of bone remodeling. The development of osteoclasts and osteoblasts is controlled by growth factors and cytokines produced in the bone marrow microenvironment and is modulated by systemic hormones and immunological mechanisms [27–30]. Certain signaling pathways, systemic hormones, pro-inflammatory cytokines, and growth factors are considered as fundamental regulators of bone remodeling.

Taken together, positive stimulator of osteoblast activity includes PTH, vitamin D3, IGFs, BMPs, and Wnt signaling, while those that promote osteoclast activation are monocyte-macrophage colony-stimulating factor M-CSF, RANKL, IL-1, and IL-6.

Eventually, the recent discovery of osteoprotegerin (OPG) and the subsequent identification of its cognate ligand, OPG ligand (OPGL or RANKL), have illuminated our understanding of the molecular basis that links between osteoblastogenesis and osteoclastogenesis and thereby the rate of bone remodeling upon which other inputs (hormonal, biomechanical, etc.) operate.

10.4.4 RANK/RANKL/OPG System

Despite that the principal function of the osteoblasts is to synthesize bone matrix proteins and to enhance bone mineralization, osteoblasts also play a crucial role in osteoclast biology that has been clearly demonstrated by the release of key molecules, which regulate osteoclastogenesis and bone resorption. Of these regulators are RANKL which is expressed on the surface of the osteoblast and interact with its receptor RANK [22] to mediate signals for osteoclast proliferation, differentiation, activation, and function [31] (Fig. 10.4), while OPG is acting as a decoy receptor for RANKL [32], noting that the OPG/RANK/RANKL system accounts only for signaling of osteoblasts to osteoclasts.

The human *RANK* is a polypeptide of 616 amino acids, related to the type 1 transmembrane protein class [33], and is expressed in various tissues such as the skeletal muscle, liver, and small and large intestines. Among bone cells RANK-mRNA is exclusively expressed in osteoclast precursor cells [22, 32]. On the other hand, *RANKL* is a TNF-related cytokine that exists in both transmembrane, the predominant form, and soluble (cleaved) forms [22]. The gene expression of RANKL can be found abundantly in the skeleton and lymphoid tissues and is produced by osteoblasts, bone marrow stromal cells, and other cells under the control of various pro-resorptive growth factors, hormones, and cytokines. Moreover, osteoblasts and stromal cells produce OPG, which binds to and thereby inactivates RANKL.

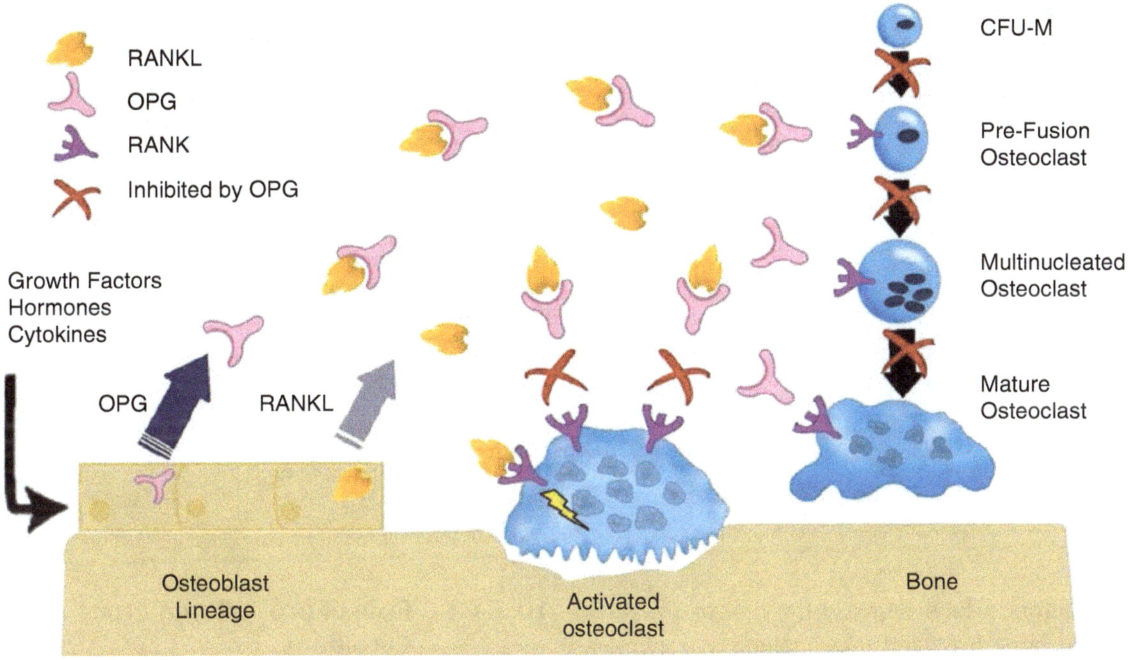

Fig. 10.4 Mechanisms of action for OPG, RANKL, and RANK [34]

Collectively, RANKL is of great importance for the development and function of osteoclasts through binding to its transmembrane-signaling receptor RANK [35]. RANK-RANKL interactions lead to pre-osteoclast recruitment, fusion into multinucleated osteoclasts, osteoclast activation, and osteoclast survival. These effects are very selective to bone and can be inhibited by the natural, soluble, decoy receptor OPG [32].

OPG is considered as a humoral regulator of bone resorption. It blocks osteoclast maturation and differentiation, and subsequently it can protect the bone from both normal osteoclast remodeling and ovariectomy-associated bone loss [36].

Certain human adult tissues showed a high level of OPG mRNA expression, namely, the heart, the bone, the placenta, and the thyroid gland [37]. It has been demonstrated that OPG expression is upregulated in various human osteoblastic cell systems by 1,25-dihydroxyvitamin D3, bone morphogenetic protein-2 (BMP-2), pro-inflammatory cytokines such as interleukin-1 (IL-1) [38], estrogen [39], as well as transforming growth factor-β (TGF-β) [40]. However, some discrepancies were noticed in the effect of these modulators on the expression of the OPG mRNA and OPG protein levels depending on the species of the cells used and on the stage of osteoblastic differentiation. In contrast, it has been established that glucocorticoids downregulate the OPG transcript in human osteoblast and in human marrow stromal cells [41, 42], and they can suppress OPG production resulting in acceleration of osteoclastic bone resorption [43].

10.5 Mediators of Bone Loss in Rheumatic Diseases

Systemic bone loss in rheumatic diseases occurs as a result of several factors including direct effects of inflammation, poor nutrition, reduced lean body mass, immobility, and the effects of therapeutic agents, specifically glucocorticoids. These mechanisms are complex and interrelated but are eventually mediated through influencing on the bone remodeling cycle and may result in increasing bone resorption, decreasing bone formation, but most commonly affecting both of these processes.

Adding to the referred mechanisms that cause bone loss, there are background predispos-

Fig. 10.5 Risk factors for osteoporosis and fractures in inflammatory rheumatic diseases [44]

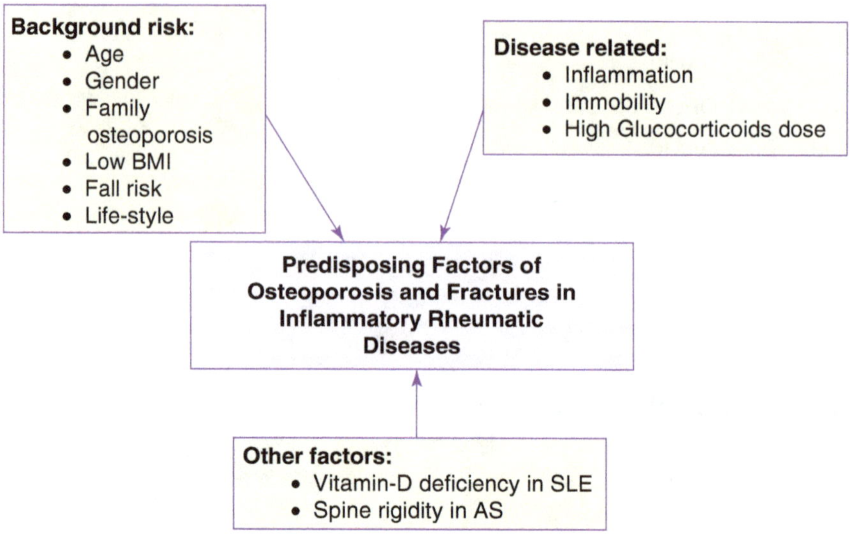

ing factors, which increase the risk of fractures due to bone loss, and they include age, gender, family history of osteoporosis, low body mass index (BMI), falling risk, and sedentary lifestyle (Fig. 10.5) [44].

The following sections will discuss the main underlying mechanisms that cause bone destruction in different rheumatic conditions, namely, the disease activity (inflammation), immobility, and treatment with glucocorticoids are considered. Noting that each rheumatic disease has a unique effect on articular bone or on other site on skeleton whether local or generalized bone loss, however, they remarkably share common pathways of skeletal remodeling (the RANKL/OPG pathway), which is involved in the regulation of bone resorption. In addition, most human and animal studies in the field of rheumatic arthritis have referred to the osteoclast as the principal cell type mediating bone loss in arthritis [45].

10.5.1 Effects of Systemic Inflammation

Inflammatory process in rheumatic diseases is usually associated with skeletal destruction. The effects of inflammation in induction bone loss involve two mechanisms, the role of pro-inflammatory cytokines and/or the role of inflammatory cells.

10.5.1.1 Role of pro-Inflammatory Cytokines

- Many of the pro-inflammatory cytokines and growth factors (Fig. 10.6) [46] involved in the inflammatory processes in rheumatic diseases have been found to have a great impact on osteoclast differentiation and activation either directly, by acting on cells of the osteoclast lineage, or indirectly, by modulating the expression of the key osteoclastogenic factor (RANKL) and/or its inhibitor, OPG [47].
- Because a wide range of cytokines have positive and negative impact on OPG/RANKL system or directly on osteoclastogenesis, they are usually kept in balance in healthy subjects. However, imbalance of these cytokines occurs during inflammation but varies between disease states, and this variation would account for differences in predisposition to bone loss.
- The cytokines that have positive (stimulatory) effects on osteoclastogenesis include TNF-α, IL-1b, IL-6, IL-11, and IL-17, whereas those that have negative (inhibitory) effects include interferon (IFN)-γ, IL-4, and transforming growth factor-β (TGF-β) [48].
- For instance, tumor necrosis factor-alpha (TNF-α) can increase the expression of RANKL by osteoblasts and hence induce osteoclastogenesis and the bone-resorbing activity. However, TNF-α and interleukin-1 (IL-1) can synergize with RANKL to directly enhance bone resorption by osteoclasts.

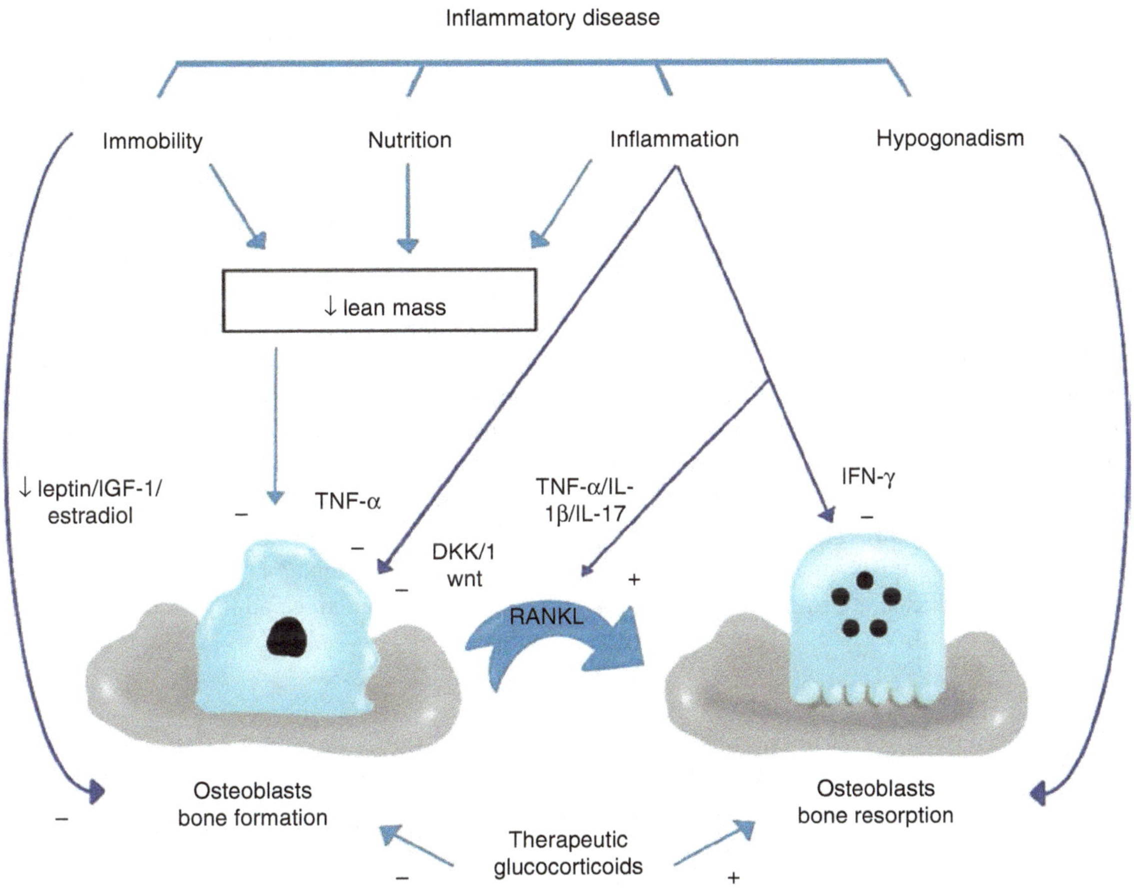

Fig. 10.6 Illustration of the impacts of chronic inflammatory disease on bone formation and resorption. A stimulatory effect is indicated by C and an inhibitory effect by K [46]

10.5.1.2 Role of Inflammatory Cells

- Under normal conditions, RANKL is derived from osteoblasts; however, during inflammation, a variety of inflammatory cells can also produce RANKL including lymphocytes and fibroblasts, which have been found in the inflamed synovium in various studies [49–51]. The expression or production of RANKL on/from non-osteoblastic cells causes a direct osteoclastogenic effect independent of osteoblasts.
- An example of these cells is T lymphocytes that are derived from Th17 subset, which has been called so after the ability of these lymphocytes to secrete IL-17, and hence they are considered to have an osteoclastogenic cytokine profile [52]. The presence of this lymphocyte subset prominently in inflammatory arthritis could explain the tendency to local osteoclastogenesis and thus bone destruction in this condition [53].
- A subsequent to the increased bone resorption, there should be also a stimulation of bone formation because the processes of bone resorption and formation are normally tightly coupled. However, during chronic inflammation, "uncoupling" of bone formation from resorption occurs with a suppressed or decreased bone formation relative to the high degree of resorption.

10.5.1.3 Causes of Uncoupling Process

The Wnt Signaling and its Antagonist, DKK1

Studying animal models of inflammatory arthritis could explain the uncoupling process via the implication of the Wnt-signaling pathway and precisely the Wnt antagonist dickkopf-1 (DKK1), in this process [54].

The canonical Wnt-signaling pathway is essential for bone development, directing differentiation of mesenchymal precursor cells into mature osteoblasts, as well as having a major role in the normal development of the skeleton in the embryo [55, 56]. The naturally occurring soluble Wnt antagonists such as DKK1, which suppress this process, are important during normal bone remodeling. This finding has been supported by that the DKK1 knockout mice develop an increased bone mass [57] and conversely myeloma cells with aberrant DKK1 expression are associated with purely lytic lesions with little evidence of bone formation [58].

The synovial fibroblast can secrete DKK1; however, in rheumatoid arthritis, the secretion is enhanced by TNF-α, and thus the circulating levels of DKK1 have been found much elevated in those patients [54]. Thus, the secreted DKK1 from the synovium would have a suppressive effect on osteoblast maturation and on OPG function leading to inhibition of local bone formation and increased bone resorption, respectively. Understanding the mechanism of Wnt signaling and its antagonist, DKK1 (Fig. 10.7), is very important, since administration of DKK1

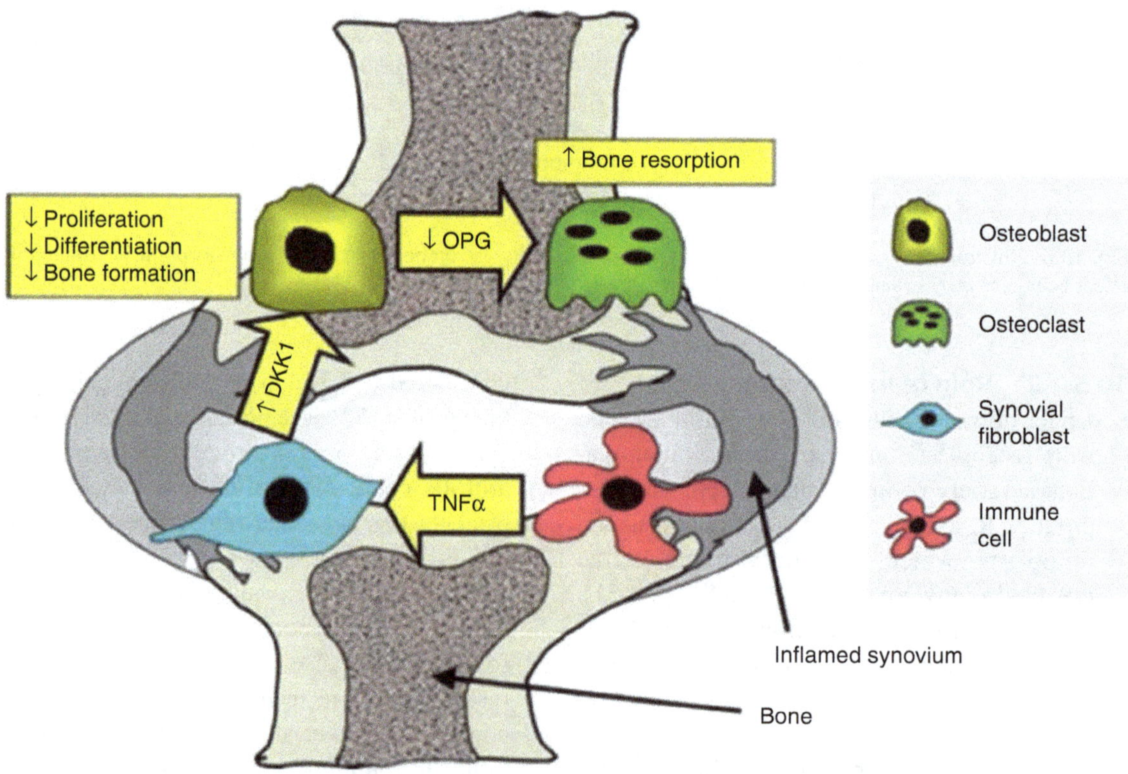

Fig. 10.7 Schematic illustration of the possible role of DKK1 in the bone remodeling imbalance in inflammatory joint disease. Production of DKK1 in response to TNF-α production by inflammatory cells is proposed to inhibit bone formation but increase bone resorption by osteoclasts through a suppression of OPG production by osteoblasts [46]

antibody would be able to prevent bone erosions and reverse this block on osteoblast formation which resulted in a paradoxical excess of bone formation during inflammation as proved by the development of new osteophytes [54].

Alteration of Glucocorticoid Signaling

The effects of glucocorticoids will be explained later in the following sections, but the current paragraph will discuss the influence of inflammation on glucocorticoid action in bone cells. Because of the intracellular metabolism of glucocorticoids by 11b-hydroxysteroid dehydrogenases (11β-HSDs) [59], it has become known that the levels of active glucocorticoids present within the circulation differ from that in the tissues. Specifically, 11β-HSD1 enzyme is expressed on osteoblast and can increase local glucocorticoid action in these cells by converting the inactive glucocorticoids such as cortisone and prednisone to their active counterparts' cortisol and prednisolone, respectively.

Overexpression of the enzyme in osteoblasts reduces proliferation and the synthesis of bone-specific proteins such as osteocalcin when cells are exposed to inactive glucocorticoids [60, 61]. It was reported previously by [62] that pro-inflammatory cytokines such as TNF-α or IL-1b can effectively induce the expression and activity of this enzyme in osteoblasts. Thus, during inflammation, osteoblasts at the site of bone exposed to pro-inflammatory cytokines are likely to also be exposed to high doses of locally active glucocorticoid [62, 63]. This is potentially a major mechanism by which the uncoupling process of osteoblasts and osteoclasts occurs. Overall, a high glucocorticoid level in osteoblasts will decrease bone formation through direct effects on osteoblasts [64], but it can also induce osteoclastogenesis due to upregulation of RANKL and downregulation of OPG in osteoblast precursors [42].

Studying the correlation of locally generated glucocorticoids with other proposed mechanisms of uncoupling such as DKK1 induction is essentially needed for therapeutic purposes of rheumatic diseases.

10.5.2 Effects of Immobility

Immobility has consequences on all inflammatory diseases specifically neuromuscular and joint disease. The major impact on bone occurs due to uncoupling process that results in reduced bone formation and increased bone resorption [65] with overall bone loss. It has been found that osteocytes mediates mechanosensing, which means they can response to mechanical strain and maintain bony matrix via modulation of the major pathways such as the Wnt pathway that couple bone formation and resorption [66]. This effect may partly be dependent on estrogen receptor signaling, and thus hypogonadism would reduce the mechanosensing [67].

Regular exercises can maintain force on bone and thus control bone loss through mechanical stimulation. However, a more advanced approach is the administration of a vibration signal that could stimulate mechanosensing effects, which in turn will induce an anabolic response to bone [46].

10.5.3 Effects of Glucocorticoids

Glucocorticoids (GCs) are frequently prescribed for patients with variety of chronic inflammatory diseases such as rheumatic diseases. An excess of circulating GCs has a major negative effects on bone [64, 68, 69]. These adverse effects on bone are owing to reduced bone formation, characterized by a low mineral apposition rate that is explained by decreased numbers of osteoblasts, while bone resorption is unchanged or even elevated [70], leading to the development of glucocorticoid-induced osteoporosis (GIOP).

Overall negative effects of GCs on bone are either directly on bone cells or indirectly by affecting the bone metabolism. The underlying molecular mechanisms of GIOP include the increased apoptosis of osteoblasts and osteocytes and increased half-life time of osteoclasts, i.e., the direct effects on bone cells (Fig. 10.8) [71]. It has been reported that the increased osteoblast apoptosis results in a significant reduction in bone formation, while decreased osteocyte num-

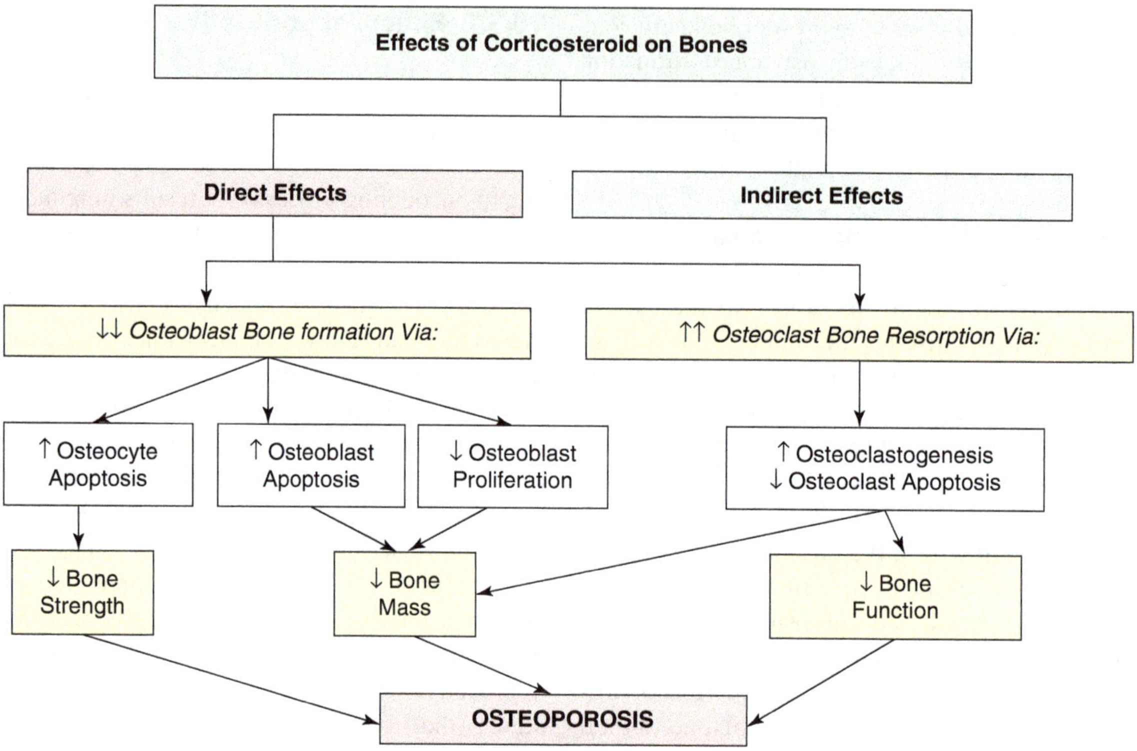

Fig. 10.8 The direct effects of glucocorticoids on bone [71]

bers result in a disturbed osteocyte-canalicular network and thus failure to respond to bone damage [72].

The process of apoptosis is induced by activating caspase-3 [73] and glycogen synthases kinase 3β (GSK3β), which suppresses the Wnt-signaling pathway by increasing the production of DKK-1, the Wnt pathway inhibitor [74, 75].

In addition to the increased apoptosis of osteoblasts, GCs impair osteoblast function by suppressing osteoblast differentiation [76] via interfering with both the bone morphogenetic protein (BMP) pathway and the Wnt-signaling pathway.

Moreover, recent studies proposed that high doses of GCs cause a shift of bone marrow stromal cells, the precursor cells of osteoblasts, to differentiate toward adipocytes instead of osteoblasts. This is mainly achieved either through an increased expression of the peroxisome proliferator-activated receptor-γ2 (PPR- γ2) and repression of the osteogenic transcription factor Runt-related protein 2 [77] or via suppression of AP-1, a process that not only mediates anti-inflammatory actions but also reduces bone strength [78].

In contrast to increased apoptosis of osteoblasts and osteocytes, GCs therapy would reduce the apoptosis of osteoclasts by extending their life span through upregulation of RANKL and suppression of OPG [42].

Likewise direct effects on osteoblasts, osteocytes, and osteoclasts, GCs have indirect effects on bone (Fig. 10.9). Previous studies asserted that GCs impair bone metabolism by inhibiting both the gastrointestinal absorption and the renal tubular reabsorption of calcium, leading to hypocalcaemia and the subsequent hyperparathyroidism [71]. Recent reports referred that GCs have influenced the bone mineralization by decreasing the production of important proteins for matrix formation, namely, osteocalcin and type 1 collagen [69]. Furthermore, GCs can cause steroid myopathy [79] [4] that may increase the risk of falling and thus indirectly increase the fracture risk.

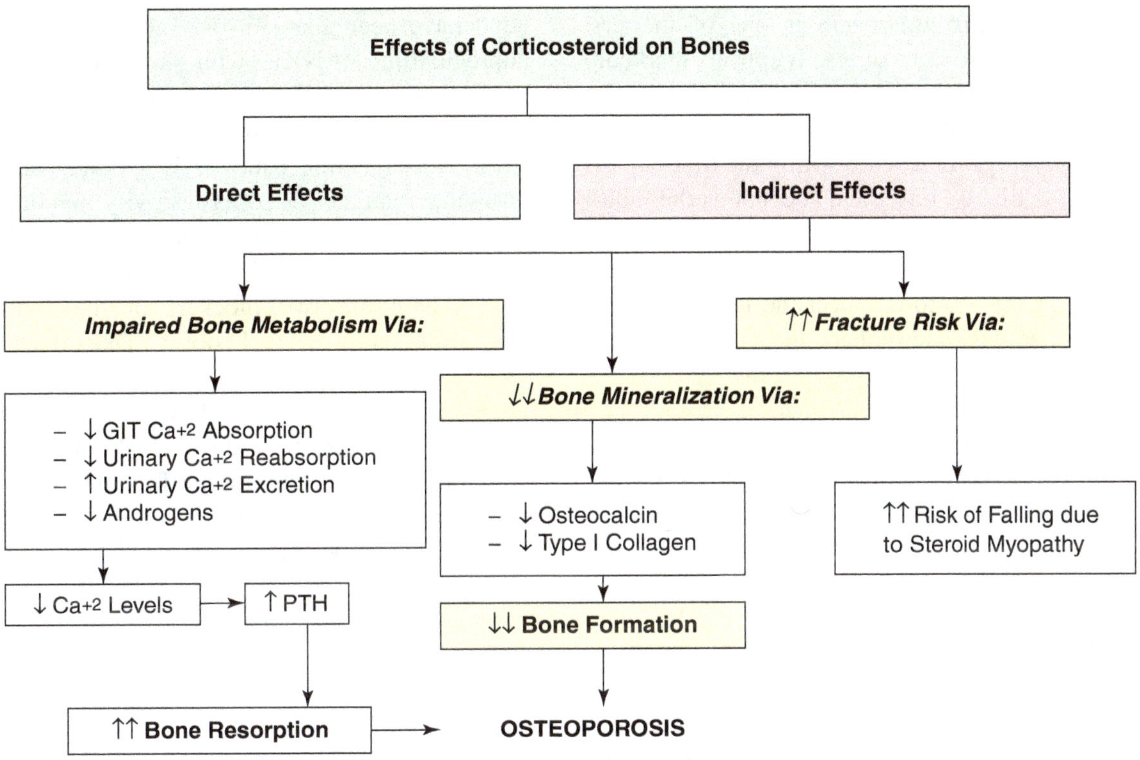

Fig. 10.9 The indirect effects of glucocorticoids on bone [71]

10.6 Common Bone Diseases Associated with Rheumatic Disease

Osteoporosis-related fragility fractures represent one of the most important complications that may occur in patients with rheumatic diseases; obviously, these fractures may contribute to an important decrease in quality of life, and hence osteoporosis becomes increasingly recognized as an eminent public health problem.

Osteoporosis is a metabolic bone disease characterized by both low bone density (mass) and low bone quality, which includes not only microarchitecture deterioration of bone tissue but also alterations in bone remodeling, damage accumulation (e.g., microfractures), and mineralization. These changes in bone density and quality enhance bone fragility with a consequent increase in fracture risk after minimal trauma. Osteoporosis is caused by an imbalance between bone formation and resorption with in favor of bone resorption over bone formation, leading to altered bone remodeling.

The reduction in bone mass can be quantified by measurement of bone mineral density (BMD) using dual-energy x-ray absorptiometry (DXA), which is the diagnostic method of osteoporosis [80]. Therefore, osteoporosis can be defined by DXA result when T score is ≤ 2.5 (i.e., bone density is 2.5 standard deviation below estimated peak BMD for the population), whereas osteopenia is defined when a T score is between -1 and -2.5.

10.6.1 Rheumatoid Arthritis and Bone Loss

Rheumatoid arthritis (RA) is characterized by three types of bone lesions: periarticular osteopenia, bone erosions, and osteoporosis:

- *Periarticular osteopenia* is one of the first radiographic signs of RA. It appears markedly in early disease and is mainly associated with disease activity.
- *Bone erosions* develop within the first months of the disease onset and account as the radiographic sign of RA and reflect undesirable prognosis of RA. Hence, the extent and severity of the erosions reflect the increasing disease activity and indicate the disability of the disease.

Within 6 months of disease onset, less than 50% of patients showed radiographic erosions, while almost 70% of the patients have erosions detected by MRI [81–83] and may be accompanied by bone edema, where CD34+ cells and potential osteoclast precursors [84] can be found during joint aspiration.

- *Osteoporosis* in RA is mainly characterized by marked loss of bone in the hip and the radius, while the axial bone is scarce, a pattern not similar to that of postmenopausal osteoporosis. In addition, several cross-sectional studies reported a lower bone mineral density (BMD) in patients with RA, with a twofold increase in osteoporosis compared to age- and sex-matched controls.

10.6.1.1 Predisposing Factor of Osteoporosis in RA

In addition to the risk factors of osteoporosis (Fig. 10.5), other factors may also contribute in RA, such as muscle wasting, glucocorticoids therapy, and disease duration. Interaction between several factors should be considered, for example, additional muscle wasting contributes to increased immobilization [85].

10.6.1.2 Pathological Process

- Several evidences suggested the presence of osteoclasts at the site of bone erosions, indicating the increased of bone resorption [86, 87].
- In RA, the local and generalized bone loss share common pathways: the RANKL/OPG pathway. The main inflammatory cytokines that have been found in RA and involve in upregulating RANKL, with subsequent activation of osteoclastogenesis, include TNF-α, IL-1, IL-6, and IL-17 [88, 89].
- The Wnt-signaling pathway is another pathway that regulates osteoblast activity, and thus the activation of the Wnt/β-catenin pathway is crucial for osteoblastic differentiation [90, 91]. There are two blockers of the Wnt-signaling pathway, dickkopf-1 (Dkk-1) and sclerostin, both of which play an important role in the pathogenesis of RA. TNF-α can induce both sclerostin and Dkk-1 [89], leading to inhibition of osteoblastic differentiation.
- Further studies in RA patients confirmed these pathological processes and revealed that OPG/RANKL ratio was lower than in healthy controls, while Dkk-1 and sclerostin were higher. After treatment with anti-IL-6, OPG/RANKL increased, Dkk-1 decreased, and sclerostin increased [92].

10.6.1.3 Management of Bone Loss in RA

- Recent treatments with biological agents were introduced in patients with rheumatoid arthritis. All available TNF-alpha blocking agents are quite successful in the prevention of erosion formation.
- However, progression of structural damage in RA patients treated with methotrexate can be avoided by denosumab, a fully human monoclonal IgG2 antibody that binds RANKL [93].
- It has also been found that in patients with RA treated with infliximab, the bone loss was abolished in the spine and hip, but not in the metacarpal cortical hand [94].
- Moreover, preventing the loss of vertebral strength in patients with RA can be principally achieved by treatment with alendronate [95].
- After this extensive review, here comes the value of early diagnosis of RA and early and aggressive intervention with disease-modifying anti-rheumatic drugs (DMARDs) to prevent bone destruction, osteoporosis, and erosions.

10.6.2 Systemic Lupus Erythematosus and Bone Loss

10.6.2.1 Predisposing Factors of Bone Loss in SLE

- In addition to the traditional background factors, there are also disease-related factors (Fig. 10.5) such as inflammation, metabolic factors, hormonal factors, serologic factors, and medication-induced adverse effects [96].
- Another factor that may contribute in decreased BMD in SLE is the associated high frequency of vitamin D deficiency [97–99], a metabolic condition that induces bone loss. Vitamin D deficiency might induce bone loss in SLE via several factors including (a) photosensitivity (so patients avoid exposure to the sun and use sunscreens), (b) dark skin pigment, (c) renal failure, and (d) treatment with GC (has a dual action, it can induce bone loss, but also it has a beneficial effect on bone mass by suppressing inflammation) and possibly hydroxychloroquine (HCQ) (via inhibiting hydroxylase α1 that form active vitamin D), which showed a controversial results [98, 100]. Due to these inconsistent results of HCQ, further studies in large groups of SLE patients and patients with other diseases treated with HCQ are needed to clarify the relationship between HCQ uses and bone metabolism.
- Changes in hormonal pattern may also negatively influence the BMD in patients with SLE, where a relatively high estrogenic and low androgenic state and a decrease in dehydroepiandrosterone (DHEA) have been demonstrated and associated with low BMD [101].
- Collectively, the factors that may adversely affect bone mass, resulting in osteoporosis and possible fracture risk in SLE, have been summarized in Table 10.1.

Table 10.1 Summary of risk factors for osteoporosis in patients with SLE [101]

Risk factors for osteoporosis in patients with SLE
Non-modifiable risk factors
• Caucasian or Asian ethnicity. • Female sex. • Advanced age. • Personal or family history of osteoporotic fractures. • High risk of falls. • Premature menopause.
Modifiable risk factors
• Weight < 127 lb. (58 kg). • Inadequate calcium and vitamin D intake. • Lifestyle habits: Smoking, alcohol use, high number of sedentary hours daily.
Risk factors specific for systemic lupus erythematosus
• **Medication use** [glucocorticoids, gonadotropin-releasing hormone agonists, cytotoxic drugs, antimalarial agent (HCQ)]. • Metabolic causes. – High frequency of vitamin D deficiency. – High homocysteine level. – Hormonal changes in SLE, a relatively high estrogen and low dehydroepiandrosterone (DHEA) [100] • Prolonged active SLE. • Systemic and localized inflammation.

10.6.2.2 Pathological Process

- Chronic systemic inflammation is a cause of bone loss in SLE, where the activated inflammatory cells at sites of inflammation produce a wide spectrum of cytokines that stimulate local and generalized bone resorption.
- Researchers have revealed increased serum levels of tumor necrosis factor (TNF) [103] and oxidized low-density lipoprotein (LDL) [104] in patients with active lupus. Oxidized LDL stimulates the activation of T cells, which in turn can increase the production of RANKL and TNF. Consequently, TNF and RANKL will induce the maturation and activation of osteoclasts [103]. In addition, oxidized LDL has the ability to inhibit osteoblast maturation, and hence it can negatively influence bone formation [105].
- Moreover, high levels of homocysteine (caused by inflammation) have been reported in patients with SLE, and this might be attributed to the accelerated bone loss [106, 107] via enhancing the bone resorption and reduction of bone formation.
- Until recently, the previous clinical studies have not been able to demonstrate the association between bone loss in SLE and the disease activity score [108–110]. However, several

studies showed an association between organ damage and reduced BMD [111], and because prolonged active SLE usually causes organ damage in the patients, this finding suggests that disease activity contributes to reduced BMD in SLE. Moreover, the Hopkins Lupus Cohort study [112] has established that low complement C4 levels (a measure of active disease) were a predictor of low spine BMD among patients with SLE.

10.6.2.3 Management of Bone Loss in SLE

- To approach bone health in SLE patients, the underlying risk factors for bone loss should be evaluated. For instance, evaluation of calcium and vitamin D levels and homocysteine status is recommended. Although there is not enough data relating the low levels of vitamin D and SLE activity, the possible association would suggest that replacement of vitamin D may have benefits beyond bone health for those patients [113].
- Supplementation with vitamin D should aim to keep the serum 25-hydroxyvitamin D [25(OH)D] level above 25 ng/mL, and calcium supplementation should be at the recommended daily allowance for the age of the patient (Table 10.2).
- Bear in mind that it takes approximately 3 months to achieve a steady state of 25(OH)D level once vitamin D supplementation is started, so rechecking a 25(OH)D should not be done earlier than 3 months [114, 115].
- Moreover, if homocysteine levels are elevated, folic acid should be initiated at 1 mg daily [116].
- Patients with SLE are at increased risk of bone loss due to the synergistic effect of the inflammatory process and its treatment with corticosteroids; therefore adequate management is essential to prevent osteoporotic fractures and maintain BMD. However, all preventative measures and pharmacological therapy will be mentioned later on under the section of "Glucocorticoid-Induced Osteoporosis" according to ACR 2010 recommendations.

Table 10.2 ACR 2010 Recommendations on counseling for lifestyle modification and assessment of patients starting glucocorticoids at any dose of >3 months duration

ACR 2010 recommendations on counseling for lifestyle modification
• Weight-bearing activities
• Smoking cessation
• Avoidance of excessive alcohol intake (>2 drinks per day).
• Nutritional counseling on calcium and vitamin D intake.
• Fall risk assessment .
• Baseline dual x-ray absorptiometry .
• Serum 25-hydroxyvitamin D level .
• Baseline height .
• Assessment of prevalent fragility fractures .
• Consider radiographic imaging of the spine or vertebral fracture assessment for those initiating or currently receiving prednisone 5 mg/day or its equivalent.
• Calcium intake (supplement plus oral intake) 1200–1500 mg/day[a].
• Vitamin D supplementation[a].

[a]Recommendations for calcium and vitamin D supplementation are for any dose or duration of glucocorticoids, rather than a duration of 3 months

10.6.3 Ankylosing Spondylitis and Bone Loss

Inflammation in ankylosing spondylitis (AS) is characterized by **subchondral bone marrow edema with subchondral bone** *erosive lesions* and eventually to **subchondral new** *bone formation* through the articular cartilage and ossification of the periarticular ligaments [85].

Bone edema is accounted as a sign of inflammatory activity and may affect limited or extensive parts of vertebrae (Fig. 10.10). Recent studies suggested a possible sequence of events of new bone formation in AS, as follows: first erosions at the site of inflammation, followed by repair reaction, and subsequently ended by new bone formation (10).

- *For instance*, at the corners of the vertebral bodies, there might be *marginal erosive lesions* with adjacent subchondral edema and sclerosis (Romanus lesion). Also, a new periosteal intraosseous *bone formation* was found and provided the typical picture of squaring of the vertebrae [85].

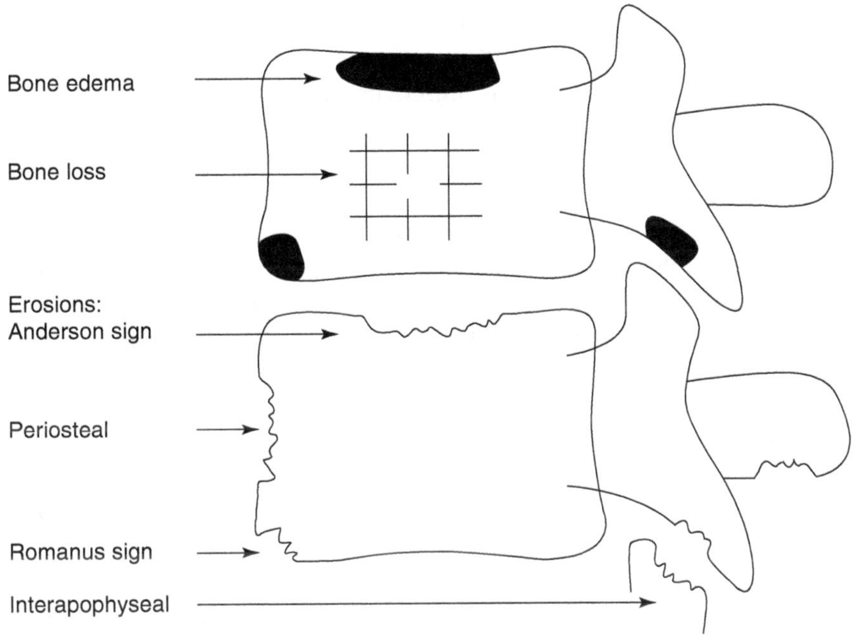

Fig. 10.10 Sites of bone edema, bone loss, and bone erosion in AS [85]

10.6.3.1 Fracture Risk in AS

Subsequent results to bone changes in AS lead to an increase in bone loss (osteoporosis) and bone fragility and therefore increased the risk of bone fractures.

- AS is associated with an elevated risk of vertebral fractures, which are six to seven times higher than in healthy population [117, 118], and these fractures are often accompanied by neurological signs and symptoms [119]. However, the increased in morphometric and clinical vertebral fractures [120] but not in peripheral (forearm or hip) fractures indicates a more local effect of AS on bone, unlike RA, where the inflammatory effects are more systemic. Furthermore, despite sharing similar pathogenesis of osteoporosis but with different clinical phenotypes, bone loss in AS is accompanied by new bone formation contrasting to RA and postmenopausal conditions,
- Of most important types of spinal fractures in AS includes wedging fracture, which contributes to spine rigidity and hyperkyphosis of upper part of the spine and impaired physical function [119, 121, 122]. In addition to wedging fracture, structural damage of the spine and the disease activity are other significant contributors to hyperkyphosis [123].

10.6.3.2 Management of Bone Loss in AS

- Because of the concomitant bone loss and the new abnormal bone formation and the presence of syndesmophytes, the reliability of BMD measurement is affected, and there would be a large variation in the prevalence of osteoporosis in patients with AS [124, 125].
- Taken together, AS is characterized by bone and cartilage degradation. The bone destruction reflects the systemic inflammatory effects on bone density and can be inhibited by TNF-α blocking agent. However, the cartilage damage might be related to syndesmophyte formation, which is not influenced by anti-inflammatory therapy [120]. This highlights the suggestion that bone degradation and new bone formation are uncoupled mechanisms in AS, the reason that might make their therapeutic intervention basically different.
- A remarkable but yet not confirmed finding has shown that the risk of clinical fracture

decreased in AS patients taking NSAIDs, which could relieve the inflammatory back pain and stiffness and thus improving the physical activity that helped in maintaining bone mass and reducing the risk of falling and subsequent fracture [126, 127]. In addition, it has recently been suggested that NSAIDs may also inhibit the formation and growth of syndesmophytes of AS in the spine via interfering with the prostaglandin metabolism. Therefore, if the divergent inhibitory effects of NSAIDs on osteoporotic fractures (bone loss) and progression of syndesmophytes (bone formation) can be confirmed, this would be an important clue in further explaining pathophysiological mechanisms in AS.

- In contrast to the treatment of osteoporosis in patients with RA, treatment of osteoporosis in patients with AS is not yet common. Data supporting the efficacy of this treatment in AS are rare. Of all bisphosphonates, alendronate and risedronate are found to be effective in increasing BMD in men. Alendronate and risedronate significantly increase BMD in both vertebrae and femur, with a significant reduction of vertebral fractures [128, 129]. More recently teriparatide was tested with the same aims, but only a positive effect on BMD could be shown [130]. It is clear that there is a need for evidence-based knowledge in these fields in the near future. Our studies highlight the need to develop strategies to identify high-risk patients with AS. Research on the treatment of osteoporosis to prevent vertebral fractures in these patients is urgently needed.

10.6.4 Glucocorticoid-Induced Osteoporosis (GIOP)

Steroids are widely used in the medical practice to treat various diseases such as asthma, systemic connective tissue diseases, and other autoimmune diseases and in addition to rheumatic diseases. Treatment with GCs results in bone loss within 1 month after initiation of the therapy but primarily occurs in the trabecular bone, so that it mainly increases the risk of vertebral fracture rather than non-vertebral fractures [79]. Fractures are considered the most clinically relevant risk of prolonged steroid therapy.

GIOP is a common type of secondary osteoporosis which occurs at any age and in both men and women. It has been known that one loss in GIOP is biphasic, with a rapid reduction in BMD of 6–12%* which occurs followed by a slower annual loss of about 3%* for as long as the glucocorticoids are administered [131, 132].

10.6.4.1 Impact of GIOP

- As a consequent to the bone loss during GCs therapy, it has been reported that the relative fracture risk within the first 3 months after initiation of the therapy increases by 75% even before any BMD changes occur [133].
- Although the increase of fracture risk has appeared to be dose dependent [134], it was found to be partially reversible so that the fracture risk would gradually return to baseline [135].

10.6.4.2 Approaching Managements of Patients with GIOP

- American College of Rheumatology (ACR) have developed and updated recommendations to provide guidance for prevention and treatment of GIOP in order to be applied by the physicians in light of each patient's circumstances.
- ACR recommendation 2001 [136] has been updated and replaced by ACR recommendation 2010 [137], which had expanded the recommendations for counseling (Table 10.2) and monitoring updated pharmacological guidelines and used patient's overall clinical risk instead of T score alone.
  - Afterward, ACR 2017 recommendations have been released for GIOP prevention and treatment, based on the balance of relative benefits and harms of the treatment options and highly considering the quality

of the evidence and patients' values and preferences [138]. Therefore, due to limited evidence on the benefits and harms of interventions in GC users, most recommendations in ACR 2017 guidelines are conditional or of good clinical practice. The strength of the recommendations is based on the fracture risk categories in GC-treated patients [138].

- The ACR 2017 recommendations for GIOP prevention and treatment have addressed, in addition to all adults' categories (< 40 years and > 40 years of age), special populations categories, namely children, people with organ transplants, women of childbearing potential, and people receiving very high-dose GC treatment.
- The initial approach of patients with GIOP begins with clinical assessment of fracture risk by interpreting detailed clinical and biochemical data, together with identifying the diagnostic criteria for assessment of bone mineral density (BMD) results, as follows:

1. **Clinical Assessment**: This is concerned with having detailed medical history to identify the cumulative risk factors for bone loss (Fig. 10.11) and performing proper physical examination to detect any underlying medical conditions or evidence of osteoporosis such as fracture, kyphosis, and loss of height or determine muscle strength and size.
2. **Biochemical Assessment:** The baseline levels of the following parameters are needed to be obtained in order to rule out any underlying medical diseases that may affect the outcome of GIOP such as low levels of calcium or vitamin D; those would affect the bone formation and metabolism [137, 138]. These parameters include:
    - Complete blood cell count.
    - Serum calcium and phosphorus.
    - Serum 25-hydroxyvitamin D.
    - Serum-free testosterone in males.
    - Estradiol in premenopausal women.
    - Renal Function Tests specifically 24-hour urinary calcium and sodium.
    - Liver function test, because healthy liver is important for synthesis of sex hormones.
3. **Assessment of Bone Mineral Density (BMD):** Measuring the BMD is one of the salient determinants of bone strength. It can be measured at different sites in the body by distinct methods. For instance, dual-energy x-ray absorptiometry (DXA) measures BMD mainly at lumbar spine and proximal femur, while quantitative computed tomography (QCT) is used mostly to estimate bone density at the forearm, tibia, or lumbar spine. The World Health Organization (WHO) has defined the diagnostic criteria for assessment of BMD results (Table 10.3) [139].
4. **Assessment and Classification of Fracture Risk:** Identifying patients with increased fracture risk solely using BMD assessment has some limitations due to its age dependency and its inaccuracy in measuring bone quality. Therefore, it has been recommended that fracture risk should be assessed using tools that calculate the absolute fracture risk for a given patient. One of the available tools proposed by the World Health Organization (WHO) is called Fracture Risk Assessment (FRAX) tool [140].

    FRAX is a unique model that is considered in calculating the risk of the following factors, **age, sex, race,** family history, the BMD, and the usage of BMD, but excludes the dosage and the evaluation of the risk factors of falls and the presence or absence of prevalent vertebral deformities, although they are known as risk factors for fractures. The output of FRAX calculation is a 10-year probability of hip fracture and the 10-year probability of a major osteoporotic fracture (clinical spine, forearm, hip, or shoulder fracture) [140].

    - Based on the risk factors shown in Fig. 10.11 as well as the FRAX results, adult patients receiving GC can be classified into low-, moderate-, and high-risk categories accordingly (Fig. 10.12). The ACR 2017 recommendations for GIOP prevention and treatment have addressed, in addition to all adults' categories (< 40 years and > 40 years of age), special populations, namely children, people with organ transplants, women of childbearing potential, and people receiving very high-dose GC treatment.

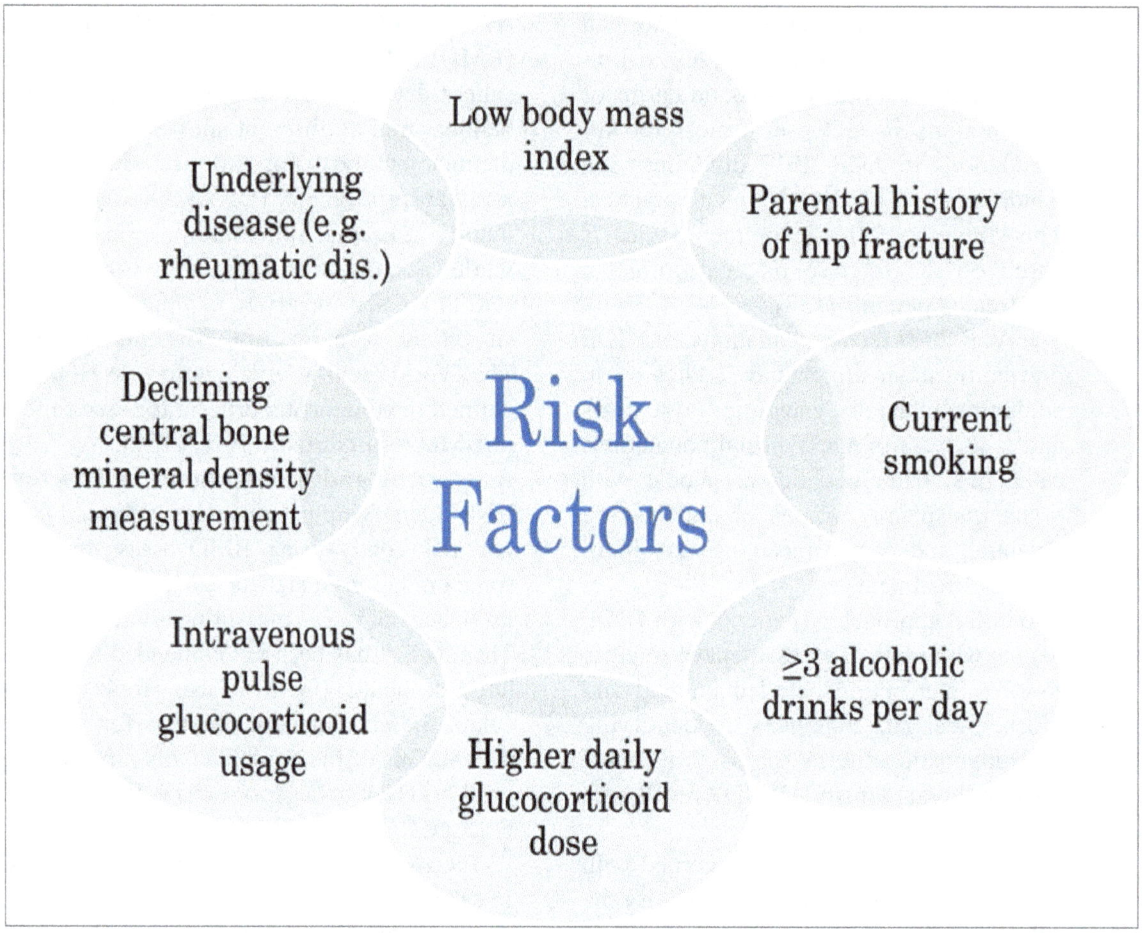

Fig. 10.11 Risk factors that may shift an individual to a greater risk category for GIOP (ACR 2010) [137]

Table 10.3 WHO criteria for assessment of BMD [139]

Diagnostic Criteria	Classification
T*= 0 to -1 SD	Normal
T = -1 to -2 SD	Osteopenia
T ≤ -2.5 SD	Osteoporosis
T ≤ -2.5 SD + fragility fractures	Severe osteoporosis

*T scores is the number of standard deviations(SD) below or above the peak bone mass in a young adult reference population of the same sex.

- Therefore, the primary implication of ACR 2017 recommendation is to clarify that all clinicians treating patients with GCs have to be aware of the GIOP risk, identify patients at high fracture risk (Fig. 10.12), and be able to provide the appropriate treatment [138].
- Moreover, the assessment of fracture risk may not only be useful in treatment decisions, but also in improving patients' treat-

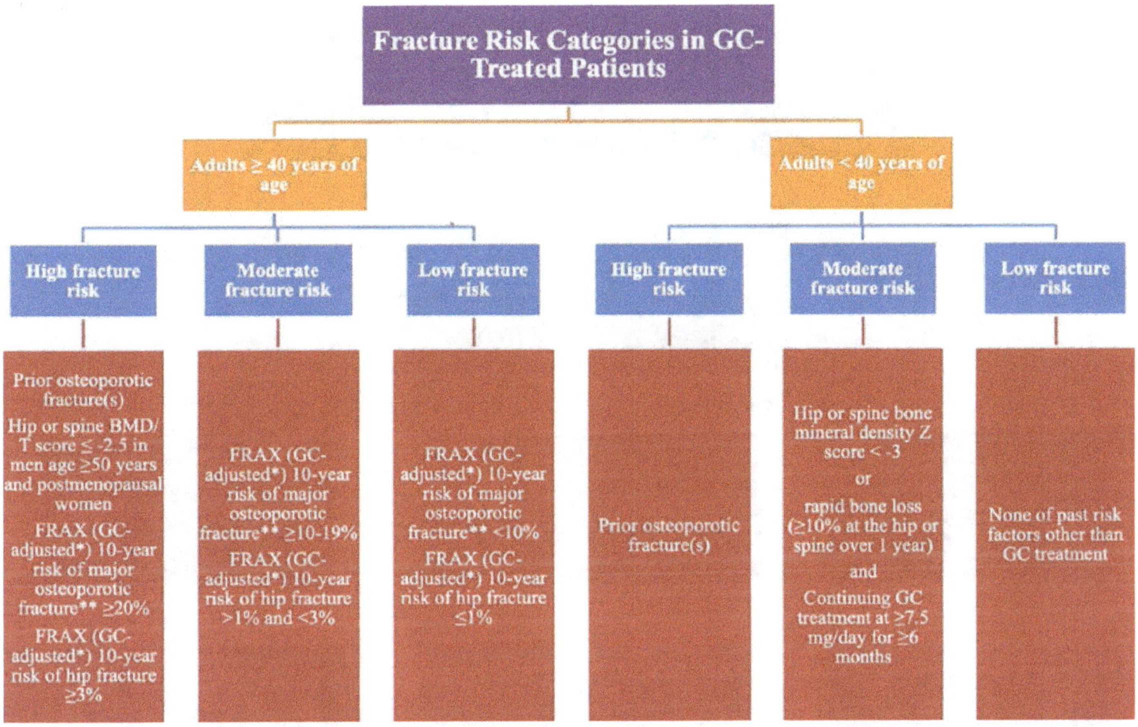

Fig. 10.12 Fracture risk categories in GC-treated patients [138]

ment compliance that would provide the patients a better insight into their future fracture risk.

10.6.4.3 Recommendations for Fracture Risk Assessment and Reassessment of Patient with GIOP

These recommendations are considered as good practice recommendations.

- Initial fracture risk assessment:

  For all adults and children, an initial clinical fracture assessment should be performed as soon within six months of the initiation of long-term GC treatment. This clinical assessment should include the following:

  – A detailed clinical history of GC use (dose, duration, mode, and pattern of use),
  – An evaluation of underlying risk factors for fracture including history of falls, fractures, frailty, others such as (malnutrition, significant weight loss or low body weight, hypogonadism, secondary hyperparathyroidism, thyroid disease, family history of hip fracture, history of alcohol use [at > 3 units/day] or smoking), and other clinical comorbidities.
  – A physical examination including measurement of weight and height, detailed examination of musculoskeletal system, and other clinical findings of undiagnosed fracture (e.g., spinal tenderness, deformity, and reduced space between lower ribs and upper pelvis).

  For adults >40 years old, the initial absolute fracture risk should be evaluated using FRAX with correction of GC dose and BMD (if available) as prompt as possible but within at least six months of starting the GC therapy (Fig. 10.13) [138].

  For adults <40 years old, BMD testing should be done as promptly as possible but at least within 6 months of starting the GC treatment if the patient has a history of previous OP fracture(s) (high risk) or if the patient has

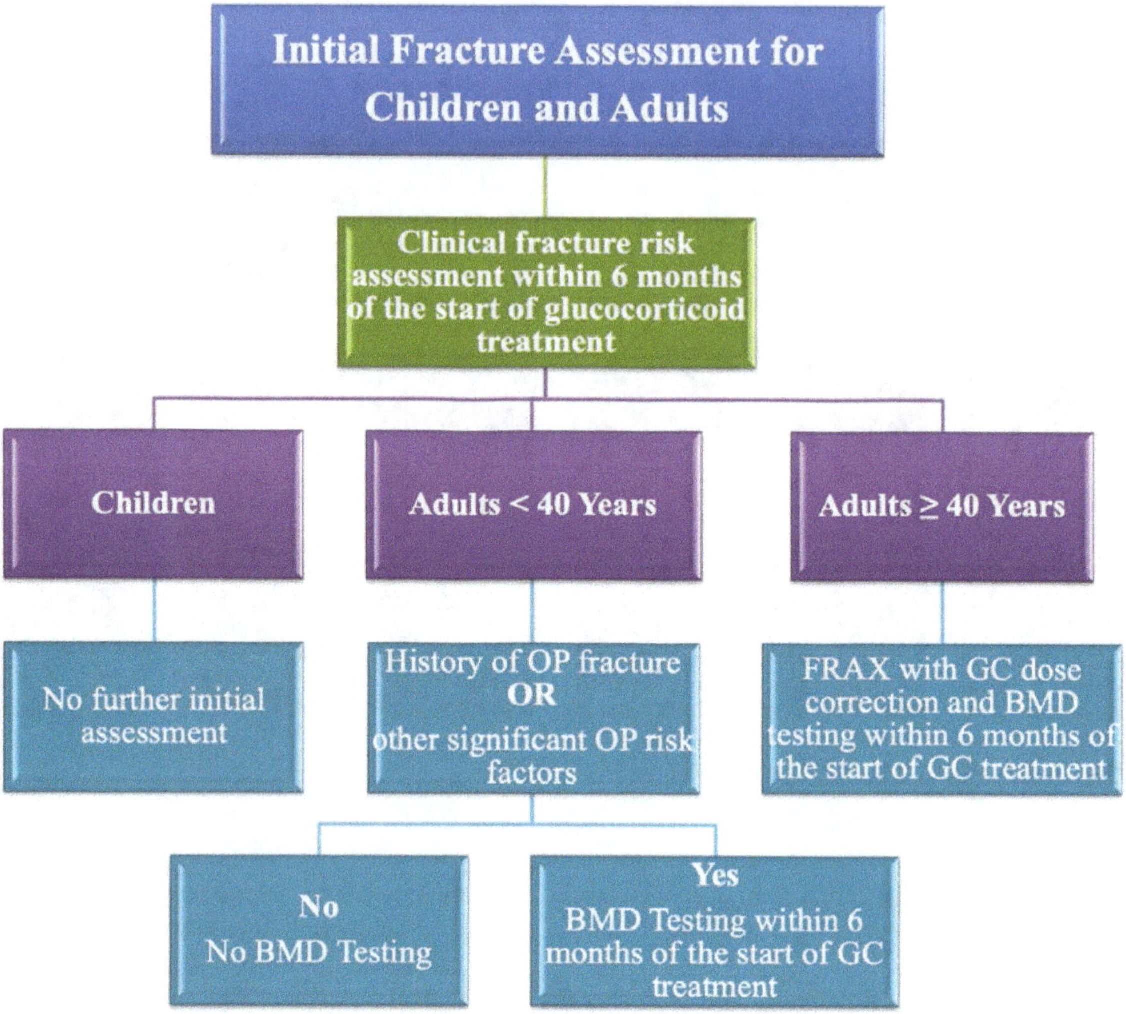

Fig. 10.13 Initial fracture risk assessment [138]

other significant OP risk factors (Fig. 10.13) [138].

- Reassessment of fracture risk:

  For all adults and children, if GC therapy is used continuously, a clinical fracture risk reassessment (as referred earlier) should be performed every 12 months. For detailed pathways of reassessment of clinical fracture risk in adults <40 and ≥40 years of age, refer to Fig. 10.14 [138].

10.6.4.4 Recommendations for Initial Treatment and Prevention of GIOP

- In addition to adjusting the pharmacologic treatment of GIOP, optimizing the dose of calcium and vitamin D uptake and counseling lifestyle modification are included within both the ACR 2010 and the ACR 2017 recommendations for treating patients with GIOP.
- A conditional recommendation is reported, generally for all adults on GC at a dose of ≥2.5 mg/day for ≥3 months, to optimize calcium intake (1000–1200 mg/day) and vitamin D intake (600–800 IU/day; serum level ≥20 ng/mL) [138, 141] alongside lifestyle modification with regard to weight, nutrition, smoking, and alcohol intake (Table 10.2).
- For children 4–17 years of age receiving GC therapy, a calcium intake of 1000 mg/day and vitamin D of 600 IU/day is recommended.

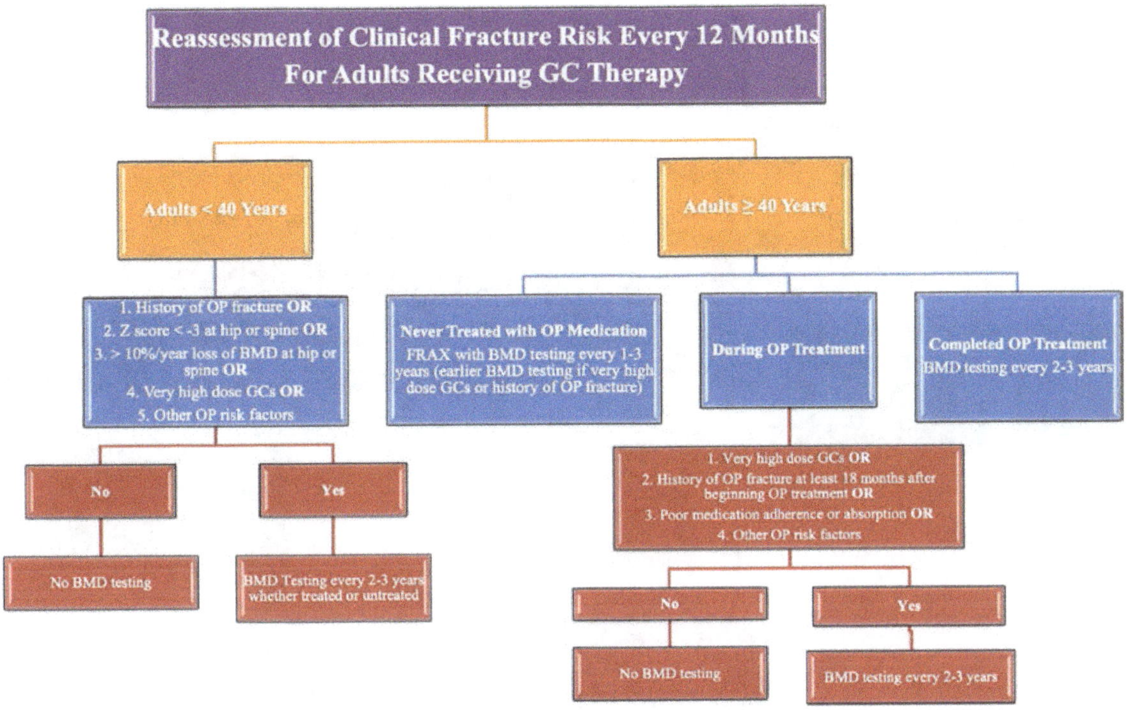

Fig. 10.14 Reassessment of fracture risk [138]

- The ACR 2017 recommendations of initial pharmacologic treatment are categorized according to the following groups and are highlighted in Fig. 10.15 and Table 10.4.
  - All adults >40 years of age, they are divided into women >40 years old but not of childbearing potential, and men >40 years old, who are at moderate to high risk of fracture (Fig. 10.15).
  - Adults <40 years of age, includes (women not of childbearing potential and men) with a history of OP fracture, or those continuing GC treatment (>6 months at a dose of >7.5 mg/day), who have either a hip or spine BMD with Z score <−3 or DXA result reveals bone loss of >10%/year at the hip or spine (Fig. 10.15).
  - Special populations that have further subgroups including (Table 10.4):

    Women who meet criteria for moderate-to-high risk of fracture and are of childbearing potential but do not plan to become pregnant within the period of OP treatment and are using effective birth control or are not sexually active.

    Adults >30 years of age who are receiving very high-dose GC treatment (initial prednisone dose of >30 mg/day [or equivalent GC exposure] and a cumulative annual dose of >5 gm) (Table 3 of main reference).

    Adults who have received an organ transplant and who are continuing treatment with GCs.

    GC-treated children at 4–17 years of age are further subdivided into two groups (Table 10.4).

10.6.4.5 Rationale of Pharmacotherapy of GIOP

- GIOP can be partially prevented by using bisphosphonates (alendronate and zoledronic acid) [142]. However, oral bisphosphonates are limited by low adherence rates, and therefore zoledronic acid provides the intravenous form of this medication and can be prescribed rather than the patient receiving no additional therapy beyond calcium and vitamin D.
- On the other hand, PTH 1-34 (teriparatide) therapy seems to be superior to oral bisphos-

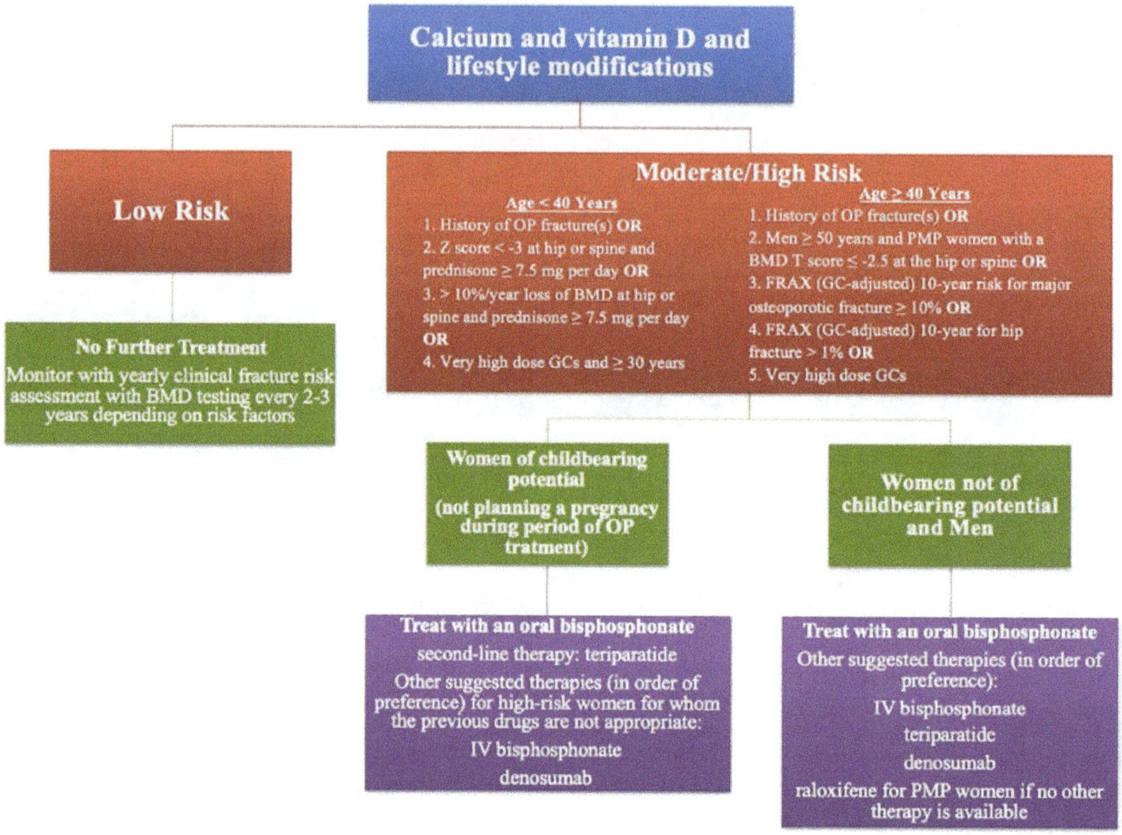

Fig. 10.15 Initial pharmacologic treatment for adults [138]. Recommended doses of calcium and vitamin D are 1000–1200 mg/day and 600–800 IU/day (serum level ≥20 ng/mL), respectively. Lifestyle modifications include a balanced diet, maintaining weight in the recommended range, smoking cessation, regular weight-bearing and resistance training exercise, and limiting alcohol intake to 1–2 alcoholic beverages/day. Very high-dose glucocorticoid (GC) treatment was defined as treatment with prednisone ≥30 mg/day and a cumulative dose of >5 gm in the past year. The risk of major osteoporotic (OP) fracture calculated with the FRAX tool should be increased by 1.15, and the risk of hip fracture by 1.2, if the prednisone dose is .7.5 mg/day (e.g., if the calculated hip fracture risk is 2.0%, increase to 2.4%)

phonates but is more expensive [143] and can be used if bisphosphonate is not appropriate.

- If neither oral nor IV bisphosphonates nor teriparatide treatment is appropriate, denosumab should be used rather than the patient receiving no additional treatment beyond calcium and vitamin D. Denosumab is a humanized monoclonal antibody to RANKL and is useful for GC-treated patients with renal insult but with stable serum Ca^{+2} levels and are not candidates for bisphosphonates or teriparatide. Denosumab has been approved for the prevention of vertebral and non-vertebral fractures, in women with postmenopausal osteoporosis [144]. Moreover, it was revealed that denosumab therapy increased spine and hip BMD and reduced bone turnover markers for 12 months in patients received GC [145]. A recent randomized, doubleblind, comparative study of denosumab and risedronate in patients ≥19 years of age taking prednisolone ≥7.5 mg/day for ≥3 months reported that denosumab significantly increased spine and femoral BMD compared to risedronate [146].
- If none of these medications is appropriate for postmenopausal women, raloxifene [selective estrogen receptor modulator (SERM)] should be used rather than the patient receiving no additional treatment beyond calcium and vitamin D. The order of the preferred treatments

Table 10.4 Recommendations for initial treatment for prevention of GIOP in special populations of patients beginning long-term GC therapy [138]

Recommendations for initial treatment for prevention of GIOP in special populations
Women of childbearing potential at moderate-to-high risk of fracture who do not plan to become pregnant within the period of OP treatment and are using effective birth control or are not sexually active
Treat with an oral bisphosphonate over calcium and vitamin D alone, teriparatide, IV bisphosphonates, or denosumab.
Oral bisphosphonates preferred for safety, cost, and because of lack of evidence of superior antifracture benefits from other OP medications.
Other therapies if oral bisphosphonates are not appropriate, in order of preference:
Teriparatide
Safety, cost, and burden of therapy with daily injections
Consider the following therapies only for high-risk patients due to lack of safety data on use of these agents during pregnancy:
IV bisphosphonates
Potential fetal risks of IV infusion during pregnancy
Denosumab
Potential fetal risks during pregnancy
Conditional recommendations because of indirect and very low-quality evidence on benefits and harms of these treatments to the fetus during pregnancy
Adults age ≥30 years receiving very high-dose GCs (initial dose of prednisone ≥30 mg/day and cumulative dose >5 gm in 1 year)
Treat with an oral bisphosphonate over calcium and vitamin D alone.
Treat with an oral bisphosphonate over IV bisphosphonates, teriparatide, or denosumab.
Oral bisphosphonates preferred for safety, cost, and because of lack of evidence of additional anti-fracture benefits from other OP medications.
If bisphosphonate treatment is not appropriate, alternative treatments are listed by age (≥40 years and <40 years) in Fig. 10.15
Conditional recommendations because of low-quality evidence on absolute fracture risk and harms in this population
Adults with organ transplant, glomerular filtration rate ≥30 mL/min, and no evidence of metabolic bone disease who continue treatment with GCs
Treat according to the age-related guidelines for adults without transplants with these additional recommendations:
An evaluation by an expert in metabolic bone disease is recommended for all patients with a renal transplant.
Recommendation against treatment with denosumab due to lack of adequate safety data on infections in adults treated with multiple immunosuppressive agents.
Conditional recommendations because of low-quality evidence on antifracture efficacy in transplant recipients and on relative benefits and harms of the alternative treatments in this population
Children ages 4–17 years treated with GCs for ≥3 months
Optimize calcium intake (1000 mg/day) and vitamin D intake (600 IU/day) and lifestyle modifications over not optimizing calcium and vitamin D intake and lifestyle modifications.
Conditional recommendation because of lack of antifracture efficacy of calcium and vitamin D in children but limited harms
Children ages 4–17 years with an osteoporotic fracture who are continuing treatment with GCs at a dose of ≥0.1 mg/kg/day for ≥3 months
Treat with an oral bisphosphonate (IV bisphosphonate if oral treatment contraindicated) plus calcium and vitamin D over treatment with calcium and vitamin D alone.
Conditional recommendation because of very low-quality antifracture data in children but moderate-quality evidence of low harms of oral bisphosphonates in children and less potential harm of oral over IV bisphosphonates

GIOP glucocorticoid (GC)-induced osteoporosis, *IV* intravenous

was established according to a comparison of efficacy (fracture reduction), toxicity, and cost.

10.6.4.6 Follow-up Treatment Recommendations

Initial treatment failure is defined if the osteoporotic fracture occurs after 18 months of treatment initiation with oral bisphosphonate or if there is significant BMD reduction (≥10%/year) at follow-up. Various categories of treatment failure of GIOP are explained in Table 10.5 with appropriate recommendations according to the reassessment of fracture risk status.

10.7 Summary

Chronic inflammatory diseases, namely, rheumatic diseases such as rheumatoid arthritis, systemic lupus erythematosus, and ankylosing spondylitis, are commonly associated with extra-articular side effects, including bone loss and fractures. Osteoporosis-related fragility fractures represent one of the most important adverse outcomes that may occur in patients with rheumatic diseases. These fractures may contribute to a significant decrease in quality of life and thus would have a great impact on the economic status of the society.

Table 10.5 Recommendations for follow up treatment for prevention of GIOP [138]

Recommendations for follow-up treatment for prevention of GIOP according to reassessment of fracture risk
Adults age ≥40 years continuing GC treatment who have had a fracture that occurred after ≥18 months of treatment with an oral bisphosphonate or who have had a significant loss of bone mineral density (≥10%/year) [Definition of Treatment Failure]
Treat with another class of OP medication (teriparatide or denosumab; or, consider IV bisphosphonate if treatment failure is judged to be due to poor absorption or poor medication adherence) with calcium and vitamin D over calcium and vitamin D alone or over calcium and vitamin D and continued oral bisphosphonate.
Conditional recommendation because of very low-quality evidence comparing benefits and harms of the compared treatment options in this clinical situation.
Adults age ≥40 years who have completed 5 years of oral bisphosphonate treatment and who continue GC treatment and are assessed to be at moderate-to-high risk of fracture:
Continue active treatment, without drug holiday, (with an oral bisphosphonate beyond 5 years or switch to IV bisphosphonate [if concern with regard to adherence or absorption] or switch to an OP treatment in another class) over calcium and vitamin D alone.
Conditional recommendation because of very low-quality data on benefits and harms in GC-treated patients, but moderate-quality data in the general OP literature on benefits and harms of continuing treatment with oral bisphosphonates past 5 years for people at high risk of fracture.
Adults age ≥40 years taking an OP medication in addition to calcium and vitamin D who discontinue GC treatment and are assessed to be at low risk of fracture:
Discontinue the OP medication but continue calcium and vitamin D over continuing the OP medication.
Conditional recommendation made by expert consensus; evidence informing it too indirect for the population and very low-quality.
Adults age ≥40 years taking an OP medication in addition to calcium and vitamin D who discontinue GC treatment and are assessed to be at moderate-to-high risk of fracture:
Complete the treatment with the OP medication over discontinuing the OP medication.
Strong recommendation for high-risk patients based on expert consensus that patients who are at high risk should continue an OP treatment in addition to calcium and vitamin D.
Conditional recommendation for moderate-risk patients because of lower fracture risk compared to potential harms.

The concept of osteoimmunology elucidates in depth the links between the immune system and bone physiology. The predisposing factors that cause the underlying pathology of bone loss in rheumatic patients are multifactorial. In addition to the traditional background fracture risks, such as age, BMI, and gender, there are potential bone loss mediators that substantially increase fracture risk in these patients. Of these common mediators are inflammation (high disease activity), immobility, and treatment with glucocorticoids. Other mediators would contribute in bone loss in rheumatic patients and may include poor nutrition, the increase of catabolic state, and the decrease in reproductive hormones (hypogonadism) in both men and women.

These effector mediators appear to interact in a complex and synergistic way to reinforce each other through various mechanisms that act on a shared common pathway, the bone remodeling cycle. The net result of these mediators is the production of a wide spectrum of cytokines that stimulate local and/or generalized bone resorption and that inhibit (as in RA) or stimulate (as in AS) bone formation. For instance, during the inflammatory process, the Wnt-signaling antagonist (DKK-1) is secreted from the synovial fibroblast and inhibits osteoblast maturation and OPG function leading to suppression of local bone formation. Therefore, administration of anti DKK-1 would be useful to prevent bone erosions and reverse the inhibition on bone formation. However, immobility will suppress the mechanosensing process of osteocytes leading to uncoupling of bone formation and bone resorption through the Wnt-signaling pathway.

Although GCs are frequently prescribed for the rheumatic patients, they have a great adverse impact on bone quality leading to GIOP. The overall effects of GCs on bone are either directly on bone cells or indirectly by affecting the bone metabolism, both of which result in enhancing bone resorption and decreasing bone formation. Inhibition of bone formation by GCs occurs by increasing the osteoblast and osteocyte apoptosis and/or impairing osteoblast function via suppressing the BMP pathway and the Wnt-signaling pathway. On the other hand, GCs can stimulate bone resorption by reducing osteoclast apoptosis via upregulation of RANKL and inhibition of OPG.

GIOP is a significant clinical complication that occurs as a result of adverse effects of the prescribed GCs for patients with rheumatic disease. ACR 2010 had set several recommendations updated that of ACR 2001 for evaluating and monitoring patients, who has just initiated or received GCs for/or more than 3 months duration. However later, ACR 2017 recommendations have been released and aimed to standardize the classification of patients at risk of GC induced fracture (Fig. 10.12). So that the appropriate recommendations can be applied on each category, while reducing the risk and burden of radiological testing and the anti-fracture therapy. Therefore, all clinicians treating patients with GCs should be aware of these fracture risks and identify the patient's level of fracture risk according to the ACR 2017 guidelines for assessment and reassessment of fracture risks. The recommendations of anti-fracture pharmacotherapy in order of preference, for prevention and treatment of GIOP, were based on their efficacy, potential harms, and cost. Hence, oral bisphosphonates were recommended as preferred first-line therapy over other recommended anti-fracture therapies.

Taking together, the salient approach for early diagnosis of rheumatic diseases would be very crucial and of great help in diminishing the magnitude of bone destruction that occur during the pathogenesis of these diseases and therefore preventing further bone erosion and osteoporosis. Finally, GIOP is a medical problem that patients should be aware of its fracture risk and clinicians should consider evaluating the fracture risks for all GC-treated patients and actively prevent reduction of bone mass.

Acknowledgments The author of this chapter is grateful to the medical student Somayya Khan for her efforts in drawing some of this chapter's figures. The authors also would like to thank Dr. Waleed Hafiz for his assistance in the development of this chapter.

References

1. Spector TD, Hall GM, McCloskey EV, Kanis JA. Risk of vertebral fracture in women with rheumatoid arthritis. BMJ. 1993;306:558.

2. Gough AK, Lilley J, Eyre S, Holder RL, Emery P. Generalised bone loss in patients with early rheumatoid arthritis. Lancet. 1994;344:23–7.
3. Bernstein CN, Blanchard JF, Leslie W, Wajda A, Yu BN. The incidence of fracture among patients with inflammatory bowel disease. A population based cohort study. Ann Intern Med. 2000;133:795–9.
4. Bultink IE, Lems WF, Kostense PJ, Dijkmans BA, Voskuyl AE. Prevalence of and risk factors for low bone mineral density and vertebral fractures in patients with systemic lupus erythematosus. Arthritis Rheum. 2005;52:2044–50.
5. Schett G, Kiechl S, Weger S, et al. High sensitivity C-reactive protein and risk of nontraumatic fractures in the Bruneck study. Arch Intern Med. 2006;166:2495–501.
6. Sinigaglia L, Varenna M, Girasole G, Bianchi G. Epidemiology of osteoporosis in rheumatic diseases. Rheum Dis Clin N Am. 2006;32:631–58.
7. Glimcher MJ. Composition, structure and organization of bone and other mineralized tissues and the mechanism of calcification. In: Aurbach GD, editor. *Handbook of Physiology-Endocrinology*, (Vol. 7/sec. 7). DC: American Physiological Society. Washington; 1976. p. 25–116.
8. Junqueira LC, Carneiro J, Kelley RO., "Bone", in basic histology (9th edition)., Appleton & Lange, (1998).
9. Manolagas SC, Jilka RL. Bone marrow, cytokines, and bone remodeling: emerging insights into the pathophysiology of osteoporosis. N Engl J Med. 1995;332(5):305–11.
10. Caplan AI. Mesenchymal stem cells. J Orthop Res. 1991;9:641–50.
11. Owen M. Marrow stromal stem cells. J Cell Sci Suppl. 1988;10:63–76.
12. Danen EH, Lafrenie RM, Miyamoto S, Yamada KM. Integrin signaling: cytoskeletal complexes, MAP kinase activation, and regulation of gene expression. Cell Adhes Commun. 1998;6:217–24.
13. Komori T. Regulation of osteoblast differentiation by transcription factors. J Cell Biochem. 2006;99(5):1233–9.
14. Day TF, Guo X, Garrett-Beal L, Yang Y. Wnt/β-catenin signaling in mesenchymal progenitors controls osteoblast and chondrocyte differentiation during vertebrate skeletogenesis. Dev Cell. 2005;8:739–50.
15. Otto F, Thornell AP, Crompton T, Denzel A, et al. Cbfa1, a candidate gene for cleidocranial dysplasia syndrome, is essential for osteoblast differentiation and bone development. Cell. 1997;89:765–71.
16. Komori T, Yagi H, Nomura S, et al. Targeted disruption of Cbfa1 results in a complete lack of bone formation owing to maturational arrest of osteoblasts. Cell. 1997;89:755–64.
17. Nakashima K, Zhou X, Kunkel G, Zhang Z, Deng JM, Behringer RR, de Crombrugghe B. The novel zinc finger-containing transcription factor osterix is required for osteoblast differentiation and bone formation. Cell. 2002;108:17–29.
18. Dempster DW, Cosman F, Parisien M, Shen V, Lindsay R. Anabolic actions of parathyroid hormone on bone. Endocr Rev. 1993;14:690–709.
19. Boyce BF, Hughes DE, Wright KR, Xing L, Dai A. Recent advances in bone biology provide insight into the pathogenesis of bone diseases. Lab Investig. 1999;79:83–94.
20. Lian JB, Stein GS, Stein JL, van Wijnen AJ. Regulated expression of the bone specific osteocalcin gene by vitamins and hormones. Vitam Horm. 1999;55:443–509.
21. Ishida Y, Heersche JH. Glucocorticoid-induced osteoporosis: both in vivo and in vitro concentrations of glucocorticoids higher than physiological levels attenuate osteoblast differentiation. J Bone Miner Res. 1998;13:1822–6.
22. Lacey DL, Timms E, Tan H-L, et al. Osteoprotegerin ligand is a cytokine that regulates osteoclast differentiation and activation. Cell. 1998;93:165–76.
23. Gao Y, Grassi F, Ryan MR, Terauchi M, Page K, Yang X, et al. IFN-gamma stimulates osteoclast formation and bone loss in vivo via antigen-driven T cell activation. J Clin Invest. 2007;117:122–32.
24. Fauci AS, Kasper DL, Braunwald E, et al., Harrison's Principles of Internal Medicine, 17th Edition: http://www.accessmedicine.com, [Copyright of The McGray-Hill Companies, Inc,. (Modified from T Suda et al: Endocr Rev 20:345, 1999, with permission.)].
25. Zaidi M. Calcium receptors on eukaryotic cells with special reference to the osteoclast. Biosci Rep. 1990;10(6):493–507.
26. Teti A, Rucci N. The unexpected links between bone and the immune system. Medicographia. 2010;32(4):341–8.
27. Zhao C, Irie N, Takada Y, Shimoda K, Miyamoto T, Nishiwaki T, Suda T, Matsuo K. Bidirectional ephrinB2–EphB4 signaling controls bone homeostasis. Cell Metab. 2006;4:111–21.
28. Goldring SR, Goldring MB. Eating bone or adding it: the Wnt pathway decides. Nat Med. 2007;13:133–4.
29. Matsuo K, Irie N. Osteoclast–osteoblast communication. Arch Biochem Biophys. 2008;473:201–9.
30. Sims NA, Gooi JH. Bone remodeling: multiple cellular interactions required for coupling of bone formation and resorption. Semin Cell Dev Biol. 2008;19:444–51.
31. Wong BR, Josien R, Lee SY, Vologodskaia M, Steinman RM, Choi Y. The TRAF family of signal transducers mediates NF-kappa B activation by the TRANCE receptor. J Biol Chem. 1998s;273(43):28355–9.
32. Burgess TL, Qian Y-X, Kaufman S, et al. The ligand for Osteoprotegerin (OPGL) directly activates mature osteoclasts. J Cell Biol. 1999;145(3):527–38.
33. Anderson MA, Maraskovsky E, Billingsley WL, et al. A homologue of the TNF receptor and its ligand enhance T-cell growth and dendritic-cell function. Nature. 1997;390:175–9.
34. Kearns AE, Khosla S, Kostenuik PJ. Receptor activator of nuclear factor kappa B ligand and osteoprotegerin regulation of bone remodeling in health and

disease. Endocr Rev. 2008;29(2):155–92. Epub 2007 Dec 5. Review
35. Suda T, Takahashi N, Udagawa N, Jimi E, Gillespie MT, Martin TJ. Modulation of osteoclast differentiation and function by the new members of the tumor necrosis factor receptor and ligand families. Endocr Rev. 1999;20(3):345–57. Review
36. Simonet WS, Lacey DL, Dunstan CR, et al. Osteoprotegerin: a novel secreted protein involved in the regulation of bone density. Cell. 1997;89:309–19.
37. Yasuda H, Shima N, Nakagawa N, et al. Identity of osteoclastogenesis inhibitory factor (OCIF) and osteoprotegerin (OPG): a mechanism by which OPG/OCIF inhibits osteoclastogenesis in vitro. Endocrinology. 1998;139(3):1329–37.
38. Hofbauer LC, Dunstan CR, Spelsberg TC, Riggs BL, Khosla S. Osteoprotegerin production by human osteoblast lineage cells is stimulated by vitamin D, bone morphogenetic protein-2, and cytokines. Biochem Biophys Res Commun. 1998;250(3):776–81.
39. Saika M, Inoue D, Kido S, Matsumoto T. 17beta-estradiol stimulates expression of osteoprotegerin by a mouse stromal cell line, ST-2, via estrogen receptor-alpha. Endocrinology. 2001;142(6):2205–12.
40. Takai H, Kanematsu M, Yano K, et al. Transforming growth factor-beta stimulates the production of osteoprotegerin/osteoclastogenesis inhibitory factor by bone marrow stromal cells. J Biol Chem. 1998;273(42):27091–6.
41. Vidal NO, Brandstrom H, Jonsson KB, Ohlsson C. Osteoprotegerin mRNA is expressed in primary human osteoblast-like cells: down-regulation by glucocorticoids. J Endocrinol. 1998;159(1): 191–5.
42. Hofbauer LC, Gori F, Riggs BL, Lacey DL, Dunstan CR, Spelsberg TC, Khosla S. Stimulation of osteoprotegerin ligand and inhibition of osteoprotegerin production by glucocorticoids in human osteoblastic lineage cells: potential paracrine mechanisms of glucocorticoid-induced osteoporosis. Endocrinology. 1999;140(10):4382–9.
43. Sasaki N, Kusano E, Ando Y, Yano K, Tsuda E, Asano Y. Glucocorticoid decreases circulating osteoprotegerin (OPG): possible mechanism for glucocorticoid induced osteoporosis. Nephrol Dial Transplant. 2001;16(3):479–82.
44. Bultink IE, Vis M, van der Horst-Bruinsma IE, Lems WF. Inflammatory rheumatic disorders and bone. Curr Rheumatol Rep. 2012;14(3):224–30. Review
45. Gravallese EM, Harada Y, Wang JT, et al. Identification of cell types responsible for bone resorption in rheumatoid arthritis and juvenile rheumatoid arthritis. Am J Pathol. 1998;152:943–51.
46. Hardy R, Cooper MS. Bone loss in inflammatory disorders. J Endocrinol. 2009;201(3):309–20. https://doi.org/10.1677/JOE-08-0568. Review
47. Walsh NC, Crotti TN, Goldring SR, Gravallese EM. Rheumatic diseases: the effects of inflammation on bone. Immunol Rev. 2005;208:228–51.
48. Lorenzo J, Horowitz M, Choi Y. Osteoimmunology: interactions of the bone and immune system. Endocr Rev. 2008;29(4):403–40.
49. Kong YY, Feige U, Sarosi I, et al. Activated T cells regulate bone loss and joint destruction in adjuvant arthritis through osteoprotegerin ligand. Nature. 1999;402:304–9.
50. Gravallese EM, Manning C, Tsay A, et al. Synovial tissue in rheumatoid arthritis is a source of osteoclast differentiation factor. Arthritis Rheum. 2000;43:250–8.
51. Kotake S, Udagawa N, Hakoda M, et al. 1 activated human T cells directly induce osteoclastogenesis from human monocytes: possible role of T cells in bone destruction in rheumatoid arthritis patients. Arthritis Rheum. 2004;4:1003–12.
52. Sato K, Suematsu A, Okamoto K, et al. Th17 functions as an osteoclastogenic helper T cell subset that links T cell activation and bone destruction. J Exp Med. 2006;203:2673–82.
53. Lundy SK, Sarkar S, Tesmer LA, Fox DA. Cells of the synovium in rheumatoid arthritis. T lymphocytes. Arthritis Res Ther. 2007;9(1):202.
54. Diarra D, Stolina M, Polzer K, et al. Dickkopf-1 is a master regulator of joint remodeling. Nat Med. 2007;13:156–63.
55. Johnson ML, Harnish K, Nusse R, Van HW. LRP5 and Wnt signaling: a union made for bone. J Bone Miner Res. 2004;19:1749–57.
56. Westendorf JJ, Kahler RA, Schroeder TM. Wnt signaling in osteoblasts and bone diseases. Gene. 2004;341:19–39.
57. Morvan F, Boulukos K, Clement-Lacroix P, et al. Deletion of a single allele of the Dkk1 gene leads to an increase in bone formation and bone mass. J Bone Miner Res. 2006;21:934–45.
58. Tian E, Zhan F, Walker R, Rasmussen E, et al. The role of the Wnt-signaling antagonist DKK1 in the development of osteolytic lesions in multiple myeloma. N Engl J Med. 2003;349:2483–94.
59. Tomlinson JW, Walker EA, Bujalska IJ, Draper N, et al. 11b-hydroxysteroid dehydrogenase type 1: a tissue-specific regulator of glucocorticoid response. Endocr Rev. 2004;25:831–66.
60. Cooper MS, Walker EA, Bland R, Fraser WD, et al. Expression and functional consequences of 11b-hydroxysteroid dehydrogenase activity in human bone. Bone. 2000;27:375–81.
61. Rabbitt E, Lavery GG, Walker EA, Cooper MS, et al. Pre-receptor regulation of glucocorticoid action by 11b-hydroxysteroid dehydrogenase: a novel determinant of cell proliferation. FASEB J. 2002;16:36–44.
62. Cooper MS, Bujalska I, Rabbitt E, Walker EA, et al. Modulation of 11b-hydroxysteroid dehydrogenase isozymes by proinflammatory cytokines in osteoblasts: an autocrine switch from glucocorticoid inactivation to activation. J Bone Miner Res. 2001;16:1037–44.
63. Canalis E, Delany AM. 11b-hydroxysteroid dehydrogenase, an amplifier of glucocorticoid action in osteoblasts. J Bone Miner Res. 2002;17:987–90.
64. Cooper MS. Sensitivity of bone to glucocorticoids. Clin Sci. 2004;107:111–23.
65. Carmeliet G, Bouillon R. The effect of microgravity on morphology and gene expression of osteoblasts in vitro. FASEB J. 1999:13 S129–34.

66. Bonewald LF, Johnson ML. Osteocytes, Mechanosensing and Wnt signaling. Bone. 2008;42:606–15.
67. Armstrong VJ, Muzylak M, Sunters A, Zaman G, et al. Wnt/beta-catenin signaling is a component of osteoblastic bone cell early responses to load-bearing and requires estrogen receptor alpha. J Biol Chem. 2007;282:20715–27.
68. Manolagas SC, Weinstein RS, Bellido T, Bodenner DL. Opposite effects of estrogen on the life span of osteoblasts/osteocytes versus osteoclasts in vivo and in vitro An explanation of the imbalance between formation and resorption in estrogen deficiency. Journal Of Bone & Mineral Research. 1999;14(suppl. 1):S169.
69. Canalis E, Mazziotti G, Giustina A, Bilezikian JP. Glucocorticoid-induced osteoporosis: pathophysiology and therapy. Osteoporos Int. 2007;18(10):1319–28. Epub 2007 Jun 14. Review
70. Weinstein RS, Jilka RL, Parfitt AM, Manolagas SC. Inhibition of osteoblastogenesis and promotion of apoptosis of osteoblasts and osteocytes by glucocorticoids. Potential mechanisms of their deleterious effects on bone. J Clin Invest. 1998;102:274–82.
71. den Uyl D, Bultink IE, Lems WF. Advances in glucocorticoid-induced osteoporosis. Curr Rheumatol Rep. 2011;13(3):233–40. https://doi.org/10.1007/s11926-011-0173-y. Review
72. O'Brien CA, Jia D, Plotkin LI, et al. Glucocorticoids act directly on osteoblasts and osteocytes to induce their apoptosis and reduce bone formation and strength. Endocrinology. 2004;145:1835–41.
73. Liu Y, Porta A, Peng X, et al. Prevention of glucocorticoid-induced apoptosis in osteocytes and osteoblasts by calbindin-D28k. J Bone Miner Res. 2004;19:479–90.
74. Ohnaka K, Tanabe M, Kawate H, Nawata H, et al. Glucocorticoid suppresses the canonical Wnt signal in cultured human osteoblasts. Biochem Biophys Res Commun. 2005;329:177–81.
75. Wang FS, Ko JY, Yeh DW, Ke HC, et al. Modulation of Dickkopf-1 attenuates glucocorticoid induction of osteoblast apoptosis, adipocytic differentiation, and bone mass loss. Endocrinology. 2008;149:1793–801.
76. Pereira RC, Delany AM, Canalis E. Effects of cortisol and bone morphogenetic protein-2 on stromal cell differentiation: correlation with CCAAT-enhancer binding protein expression. Bone. 2002;30:685–91.
77. Shi XM, Blair HC, Yang X, McDonald JM, et al. Tandem repeat of C/EBP binding sites mediates PPARgamma2 gene transcription in glucocorticoid-induced adipocyte differentiation. J Cell Biochem. 2000;76:518–27.
78. Carcamo-Orive I, aztelumendi A, Delgado J, et al. Regulation of human bone marrow stromal cell proliferation and differentiation capacity by glucocorticoid receptor and AP-1 crosstalk. J Bone Miner Res. 2010;25:2115–25.
79. Natsui K, Tanaka K, Suda M, et al. High-dose glucocorticoid treatment induces rapid loss of trabecular bone mineral density and lean body mass. Osteoporos Int. 2006;17:105–8.
80. Kanis JA. Diagnosis of osteoporosis and assessment of fracture risk. Lancet. 2002;359:1929–36.
81. Van Der Heijde DMFM. Joint erosions and patients with early rheumatoid arthritis. Br J Rheumatol. 1995;34(Suppl. 2):74–8.
82. McQueen FM, Stewart N, Crabbe J, et al. Magnetic resonance imaging of the wrist in early rheumatoid arthritis reveals a high prevalence of erosions at four months after symptom onset. Ann Rheum Dis. 1998;57:350–6.
83. McGonagle D, Conaghan PG, O'Connor P, et al. The relationship between synovitis and bone changes in early untreated rheumatoid arthritis: a controlled magnetic resonance imaging study. Arthritis Rheum. 1999;42:1706–11.
84. Boyle WJ, Simonet WS, Lacey DL. Osteoclast differentiation and activation. Nature. 2003;423:337–42.
85. Vosse D, de Vlam K. Osteoporosis in rheumatoid arthritis and ankylosing spondylitis. Clin Exp Rheumatol. 2009;27(4 Suppl 55):S62–7.
86. Romas E, Bakharevski O, Hards DK, Kartsogiannis V, et al. Expression of osteoclast differentiation factor at sites of bone erosion in collagen-induced arthritis. Arthritis Rheum. 2000;43:821–6.
87. Leisen JCC, Duncan H, Riddle JM, Pitchford WC. The erosive front: a topographic study of the junction between the pannus and the subchondral plate in the macerated rheumatoid metacarpal head. J Rheumatol. 1988;15:17–22.
88. Geusens PP, Lems WF. Osteoimmunology and osteoporosis. Arthritis Res Ther. 2011;13(5):242. Epub. This is a large overview on osteoimmunology in rheumatic diseases
89. Schett G, Saag KG, Bijlsma JWJ. From bone biology to clinical outcome: state of the art and future perspectives. Ann Rheum Dis. 2010;69:1415–9. This is an outstanding state-of-the-art article on bone biology
90. Rachner TD, Khosla S, Hofbauer LC. Osteoporosis: now and the future. Lancet. 2011;377:1276–87.
91. Lories RJ, Luyten FP"O. Wnt antagonists: for better or worse? Nat Rev Rheumatol. 2009;5:420–1.
92. Terpos E, Fragidaki K, Konsta M, et al. Early effects of Il-6 receptor inhibition on bone homeostasis. Clin Exp Rheumatol. 2011;29:921–5.
93. Cohen SB, Dore RK, Lane NE, et al. Denosumab treatment effects on structural damage, bone mineral density, and bone turnover in rheumatoid arthritis: a twelvemonth, multicenter, randomized, double blind, placebo-controlled, phase II clinical trial. Arthritis Rheum. 2008;58:1299–309.
94. Vis M, Havaardsholm EA, Haugeberg G, et al. Evaluation of bone mineral density, bone metabolism, osteoprotegerin and receptor activator of the NF kappa B ligand serum levels during treatment with infliximab in patients with rheumatoid arthritis. Ann Rheum Dis. 2006;65:1495–9.

95. Mawatari T, Miura H, Hamai S, et al. Vertebral strength changes in rheumatoid arthritis patients treated with alendronate, as assessed by finite element analysis of clinical computed tomography scans: a prospective randomized clinical trial. Arthritis Rheum. 2008;58:3340–9.
96. Bultink IE. Osteoporosis and fractures in systemic lupus erythematosus. Arthritis Care Res. 2012;1:2–8. This is an outstanding overview on the multifactorial pathogenesis of osteoporosis and fractures in SLE
97. Borba VZ, Vieira JG, Kasamatsu T, et al. Vitamin D deficiency in patients with active systemic lupus erythematosus. Osteoporos Int. 2009;20:427–33.
98. Huisman AM, White KP, Algra A, et al. Vitamin D levels in women with systemic lupus erythematosus and fibromyalgia. J Rheumatol. 2001;28:2535–9.
99. Toloza SM, Cole DE, Gladman DD, et al. Vitamin D insufficiency in a large female SLE cohort. Lupus. 2010;19:13–9.
100. Ruiz-Irastorza G, Egurbide MV, Olivares N, et al. Vitamin D deficiency in systemic lupus erythematosus: prevalence, predictors and clinical consequences. Rheumatology (Oxford). 2008;47:920–3.
101. Formiga F, Moga I, Nolla JM, et al. The association of dehydroepiandrosterone sulphate levels with bone mineral density in systemic lupus erythematosus. Clin Exp Rheumatol. 1997;15:387–92.
102. Lee C, Ramsey-Goldman R. Bone health and systemic lupus erythematosus. Curr Rheumatol Rep. 2005;7:482–9.
103. Svenungsson E, Fei GZ, Jensen-Urstad K, et al. TNF-α: a link between hypertriglyceridaemia and inflammation in SLE patients with cardiovascular disease. Lupus. 2003;12:454–61.
104. Frostegard J, Svenungsson E, Wu R, et al. Lipid peroxidation is enhanced in patients with systemic lupus erythematosus and is associated with arterial and renal disease manifestations. Arthritis Rheum. 2005;52:192–200.
105. Moerman EJ, Teng K, Lipschitz DA, et al. Aging activates adipogenic and suppresses osteogenic programs in mesenchymal marrow stroma/stem cells: the role of PPAR-γ2 transcription factor and TGF-β/BMP signaling pathways. Aging Cell. 2004;3:379–89.
106. McLean RR, et al. Homocysteine as a predictive factor for hip fracture in older persons. N Engl J Med. 2004;350:2042–9.
107. Yesilova Z, et al. Hyperhomocysteinemia in patients with Behcet's disease: is it due to inflammation or therapy? Rheumatol Int. 2005;25:423–8.
108. Lakshminarayanan S, Walsh S, Mohanraj M, et al. Factors associated with low bone mineral density in female patients with systemic lupus erythematosus. J Rheumatol. 2001;28:102–8.
109. Almehed K, Forsblad DH, Kvist G, et al. Prevalence and risk factors of osteoporosis in female SLE patients: extended report. Rheumatology (Oxford). 2007;46:1185–90.
110. Mendoza-Pinto C, Garcia-Carrasco M, Sandoval-Cruz H, et al. Risk factors of vertebral fractures in women with systemic lupus erythematosus. Clin Rheumatol. 2009;28:579–85.
111. Lee C, Almagor O, Dunlop DD, et al. Disease damage and low bone mineral density: an analysis of women with systemic lupus erythematosus ever and never receiving corticosteroids. Rheumatology (Oxford). 2006;45:53–60.
112. Petri M. Musculoskeletal complications of systemic lupus erythematosus in the Hopkins lupus cohort: an update. Arthritis Care Res. 1995;8:137–45.
113. Kamen D, Aranow C. Vitamin D in systemic lupus erythematosus. Curr Opin Rheumatol. 2008;20:532–7.
114. Hollis BW, Wagner CL. Assessment of dietary vitamin D requirements during pregnancy and lactation. Am J Clin Nutr. 2004;79(5):717–26.
115. Kamen DL. Vitamin D in lupus - new kid on the block? Bull NYU Hosp Jt Dis. 2010;68(3):218–22. Review
116. Lane NE. Therapy Insight: Osteoporosis and osteonecrosis in systemic lupus erythematosus. Nat Clin Pract Rheumatol. 2006;2(10):562–9. Review
117. Cooper C, Carbone L, Michet CJ, et al. Fracture risk in patients with AS: a population based study. J Rheumatol. 1994;10:1887–2.
118. Vosse D, Landewé R, van der Heijde D, et al. AS and the risk of fracture: results from a large primary care based nested case–control study. Ann Rheum Dis. 2009;68:1839–42.
119. Vosse D, Feldtkeller E, Erlendsson, et al. Clinical vertebral fractures in patients with Ankylosing spondylitis. J Rheumatol. 2004;10:1981–5.
120. Ralston SH, Urquhart GDK, Brzeski M, Sturrock RD. Prevalence of vertebral compression fractures due to osteoporosis in ankylosing spondylitis. BMJ. 1990;300:563–5.
121. Mitra D, Elvins DM, Speden DJ, Collins AJ. The prevalence of vertebral fractures in mild ankylosing spondylitis and their relationship to bone mineral density. Rheumatology. 2000;39:85–9.
122. Nguyen HV, Ludwig S, Gelb D. Osteoporotic vertebral burst fractures with neurologic compromise. J Spin Dis Techn. 2003;16:10–9.
123. Voss D, Van Der Heijde DM, Landewe R, et al. Determinants of hyperkyphosis in patients with Ankylosing spondylitis. Ann Rheum Dis. 2006;65:770–4.
124. Bessant R, Keat A. How should clinicians manage osteoporosis in ankylosing spondylitis? J Rheumatol. 2002;29:1511–9.
125. Gran JT, Husby G. Clinical, epidemiological, and therapeutic aspects of ankylosing spondylitis. Curr Opin Rheumatol. 1998;10:292–8.
126. Gillespie LD, Gillespie WJ, Robertson MC, Lamb SE, et al. Interventions for preventing falls in elderly people. Cochrane Database Syst Rev. 2003;4:CD000340.
127. Wolf SL, Sattin RW Kutner M, O'Grady M, Greenspan AI, et al. Intense tai chi exercise training and fall occurrences in older, transitionally frail adults: a randomized, controlled trial. J Am Geriatr Soc. 2003;51:1693–701.

128. Orwoll E, Ettinger M, Weiss S, Miller P, et al. Alendronate for the treatment of osteoporosis in men. N Engl J Med. 2000;343:604–10.
129. Ringe JD, Faber H, Farahmand P, Dorst A. Efficacy of risedronate in men with primary and secondary osteoporosis\: results of a 1-year study. Rheumatol Int. 2006;26:427–31.
130. Kaufman JM, Orwoll E, Goemaere S, San Martin S, et al. Teriparatide effects on vertebral fractures and bone mineral density in men with osteoporosis: treatment and discontinuation of therapy. Osteoporos Int. 2005;16:510–6.
131. LoCascio V, Bonucci E, Imbimbo B, et al. Bone loss in response to long-term glucocorticoid therapy. Bone Miner. 1990;8:39–51.
132. Reid DM, Devogelaer JP, Saag K, et al. Zoledronic acid and risedronate in the prevention and treatment of glucocorticoid-induced osteoporosis (HORIZON): a multicentre, double-blind, double-dummy, randomised controlled trial. Lancet. 2009;373:1253–63.
133. van Staa TP, Laan RF, Barton IP, et al. Bone density threshold and other predictors of vertebral fracture in patients receiving oral glucocorticoid therapy. Arth Rheum. 2003;48:3224–9.
134. van Staa TP, Geusens P, Pols HA, de Laet C, et al. A simple score for estimating the long-term risk of fracture in patients using oral glucocorticoids. QJM. 2005;98:191–8.
135. De Vries F, Bracke M, Leufkens HG, et al. Fracture risk with intermittent high-dose oral glucocorticoid therapy. Arthritis Rheum. 2007;56:208–14.
136. American College of Rheumatology Ad Hoc Committee on Glucocorticoid-Induced Osteoporosis. Recommendations for the prevention and treatment of glucocorticoid-induced osteoporosis: 2001 update. Arthritis Rheum 2001;44:1496–1503.
137. Grossman JM, Gordon R, Ranganath VK, Deal C, et al. American College of rheumatology 2010 recommendations for the prevention and treatment of glucocorticoid-induced osteoporosis. Arthritis Care Res (Hoboken). 2010;62(11):1515–26. https://doi.org/10.1002/acr.20295. *Epub* 2010 Jul 26. Review. Erratum in: Arthritis Care Res (Hoboken). 2012 Mar;64(3):464. PubMed PMID: 20662044].
138. Buckley L, Guyatt G, Fink HA, et al. American College of Rheumatology Guideline for the Prevention and Treatment of Glucocorticoid-Induced Osteoporosis. Arthritis Rheumatol. 2017;69(8):1521–1537. https://doi.org/10.1002/art.40137. Epub 2017 Jun 6. Erratum in: Arthritis Rheumatol. 2017;69(11):2246. PMID: 28585373.
139. Assessment of fracture risk and its application to screening for postmenopausal osteoporosis. Report of a WHO Study Group. Geneva, World Health Organization, 1994 (WHO Technical Report Series, No. 843).
140. FRAX: (https://www.shef.ac.uk/FRAX/tool.jsp).
141. Ross AC, Manson JE, Abrams SA, Aloia JF, Brannon PM, Clinton SK, et al. The 2011 report on dietary reference intakes for calcium and vitamin D from the Institute of Medicine: what clinicians need to know. J Clin Endocrinol Metab 2011;96:53–8.
142. Weinstein RS. "Clinical Practice: Glucocorticoid-induced bone disease". N Engl J Med. 2011;365:62–70. [PubMed: 21732837].
143. Weinstein RS, Jilka RJ, Roberson PK, et al. "Intermittent parathyroid hormone administration prevents glucocorticoid-induced osteoblast and osteocyte apoptosis, decreased bone formation, and reduced bone strength in mice". Endocrinol. 2010;151:2641–649.
144. Cummings SR, San Martin J, McClung MR, et al. Denosumab for prevention of fractures in postmenopausal women with osteoporosis. N Engl J Med. 2009;361:756–65. [PubMed: 19671655].
145. Dore RK, Cohen SB, Lane NE, et al. Effects of denosumab on bone mineral density and bone turnover in patients with rheumatoid arthritis receiving concurrent glucocorticoids or bisphosphonates. Ann Rheum Dis. 2010;69:872–5.
146. Saag KG, Wagman RB, Geusens P, et al. Denosumab versus risedronate in glucocorticoid-induced osteoporosis: a multicentre, randomised, double-blind, active-controlled, double-dummy, non-inferiority study. Lancet Diabetes Endocrinol. 2018;6:445–54.

11

Rheumatic Diseases and Fever

Mohamed Cheikh and Nezar Bahabri

11.1 Introduction

In all the patients with rheumatic diseases, fever should prompt an immediate and thorough evaluation. There are different disorders that can cause fever and arthritis. Fever that is thought to be due to active rheumatic disease is seen in over 50% of patients with SLE30. However, it can be also related to or a sequel of an infectious process. There are many infectious diseases with rheumatological manifestations. The aim of this chapter therefore is to address variable relationships of fever with patients with arthritis. Fever of unknown origin will be addressed as some systemic rheumatic disease may present with fever. It is always a dilemma when an established patient with arthritis presents with fever. What should you do? This issue is addressed with a suggested diagnostic approach that guides you in a stepwise manner until you reach to the definitive diagnosis.

A quick review of rheumatological manifestations of some infections is presented. This is to widen your knowledge about this area in medicine and not to ignore common viruses, for example, in your differential diagnosis of fever and arthritis. Vaccination is quite an ignored aspect of clinical practice among patients with arthritis.

The objective of this chapter is to provide a systemic approach to patient with fever and arthritis.

Specific objectives:

By the end of the chapter the reader should be able to:

- Approach a patient with fever of unknown origin.
- Approach a patient with known rheumatological disease presenting with fever and recognize the common infections that affect immunocompromised patients.
- Recognize the rheumatological manifestations of common infectious diseases.
- Provide a safe and proper method of vaccinations to patients with rheumatological disease.

M. Cheikh (✉) · N. Bahabri
Doctor Soliman Fakeeh Hospital,
Jeddah, Saudi Arabia
e-mail: Mohamed.m.cheikh@gmail.com

11.2 Fever of Unknown Origin (FUO)

11.2.1 Definition [28]

- Temp >38.3 on several occasions.
- Duration ≥3 weeks.
- No clear diagnosis after 1 week of in-hospital investigation.

11.2.2 Epidemiology

The epidemiology of FUO has changed over time due to scientific and technologic advances (better imaging, more advanced organism isolation, and more understanding of connective tissue disease). A prospective multicenter study on fever of unknown origin showed the following distribution: connective tissue diseases 22%, infection 16%, malignancy 7%, miscellaneous 4%, no diagnosis 51%.

Box 11.1 Initial evaluation for FUO

- Comprehensive History (Table 11.2)
- Detailed Physical examination (Table 11.2)
- CBC with differential & Blood film
- U&E–LFTs–LDH–ESR - CRP
- hepatitis A, B, and C serologies if LFTs are abnormal
- Blood cultures (X3 - different sites - several hours between each set - off antibiotics)
- HIV antibody assay and HIV viral load for patients at high risk
- Urinalysis + microscopic examination + urine culture
- CXR

Epidemiology: Table 11.1 shows the etiologies of FUO.

11.2.3 General Principles in the Treatment of FUO (Table 11.2)

Physician should explain to the patient that FUO is a well-known entity, and it needs time for investigation to decrease anxiety of the patient. Empiric therapy with antimicrobial or glucocorticoids *should not* be given to stable patients with FUO because it often obscure or delay the diagnosis [29]:

- The diagnostic yield of some investigation like cultures will be reduced after starting antimicrobial.
- Empiric treatment of a certain infection can affect other infection (e.g., therapeutic trial for tuberculosis with rifampicin may suppress staphylococcal osteomyelitis or diminish the ability to detect difficult to isolate organisms causing endocarditis.
- The duration of a therapeutic trial is also unclear.
- Initiation of glucocorticoid without rolling out infection can lead to severe life-threatening infections.

There are some exceptions where patient with FUO should be treated empirically. The exceptions are:

1. Septic or hemodynamically unstable patient → empirical treatment.
2. Immunocompromised or neutropenic patient→ empirical treatment.
3. Query giant cell arteritis → treat with corticosteroids until biopsy result → risk of visual loss.

Figure 11.1 shows a suggested algorithm to approach a patient with FUO.

Table 11.1 Etiologies of FUO [1–27]

Infection	• **Tuberculosis**: *require high clinical suspicion as patient can have normal PPD or interferon gamma release assay and may require biopsy to yield diagnosis.* • **Abscesses**: *Intra-abdominal, pelvic, dental, or paraspinal.* • **Osteomyelitis**: *some sites can have no localized symptoms like vertebral and mandibular osteomyelitis.* • **Endocarditis**: *consider culture negative organism→ HACK, Coxiella, Bartonella, T. whipplei, Brucella, Mycoplasma, Chlamydia, Histoplasma, and Legionella.* • Other causes: **Brucellosis**, **HIV**, *sinusitis, CMV, EBV, secondary syphilis, Lyme disease, prostatitis, visceral leishmaniasis, Q fever, leptospirosis, psittacosis, tularemia, melioidosis, disseminated gonococcemia, chronic meningococcemia, Whipple's disease, and yersiniosis.*
Connective tissue disease	• **Adult Still's disease**: *evanescent rash, arthritis, lymphadenopathy, and high ferritin.* • **Giant cell arteritis:** >50y, *headache, scalp pain, visual disturbances, myalgias, arthralgias, high ESR.* • Other: *polyarteritis nodosa, granulomatosis with polyangiitis, RA, SLE, psoriatic or reactive arthritis, PMR, Takayasu's arteritis, mixed cryoglobulinemia.*
Malignancy	• Lymphoma (especially non-Hodgkin's). • Leukemia. • Myelodysplasia. • Renal cell carcinoma (*increase HCT, microscopic hematuria*). • Hepatocellular carcinoma or other tumors metastatic to the liver. • Multiple myeloma. • Pancreatic and colon cancers, sarcomas, mastocytosis. • Atrial myxomas (*arthralgias, emboli, and hypergammaglobulinemia*).
Miscellaneous	• Drug-induced fever. • DVT/PE. • Hematoma. • Thyroid storm, thyroiditis, adrenal insufficiency, pheochromocytoma. • Sarcoidosis. • Alcohol or granulomatous hepatitis. • Hereditary periodic fever syndromes: FMF, TRAPS, hyper-IgD syndrome, muckle-Wells syndrome, and familial cold autoinflammatory syndrome.

Table 11.2 Initial evaluation for FUO

History	Physical examination
Carefl and through history including: • Any localizing symptoms. • Travel Hx (TB, malaria, hepatitis, typhoid fever, parasitic infections, Rocky Mountain spotted fever, or Lyme disease). • Exposure to TB patient. • Unpasteurized milk and cheese, • Animal and insect exposure. • Immunosuppression (medication or diseases). • Sexual contacts. • New unusual activity. • Drug and toxin history including alcohol, illicit drug use, over-the-counter medications and recent antimicrobial. • Ethnic background.	Complete physical examination including: • Skin, mucous membranes, and lymphatic system. • Abdominal palpation for masses or organomegaly. • Joint examination and the back → Pott's disease. • Heart auscultation → new murmur (infective endocarditis). • Sinuses. • Prostate examination.

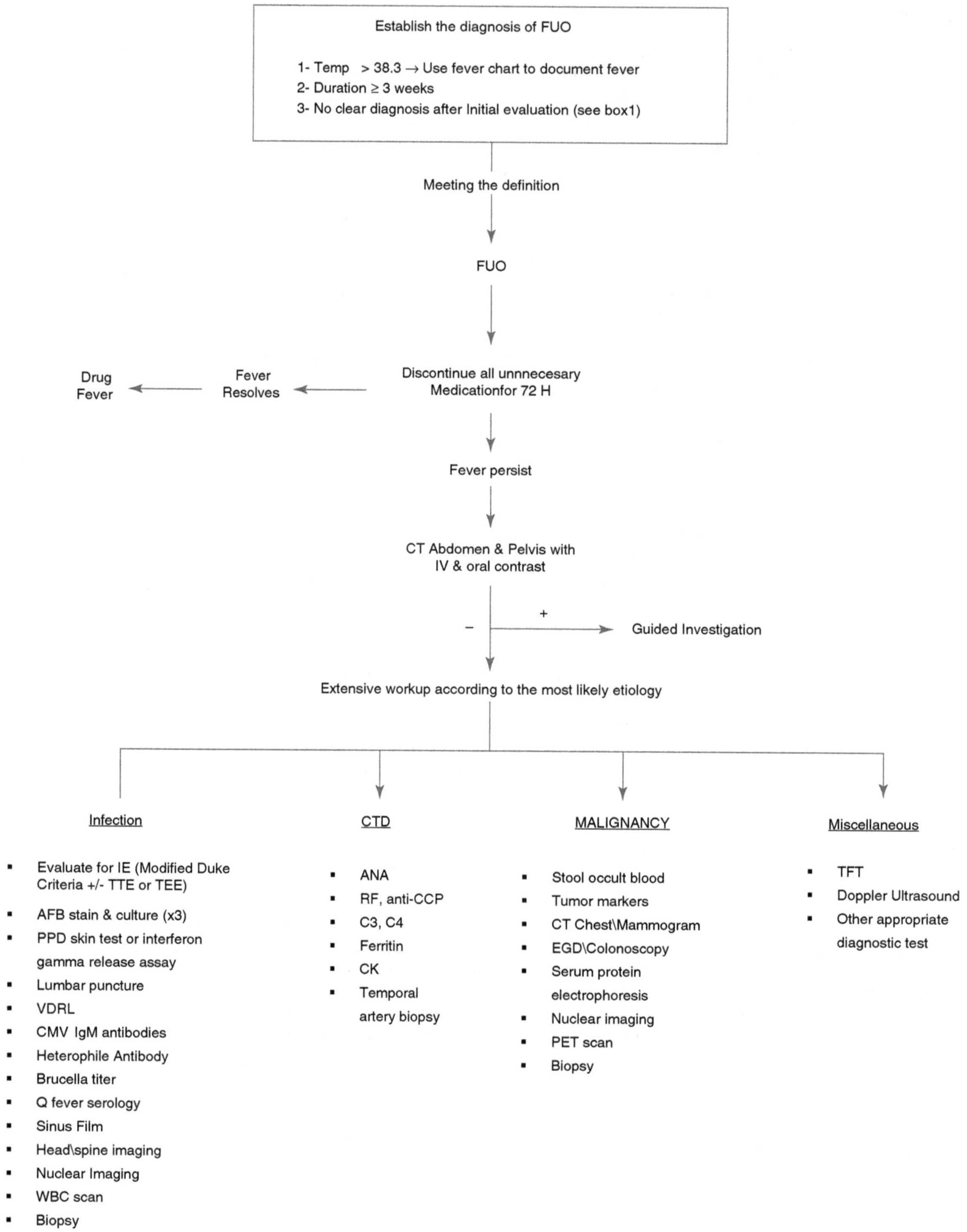

Fig. 11.1 Suggested algorithm to approach patient with FUO

11.2.4 Tips in FUO

- Think of uncommon presentations of common diseases rather than thinking of uncommon diseases.
- <40 Y → infection > rheumatological > malignancy.
- >40 Y → Infection > Malignancy > Rheumatological.
- Rheumatological disease usually present in stable condition.
- Empirical treatment not recommended unless there is an indication.
- If empiric treatment is a must avoid quinolone (TB resistance).
- Chills, rigors, night sweat (infection > rheumatological).
- Most of undiagnosed cases of FUO are related to viruses that we don't usually investigate.
- Viral infections can give a temperature up to 40–41 °C and can persist up to 3 weeks (average 9 days).

11.3 Fever and Rheumatology

11.3.1 Introduction

Approach to fever is a very challenging in a patient with rheumatic disease as it could be an infection, disease activity, or medication side effect. Fever that is thought to be due to active disease is seen in over 50% of patients with SLE [30]. On the other hand, fever is a rare presentation of RA disease activity. Infections are often difficult to diagnose and treat in this group of patient because of the following reasons:

1. Clinical manifestations of infections are often indistinguishable from the underlying disease and vice versa [52–55].
2. The typical signs and symptoms of infection may be absent because of concomitant immunosuppressive therapies [56–58].
3. The anti-inflammatory and antipyretic effects of glucocorticoids may diminish the usual systemic and localizing signs of infection.
4. With the immunosuppressive impact of the medication and the disease itself, the spectrum of potential pathogens is large, making empiric treatment difficult.

In patient with rheumatoid arthritis, bone and joints, skin, soft tissues, and the respiratory tract are the most frequently involved sites in infectious processes [33]. In patients with chronic inflammatory rheumatic or autoimmune diseases without arthritis, infections of the respiratory tract are the most common site. **Finally, ascribing fever to the underlying rheumatological disease itself in an immunosuppressed patient should be done only after reasonable and good efforts have been made to exclude infection.** Figure 11.2 shows suggested algorithm to approach a patient with rheumatic disorder presenting with fever.

Risk factors for infection in a patient with rheumatic disease include:

- Active disease.
- Long-term disease damage.
- Neutropenia.
- Lymphopenia.
- Hypocomplementemia.
- Renal involvement.
- Neuropsychiatric manifestations.
- Use of glucocorticoids and other immunosuppressive drugs.
- Arthrocentesis [23].

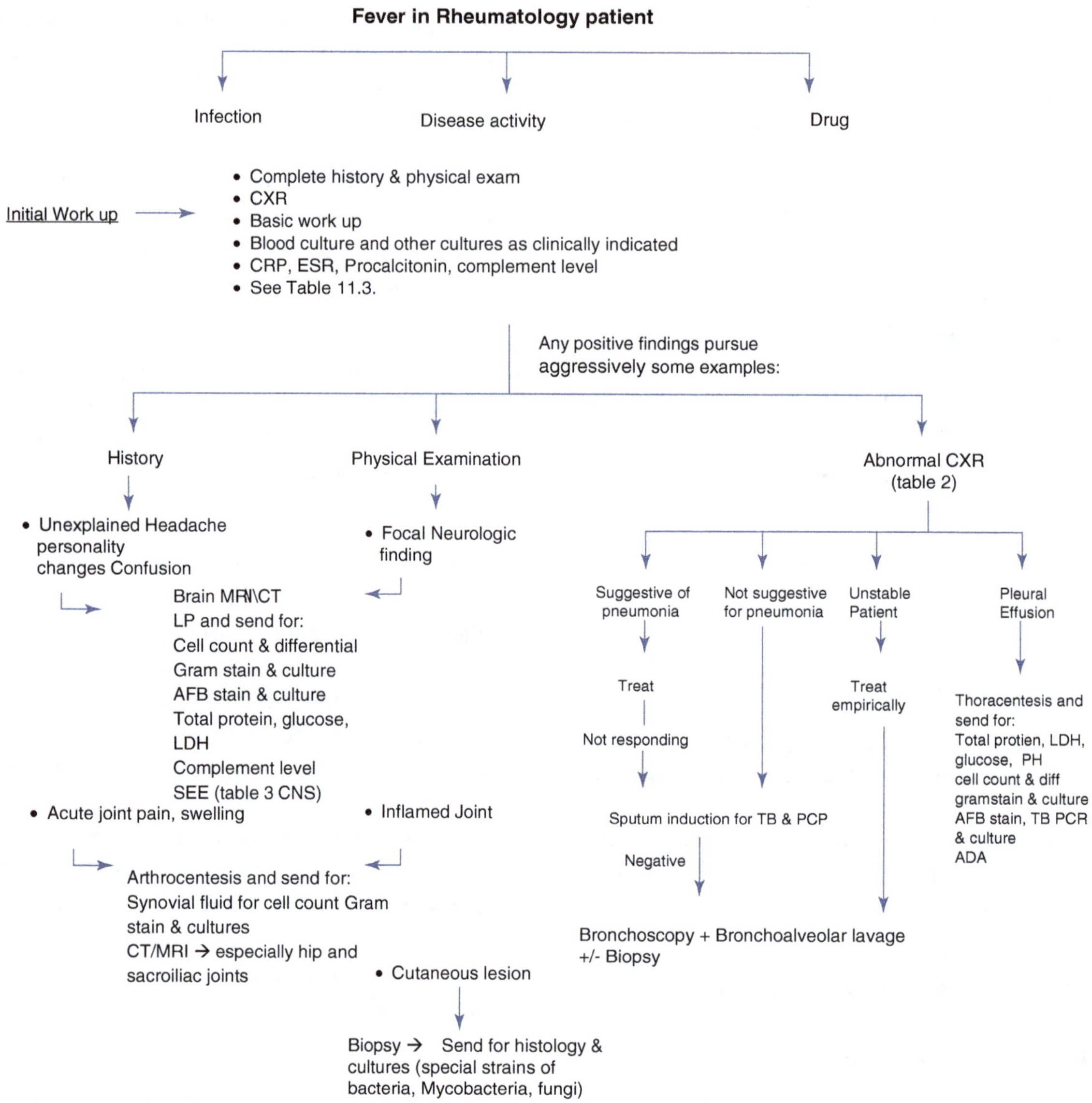

Fig. 11.2 Suggested algorithm to approach a patient with rheumatic disorder presenting with fever

Points to consider in the approach to this group of patients:

- Respiratory viral infections are the most common cause of fever in rheumatological patient as non-rheumatological patient.
- There is no single clinical or laboratory finding that can differentiate between infection, disease activity, or drug-induced insult as a cause of fever. It is rather a collective clinical and laboratory finding with good clinical judgment.
- One of the crucial points in determining the cause of fever is to know the patient's disease activity statues prior to presentation and if he is on immunosuppressive therapy or no.
- Both the patient's underlying rheumatic disease and its therapy need to be taken into con-

sideration when evaluating the white blood cell count in a febrile immunosuppressed patient because:
  - Glucocorticoids therapy can cause a neutrophilic leukocytosis.
  - Cytotoxic drug therapy can impair a patient's ability to mount a neutrophilic leukocytosis in response to infection.
  - Neutrophilic leukocytosis may be a manifestation of certain rheumatic diseases, such as active granulomatosis with polyangiitis [101].

- Recent systemic review and meta-analysis for the utility of procalcitonin as a diagnostic marker for bacterial infection in patients with autoimmune disease showed that:
  - Procalcitonin has higher diagnostic value than CRP for the detection of bacterial sepsis in patients with autoimmune disease, and the test for procalcitonin is more specific than sensitive 32.
  - Procalcitonin test is not recommended to be used in isolation as a rule-out tool 32.

11.4 Fever in Rheumatology Patient

11.4.1 History

Careful and through history including:

- Medication history → immunosuppressed (type and for how long)→ suspect new infection, particular if other signs of active disease have begun to remit.
- Onset of symptoms → few days → infection.
- Days to weeks → disease activity/opportunistic infection
- Fever pattern → episodic → disease activity/infection.
- Sustained → drug/CNS involvement
- Shaking chills occurred in significantly more patients with proven infections (68% versus 27% non-infectious).
- Contact with children (viral infection).
- Recent travel and exposure to TB.
- Vaccination history.

11.4.2 Physical Examination (Table 11.3)

Complete physical examination includes:

- Oral mucosal candidiasis →significant immunodeficiency → increased risk of opportunistic infections, such as PCP [36].
- Erythematous necrotic cutaneous lesions→? Gram-negative sepsis, in particular *P. aeruginosa*.
- Cutaneous vesicular rash → varicella.
- Pulmonary infiltrates + cutaneous lesions→? Disseminated histoplasmosis, *Cryptococcus*, and nocardiosis (Table 11.4).
- Pulmonary infiltrates + focal neurologic deficits→? Disseminated infection with mycobacteria, fungi (C. *neoformans*, *Aspergillus* spp.), or *Nocardia* spp. (Table 11.5).
- A detailed neurologic examination should be performed and repeated frequently to monitor the patient's progress.
- Each patient should undergo a careful ophthalmologic examination looking for papilledema, signs of retinal and choroid infection (e.g., cryptococcosis, toxoplasmosis), and proptosis (suggestive of orbital infection or cavernous sinus involvement).
- Parotid gland enlargement → mumps.

[39–57, 59–99].

Table 11.3 Possible pathogens by the predominant immune system defect caused by pharmacological agent used in the treatment of rheumatic disease [37–38]

Abnormality	Agent	Infection	
Qualitative defect of phagocytic function Or neutropenia	Corticosteroids Cyclophosphamide and other alkylating agents Azathioprine	Bacterial	**Gram positive** Coag (−) staph, *Staphylococcus aureus*, *Streptococcal* spp., *Corynebacterium* spp., *Bacillus* spp., *Nocardia* spp.
			Gram negative *Escherichia coli*, *Klebsiella pneumoniae*, *Pseudomonas aeruginosa*
		Viral	VZV, HSV1&2, CMV
		Fungal	*Candida* spp., *Aspergillus* spp.
Defective cell-mediated immunity	Corticosteroids Cyclophosphamide Other alkylating agents Azathioprine Methotrexate Cyclosporine A	Bacterial	*Salmonella* spp., *Campylobacter*, *Listeria*, *Yersinia*, *Legionella*, *Rhodococcus*, *Nocardia*, TB, non-TB *Mycobacterium* spp.
		Viral	CMV, EPV, VZV, HSV, JC virus, BK virus
		Fungal	*Candida*, Histo, crypto, Coccidio, *Aspergillus*, pneumocystis, *Zygomycetes* spp., and other mold
		Parasites	*Toxoplasma*, *Cryptosporidium*, *Isospora*, *Microsporidia*, *Babesia*, *Strongyloides*
Defective humoral immunity and asplenia	Cyclophosphamide Corticosteroids (high dose) Azathioprine	Bacterial	**Encapsulated bacteria:** *Streptococcus pneumoniae* *Haemophilus influenzae* *Neisseria meningitidis* **Other bacteria:** *E. coli* And GNRs
		Viral	VZV, *Echovirus*, *Enterovirus*
		Parasites	*Babesia*, *Giardia*

11.5 Rheumatologic Manifestation of Infectious Diseases

11.5.1 Introduction

Rheumatologic manifestations of infectious diseases are well-recognized and relatively common. This topic will review the most common infectious diseases associated with rheumatologic manifestations. *An overview of each infectious agent is presented separately.*

11.5.1.1 Hepatitis B Virus Arthritis [104]

Evidences have shown that four rheumatologic syndromes are linked with hepatitis B virus infection.

Clinical and laboratory features of each syndrome will be described below.

11.5.1.2 Acute Hepatitis B and Arthritis

The symptoms are abrupt in onset, and they are composed of low-grade fever, a symmetrical polyarthritis which might be additive or migratory in pattern, morning stiffness, and other constitutional symptoms. The most common joints involved are the knees and small joints of the hands, but any peripheral joint might be involved with either arthralgia or frank arthritis. It may last from several days to several months.

11.5.1.3 Chronic Active Hepatitis B

Chronic active hepatitis is linked with joint discomfort and occasional rash. The joints

Table 11.4 Causes of CXR abnormalities in patient with rheumatic disease[a]

Radiographic pattern	Infectious causes	Noninfectious causes
Localized infiltrates	Bacterial pneumonia (including *Legionella* spp.) *Mycobacteria* spp. Opportunistic fungi: *Aspergillus* spp. *Histoplasma capsulatum* *Coccidioides immitis* *Cryptococcus neoformans* *Pneumocystis jiroveci* (*uncommon*)	Granulomatosis with polyangiitis Eosinophilic granulomatosis with polyangiitis Pulmonary embolus
Diffuse infiltrates	*Pneumocystis jiroveci* Bacterial pneumonia (haematogenous spread) *Mycoplasma pneumoniae* *Chlamydia* spp. *Mycobacteria* spp. (miliary pattern) Opportunistic fungi Viral Influenzae Cytomegalovirus Varicella-zoster virus (rare)	Systemic lupus erythematosus Rheumatoid arthritis Microscopic polyangiitis Granulomatosis with polyangiitis Eosinophilic granulomatosis with polyangiitis Scleroderma Sjogren's syndrome Dermatomyositis/polymyositis Pulmonary edema **Drug induced** Methotrexate Cyclophosphamide (rare) Azathioprine (rare)
Nodules or nodular infiltrates	Septic emboli *Staphylococcus aureus* *Pseudomonas aeruginosa* *Mycobacteria* spp. *Nocardia* spp. Opportunistic fungi	Granulomatosis with polyangiitis Eosinophilic granulomatosis with polyangiitis Rheumatoid arthritis Lymphoma

[a]The appearance or progression of pulmonary disease following the initiation or intensification of immunosuppressive therapy should always prompt a thorough evaluation for a possible infectious cause

Table 11.5 Infections in rheumatological patient and most common causes [34, 35, 100, 102, 103, 133–136]

Disease	Causes	Comments
Pneumonia	• Immunocompromised patient are prone to the same pathogens acquired in the community by immunocompetent hosts. • (*S. pneumoniae, S. aureus*, and enteric GNRs) are the most common isolated pathogens • Less common organism. Fungi (*Pneumocystis jirovecii*→most common OI, *Aspergillus* spp., *C. neoformans*, *C. immitis*, and *H. capsulatum*) TB & non-TB mycobacteria *Nocardia* spp. CMV HSV	• Pneumonia is one of the most frequent life-threatening infections in patients with rheumatic diseases. • Pneumonia in immunosuppressed rheumatic patient is a challenging diagnosis because of: 1. Pulmonary manifestations of certain rheumatic diseases and medications used to treat rheumatic diseases may produce many of the same clinical and radiographic abnormalities as pneumonia. 2. The usual radiographic appearance of pulmonary infections can be dramatically altered by immunosuppressive therapy.

(continued)

Table 11.5 (continued)

Disease	Causes			Comments
CNS Involvement	Clinical syndrome	Infectious causes	Non-infectious causes	• CNS involvement occurs in many rheumatic diseases, including granulomatosis with polyangiitis, polyarteritis nodosa, Behcet's disease, and most frequently SLE. • Immunosuppressive therapy increases the risk of CNS infections which may be indistinguishable from CNS manifestation of underlying rheumatic disease. • The usual signs and symptoms of life-threatening CNS infection may be greatly diminished or absent because of the effect of immunosuppressive therapy. • In lupus cerebritis, clinical and LP findings are almost similar to bacterial meningitis with the exception of: – Less nick stiffness in lupus cerebritis. – Normal lactic acid level (↑ bacterial). – Decreased C4 level in the CSF.
	Acute meningitis	***Bacterial*** *Listeria monocytogenes* *Streptococcus pneumoniae* *Haemophilus influenzae* *Neisseria meningitides* ***Viral:*** *Enterovirus, HIV, HSV, VZV, CMV, EBV, and others*	NSAIDS Azathioprine IVIG Sarcoid SLE Behcet's disease	
	Sub-acute meningitis	*Cryptococcus neoformans* *Listeria monocytogenes* *Mycobacterium tuberculosis* *Coccidioides immitis* *Strongyloides stercoralis*		
	Focal brain lesion	*Toxoplasma gondii* *Aspergillus* spp. *Nocardia* spp. *Cryptococcus neoformans* *Mycobacterium TB* JC virus (PML)	Lymphoma	
UTI	• Usually caused by gram negative organisms and may be accompanied by septicemia. • *Candida albicans*→ immunosuppressed .			• The incidence of UTI in immunosuppressed patients other than diabetics or renal transplant recipients is not higher than the incidence in immunocompetent individuals. • Neutropenia blunts the clinical manifestations of UTI and predisposes to bacteremia.

Table 11.5 (continued)

<table>
<tr><th>Disease</th><th colspan="3">Causes</th><th>Comments</th></tr>
<tr><td rowspan="6">Skin infection</td><td colspan="3">• Staphylococcus aureus, group A streptococci, and GNR.</td><td rowspan="6"></td></tr>
<tr><td rowspan="2">Neutropenic</td><td colspan="2">Initial infection:
Gram negative and gram positive</td></tr>
<tr><td colspan="2">Subsequent infection:
Antibiotic-resistant bacteria, fungi</td></tr>
<tr><td rowspan="3">Cellular immune deficiency</td><td>Bacterial</td><td>Nocardia spp., atypical mycobacteria</td></tr>
<tr><td>Viral</td><td>VZV, HSV, CMV</td></tr>
<tr><td>Fungal</td><td>Cryptococcus species
Histoplasma species</td></tr>
<tr><td>Septic arthritis</td><td colspan="3">• Staphylococcus aureus (most common), other species Streptococcus pneumoniae, groups B, C, and G Strep, Haemophilus, and gram-negative bacilli.
• Consider →OI such as atypical mycobacteria and Pneumocystis jirovecii immunocompromised host.</td><td>• The risk of septic arthritis in RA patient, irrespective of therapy, is increased by 4–15-fold.
• Diagnosis of septic arthritis in the rheumatoid patient is often delayed.
• Use of anti-TNF therapy in RA is associated with a doubling in the risk of septic arthritis.
• DMARDS can predispose some patients with rheumatoid arthritis to septic arthritis.</td></tr>
<tr><td rowspan="3">Osteomyelitis</td><td>Haematogenous</td><td colspan="2">Usually monomicrobial →
S. aureus (most common), Mycobacteria</td><td rowspan="3"></td></tr>
<tr><td>Contiguous</td><td colspan="2">Polymicrobial or monomicrobial → Staphylococcus aureus, coagulase-negative staphylococci, and (aerobic gram
+ anaerobic GPC and GNR)</td></tr>
<tr><td colspan="3">In immunocompromised patients consider →Aspergillus spp., Candida albicans, Mycobacteria spp., Salmonella spp., or Streptococcus pneumonia</td></tr>
</table>

(continued)

Table 11.5 (continued)

Disease	Causes	Comments
Bacteremia or fungemia	• The presentation and etiology of **bacteremia or fungemia** is similar to that in other patients. • Disseminated Neisseria and non-typhoid *Salmonella* infections are more common in SLE patients.	**Salmonella:** • Can cause serious infections in SLE patients. • Most cases occur during periods of active SLE and may be the presenting illness of SLE. • Although fever at presentation is the rule but 15% to 20% of patients may be afebrile. And most patients are not toxic or septic on admission. • Clinical syndromes include gastroenteritis, arthritis, and pneumonia. Less commonly diagnoses included cellulitis, osteomyelitis, urinary tract infection, or meningitis. **Neisseria:** • Patients are often young sexually active women with renal disease and low C3 and C4 levels. • Arthritis is a common presentation of disseminated *Neisseria* infection and less commonly meningitis and endocarditis.
Viral infection	• Viruses can cause both systemic and organ-specific disease. • The most common viral infections in patients with SLE are parvovirus B19 and CMV. Other herpesviruses are common in immunosuppressed SLE patients. • Viral infection can be easily confused with a lupus flare due to significant overlap in the features induced by acute viral infections (fever, arthralgia, malaise, cutaneous rash, lymphadenopathy, and cytopenia) and those observed in active SLE. • Acute viral infections are not adequately investigated in SLE patients and are only suspected after rolling out other causes of fever. • The differential diagnosis of SLE patients presenting with fever suspected to be of infectious origin should consider not only common bacterial infections but also opportunistic viral infections, especially in patients with severe SLE involvement or those who are on immunosuppressive therapy. This group of patient should have a detailed physical examination, serologic studies, and invasive organ-specific diagnostic procedures to rule out an underlying viral infection.	

Table 11.6 Rheumatic manifestations of hepatitis B virus

	Acute hepatitis B	Chronic active hepatitis B	Polyarteritis nodosa	Mixed cryoglobulinemia
Rheumatic manifestation	Transient symmetrical polyarthritis	Transient asymmetrical arthritis or arthralgia	Symmetrical polyarthritis in 50%	Chronic polyarthralgia, rarely arthritis
Systemic involvement	Evanescent erythematous urticarial or petechial rash	Erythematous rash rarely reported	Peripheral neuropathy, CNS, muscle, liver, skin, intestines, kidneys, and heart	(skin: Purpura, ulceration), kidney, liver and neuropathy
Serum HBs antigen	Present during rheumatic prodrome	Variable	Up to 40%	Rarely present
Serum free antibody to HBs antigen	Present in convalescent phase	Not present	Rarely present	Present in 48%

abnormality usually manifest as arthralgias which have a fleeting nature which have a fleeting nature (Table 11.6).

11.5.1.4 Polyarteritis Nodosa

- The incidence of HBs antigenemia in polyarteritis nodosa is varied based on the criteria used for diagnosis and the sensitivity of the technique used for detection of the HBs antigen.
- Clinically, these patients might present with multisystem involvement of the skin, muscles, nervous system, lungs, and polyarthritis as well as liver disease.

11.5.1.5 Essential Mixed Cryoglobulinemia

It has the following clinical features: non-thrombocytopenic purpura upon exposure to cold, diffuse arthralgia, and generalized weakness and hepatosplenomegaly; rarely it is associated with neuropathy and gangrene.

11.5.2 Hepatitis C Virus Arthritis

Hepatitis C virus (HCV) is associated with many rheumatologic manifestations including those related to joints, muscles, and connective tissue resulting from the body's immune system interaction with the infectious agent antigens with the subsequent immune complex formation that will be deposited in various parts of the body eliciting an inflammatory reaction that damage the involved organs. Patients who are infected with HCV often have no symptoms. Anyone newly diagnosed with arthritis or cryoglobulinemia should be tested for HCV infection. Also, there are certain drugs used in the treatment of HCV infection, e.g., interferon can worsen a related rheumatologic disease.

Arthritis is noted in 2 to 20% of HCV patients [107, 108]. The arthritis takes the form of evanescent rheumatoid-like picture in two-thirds of the cases and an oligoarthritis pattern in the rest. Rheumatologic manifestations include painful joints and muscle and fatigue, "the first and most common complain," and less commonly patients might have joint swelling and vasculitis.

Cryoglobulinemia happens when cryoglobulins (which are abnormal immunoglobulin) precipitate in cold temperature. It may affect the blood vessels specially during cold weather leading to "'Raynaud's phenomenon." [105, 106] The diagnosis of HCV can be made by finding HCV Immunoglobulins or by detecting the virus RNA.

Table 11.7 Rheumatic manifestations of Parvovirus B19 infection

Rheumatologic manifestations	Parvovirus B19 arthropathy	
	Male	Female
	30%	59%
	Children [113]	Adults [112]
	• Occur in about 8%. • Pattern: Asymmetrical or pauciarticular • Joint involved.It affects the knee most often • At times children may meet criteria of juvenile idiopathic arthritis.	• Occur in about 60%. • Many adult have arthritis alone without other symptoms. • Typical pattern. Acute onset symmetrical polyarticular arthritis • Joints involved. Proximal interphalangeal with metacarpophalangeal most commonly

11.5.3 Parvovirus B19 Arthropathy

Parvovirus B19 is the cause of fifth disease "slapped cheeks" or erythema infectiosum. The disease manifests by rash, arthritis/arthralgia, laboratory abnormalities, and other connective tissue diseases like syndrome. It may mimic systemic lupus (SLE) both in children and adults (Table 11.7) [109, 110].

Arthritis/arthralgia may accompany or follow the skin eruption. The rheumatologic symptoms may persist for weeks to rarely months with resolution, but recurrences are reported [111, 112].

The diagnosis of acute parvovirus infection is made by finding IgM antibody, while IgG antibody is evidence of preexisting exposure. Acute phase reactant, i.e., erythrocyte sedimentation rate and C-reactive protein are occasionally elevated. The leukocyte remains normal, but in some cases, rheumatoid factor and antinuclear antibody may be present in the acute period.

11.5.4 Dengue Virus

- The classical features of dengue virus (DV) are acute febrile illness, headache, and muscle and **joint pain**. It is also referred to as "breakbone fever." [114] **Arthralgia occurs in 60 to 80% of the patients infected with DV.**

Investigations may reveal leucopenia, thrombocytopenia, and elevated liver enzymes. A small percentage of patients may have potentially lethal forms known as hemorrhagic fever and dengue shock syndrome [115].

11.5.5 Septic Arthritis

It is a bacterial infection of the joint that is usually curable with treatment, but morbidity and mortality are still significant specially in patients who have underlying rheumatoid arthritis, patients who have prosthetic joints, elderly patients, and patients who have severe and multiple comorbidities. Incidence of septic arthritis 10 cases per 100,000 patient-years in general population in Europe [116]. Incidence of septic arthritis in patients with rheumatoid arthritis.

(Based on prospective British Society for Rheumatology Biologics Register)

1.8 cases per 1,000 patient-years in 3,673 patients taking non-biologic disease-modifying antirheumatic drugs, where 4.2 cases per 1,000 patient-years in 11,881 patients taking anti-tumor necrosis factor therapy.

Usually it is monoarthritis, but up to 20% of patients have infection in >1 joint "polyarticular." [116] The joints mostly affected are knee (which is the most common affected joint approximately 50%) followed by the hip, shoulder, and then elbow [120]. In IV drug users, axial skeletal joints are mainly involved often with *Staphylococcus aureus*.

The most common causes of septic arthritis in adults are: [116]

- *Staphylococcus aureus* most frequent causative agent, followed by *Streptococcus*.
- *Neisseria gonorrhoeae*, but it is considered *separately* as disseminated gonococcal infection.
- Gram negatives, *Haemophilus*, are usually seen in older patients.

In IV drug users, septic arthritis is frequently duo to methicillin-resistant Staphylococcus (MRSA), mixed infections, fungal infections, or unusual organisms [116]. Patients may have *1–2 weeks* history of joint pain, tenderness, warmth, redness, restricted motion, loss of function, and fever. Joint-related risk factors for infection are joint prosthesis, intra-articular injection, and joint trauma [119]. **Fever** occurs in about one-third of patients [116]. "**Large joints in legs (hips and knees) are the typical sites of infection.**" [116–118] Septic arthritis is diagnosed by clinical signs (hot, red, tender, swollen, restricted) with any of the following:

- Pathogenic organism in synovial fluid detected by culture and gram stain.
- Pathogenic organism isolated in blood or other site.
- Turbid synovial fluid in patient with recent antibiotic treatment.
- Synovial WBC count **more than 30,000**.
- Leukocytosis.

11.5.6 Poncet's Disease (Reactive Arthritis Associated with Tuberculosis) [121]

There is a new pattern of reactive arthritis associated with tuberculosis (TB), identified as Poncet's disease (PD) or tuberculous rheumatism, which is a sterile reactive arthritis that can emerge during any stage of acute TB infection. In a retrospective case series study, seven cases of Poncet's disease were identified:

- The most common presentation was extrapulmonary with involvement.
  - of multiple sites.
- Six out of seven patients developed arthritis after initiation of anti-TB drugs.
- One patient developed polyarthritis after completion of anti-TB medication.
- Asymmetrical polyarthritis was the most common pattern of joints involvement.

The resolution of the arthritis was with symptomatic treatment and continuation of anti-TB drugs. PD may manifest in a variable pattern during the course of active tuberculous infection. Physicians should be aware of this rare complication associated with a common disease to prevent delay in diagnosis and initiation of appropriate treatment.

11.6 Vaccination in Adult Patient with Autoimmune Inflammatory Rheumatic Diseases (AIIRD)

11.6.1 Introduction

It is well known that vaccination is one of the most effective measures to prevent infections and as discussed earlier in this chapter patient with autoimmune inflammatory rheumatic diseases is at increased risk of infection compared to the normal population with the respiratory tract being the most affected organ [122, 123]. However, vaccination of immunocompromised patients is challenging both regarding efficacy and safety. The efficacy of vaccinations in patients with AIIRD may be reduced, and there is a potential risk of flares of the underlying AIIRD following vaccination. The two major issues to consider in vaccine administration of this group of patients are what is the expected immune response following vaccination and what are the potential for worsening the underlying disease.

Table 11.8 Vaccinations by type

Inactivated vaccines	Live vaccines
Tetanus	Adenovirus
Haemophilus influenzae type b	Herpes zoster (shingles)
Hepatitis A and B	Measles, mumps, rubella
Human papillomavirus (HPV)	Varicella
Japanese encephalitis	Rotavirus
Pneumococcal	Yellow fever
Meningococcal	BCG
Typhoid (IM)	Typhoid (oral)
Inactivated polio	Live polio (oral)
Inactivated influenza	Live influenza (nasal spray)
Diphtheria	
Rabies	
Cholera	

11.6.2 General Rules

All inactivated vaccines can be administered safely to persons with AIIRD whether the vaccine is a killed whole organism or a recombinant, subunit, toxoid, polysaccharide, or polysaccharide protein-conjugate vaccine. Live viral and bacterial vaccines should be avoided whenever possible in immunosuppressed patients with AIIRD because it might lead to severe infection in immunocompromised patients (Table 11.8). Table 11.9 shows vaccinations recommendations in adult patient with autoimmune inflammatory rheumatic diseases (AIIRD).

Table 11.9 Vaccination recommendation in AIIRD * [124–127]

Inactivated influenza vaccine	Give annually	Special consideration
Pneumococcal polysaccharide (PPV23)	• Age 19 to 64 y. (one dose + revaccination dose) • All adults ≥65 y of age.	Minimum interval of 5 y between PPSV23 doses should be maintained
Pneumococcal 13 valent conjugate (PCV13)	• Age 19 to 64 y. • No revaccination.	
Tetanus toxoid vaccine	Like general population	In case of major and/or contaminated wounds in patients who received rituximab within the last 24 W ⇨ tetanus immunoglobulin's should be administered
Human papilloma virus vaccine (HPV)	Like general population	
Hepatitis A vaccine	Only recommended in patient at increased risk	Protective antibodies against hepatitis A should be absent
Hepatitis B vaccine	EULAR/ACIP ⇨ only for patient at increased risk ACR: • Should be given before starting DMARD or biologic drug. • If not ⇨ give to patients already on DMARD or biologic drug.	Protective antibodies against hepatitis B should be absent

Table 11.9 (continued)

Inactivated influenza vaccine	Give annually	Special consideration
Herpes zoster vaccine (HZV)	Special circumstances	• Before starting DMARDS or biologic agent. • At least 14 days before initiation of immunosuppressive therapy or 3 months after immunosuppression has stopped. • The following conditions not consider sufficiently immunosuppressive to be a contraindication for HZV: – MTX (<0.4 mg/kg/week), AZA (<3.0 mg/kg/day) or 6-mercaptopurine (<1.5 mg/kg/day) [4]. – Short-term corticosteroid (<14 days). – Low to moderate doses of corticosteroids (<20 mg/day of prednisone or equivalent). – Long-term alternate-day treatment with short acting preparation. – Maintenance physiologic doses (replacement therapy). – Topical, inhaled, intra-articular, bursal, or tendon corticosteroids injections.
Asplenic/hyposplenic	Give: • Influenza vaccine. • Pneumococcal vaccine. • Meningococcal C vaccine. • Haemophilus influenzae B .	AIIRD⇨ live in or travel to areas where other meningococcal strains are endemic (A, Y, W135), vaccination for these meningococcal subtypes is also indicated
Travelers with AIIRD	Vaccinations according to the general rules with some exception	Exceptions are: • BCG vaccine. • Oral poliomyelitis vaccine. • Oral typhoid fever. • Yellow fever .
PCP prophylaxis	Special circumstance	• Patients on a glucocorticoid dose ≥20 mg of prednisone daily for month or longer who also have another cause of immunocompromised .

[a]Vaccination in patients with AIIRD should ideally be administered during stable disease. *AIIRD* autoimmune inflammatory rheumatic disease, *MTX* methotrexate, *AZA* azathioprine [31, 128, 129, 130, 131, 132]

Acknowledgments The Authors would like to thank Abdullah Sakkat, MD, for his contributions to this chapter in the previous edition.

References

1. Alt HL, Barker MH. Fever of unknown origin. JAMA. 1930;94:1457.
2. PETERSDORF RG, BEESON PB. Fever of unexplained origin: report on 100 cases. Medicine (Baltimore). 1961;40:1.
3. deKleijn EM, Vandenbroucke JP, van der Meer JW. Fever of unknown origin (FUO). I A. prospective multicenter study of 167 patients with FUO, using fixed epidemiologic entry criteria. The Netherlands FUO Study Group. Medicine (Baltimore). 1997;76:392.
4. Vanderschueren S, Knockaert D, Adriaenssens T, et al. From prolonged febrile illness to fever of unknown origin: the challenge continues. Arch Intern Med. 2003;163:1033.
5. Miller RF, Hingorami AD, Foley NM. Pyrexia of undetermined origin in patients with human immunodeficiency virus infection and AIDS. Int J STD AIDS. 1996;7:170.
6. Knockaert DC, Vanneste LJ, Bobbaers HJ. Fever of unknown origin in elderly patients. J Am GeriatrSoc. 1993;41:1187.

7. Zenone T. Fever of unknown origin in adults: evaluation of 144 cases in a non-university hospital. Scand J Infect Dis. 2006;38:632.
8. Bleeker-Rovers CP, Vos FJ, de Kleijn EM, et al. A prospective multicenter study on fever of unknown origin: the yield of a structured diagnostic protocol. Medicine (Baltimore). 2007;86:26.
9. Horowitz HW. Fever of unknown origin or fever of too many origins? N Engl J Med. 2013;368:197.
10. Knockaert DC, Dujardin KS, Bobbaers HJ. Long-term follow-up of patients with undiagnosed fever of unknown origin. Arch Intern Med. 1996;156:618.
11. Foley NM, Miller RF. Tuberculosis and AIDS: is the white plague up and coming? J Infect. 1993;26:39.
12. Greenberg SD, Frager D, Suster B, et al. Active pulmonary tuberculosis in patients with AIDS: spectrum of radiographic findings (including a normal appearance). Radiology. 1994;193:115.
13. Arnow PM, Flaherty JP. Fever of unknown origin. Lancet. 1997;350:575.
14. Metcalfe JZ, Everett CK, Steingart KR, et al. Interferon-γ release assays for active pulmonary tuberculosis diagnosis in adults in low- and middle-income countries: systematic review and meta-analysis. J Infect Dis. 2011;204(Suppl 4):S1120.
15. Tholcken CA, Huang S, Woods GL. Evaluation of the ESP culture system II for recovery of mycobacteria from blood specimens collected in isolator tubes. J Clin Microbiol. 1997;35:2681.
16. Smith MB, Bergmann JS, Woods GL. Detection of Mycobacterium tuberculosis in BACTEC 12B broth cultures by the Roche Amplicor PCR assay. J Clin Microbiol. 1997;35:900.
17. Molavi A. Endocarditis: recognition, management, and prophylaxis. Cardiovasc Clin. 1993;23:139.
18. Kamimura T, Hatakeyama M, Torigoe K, et al. Muscular polyarteritis nodosa as a cause of fever of undetermined origin: a case report and review of the literature. Rheumatol Int. 2005;25:394.
19. Mueller PS, Terrell CL, Gertz MA. Fever of unknown origin caused by multiple myeloma: a report of 9 cases. Arch Intern Med. 2002;162:1305.
20. Mackowiak PA, Le Maistre CF. Drug fever: a critical appraisal of conventional concepts. An analysis of 51 episodes in two Dallas hospitals and 97 episodes reported in the English literature. Ann Intern Med. 1987;106:728.
21. Harb GE, Alldredge BK, Coleman R, Jacobson MA. Pharmacoepidemiology of adverse drug reactions in hospitalized patients with human immunodeficiency virus disease. J Acquir Immune Defic Syndr. 1993;6:919.
22. Siminoski K. Persistent fever due to occult dental infection: case report and review. Clin Infect Dis. 1993;16:550.
23. Cohen JA, Kaplan MM. The SGOT/SGPT ratio--an indicator of alcoholic liver disease. Dig Dis Sci. 1979;24:835.
24. Simon HB, Daniels GH. Hormonal hyperthermia: endocrinologic causes of fever. Am J Med. 1979;66:257.
25. Drenth JP, van der Meer JW. Hereditary periodic fever. N Engl J Med. 2001;345:1748.
26. Palda V, Allan S. Detsky. Arch Intern Med. 2003;163(5):545–51.
27. Bleeker-Rovers CP, Vos FJ, de Kleijn EM, et al. A prospective multicenter study on fever of unknown origin: the yield of a structured diagnostic protocol. Medicine (Baltimore). 2007;86:26–38.
28. Petersdorf RG, Beeson PB. Fever of unexplained origin: report on 100 cases. Medicine (Baltimore). 1961;40:1.
29. Mourad O, Palda V, Detsky AS. A comprehensive evidence-based approach to fever of unknown origin. Arch Intern Med. 2003;163:545.
30. Cervera R, Khamashta MA, Font J, et al. Morbidity and mortality in systemic lupus erythematosus during a 10-year period: a comparison of early and late manifestations in a cohort of 1,000 patients. Medicine (Baltimore). 2003;82:299.
31. Gluck T, Muller-Ladner U. Vaccination in patients with chronic rheumatic or autoimmune disease. Clin Infect Dis. 2008;46:1459–65.
32. Use of serum procalcitonin to detect bacterial infection in patients with autoimmune diseases: a systematic review and meta-analysis. Arthritis Rheum. 2012;64(9):3034–42. https://doi.org/10.1002/art.34512.
33. Doran MF, Crowson CS, Pond GR, O'Fallon WM, Gabriel SE. Frequency of infection in patients with rheumatoid arthritis compared with controls: a population-based study. Arthritis Rheum. 2002;46:2287–93.
34. Rheumatology (Oxford). 2013;52(1):53–61. https://doi.org/10.1093/rheumatology/kes305. Epub 2012 Nov 28
35. Serious infections in a population-based cohort of 86,039 seniors with rheumatoid arthritis. Arthritis Care Res (Hoboken). 2013;65(3):353–61. https://doi.org/10.1002/acr.21812.
36. Yale SH, Limper AH. *Pneumocystis carinii* pneumonia in patients without acquired immunodeficiency syndrome: associated illness and prior corticosteroid therapy. Mayo Clin Proc. 1996;71:5.
37. Infectious complications of immunosuppressive therapy in patients, with rheumatic diseases. Rheum Dis Clin N Am. 1997;23:219–37.
38. NEJM. 2007;357:2601; Am J Med 2007;120;764; CID 2011;53:798
39. Anaya JM, Diethelm L, Ortiz LA, et al. Pulmonary involvement in rheumatoid arthritis. Semin Arthritis Rheum. 1995;24:242.
40. Duffy KN, Duffy CM, Gladman DD. Infection and disease activity in systemic lupus erythematosus: a review of hospitalized patients. J Rheumatol. 1991;18:1180.

41. Bradley JD, Brandt KD, Katz BP. Infectious complications of cyclophosphamide treatment for vasculitis. Arthritis Rheum. 1989;32:45.
42. Ginzler E, Diamond H, Kaplan D, et al. Computer analysis of factors influencing frequency of infection in systemic lupus erythematosus. Arthritis Rheum. 1978;21:37.
43. Hellmann DB, Petri M, Whiting-O'Keefe Q. Fatal infections in systemic lupus erythematosus: The role of opportunistic infections. Medicine. 1987;66:341.
44. Hoffman GS, Kerr GS, Leavitt RY, et al. Wegener's granulomatosis: An analysis of 158 patients. Ann Intern Med. 1992;116:488.
45. Jonsson H, Nived O, Sturfelt G. Outcome in systemic lupus erythematosus: a prospective study of patients from a defined population. Medicine. 1989;68:141.
46. Godeau B, Coutant-Perronne V, DLT H, et al. *Pneumocystis carinii* pneumonia in the course of connective tissue disease: Report of 34 cases. J Rheumatol. 1994;21:246.
47. Pohl MA, Lan SP. BerlT: plasmapheresis does not increase the risk for infection in immunosuppressed patients with severe lupus nephritis. Ann Intern Med. 1991;114:924.
48. Sneller MC, Hoffman GS, Talar-Williams C, et al. An analysis of forty-two Wegener's granulomatosis patients treated with methotrexate and prednisone. Arthritis Rheum. 1995;38:608.
49. Staples PJ, Gerding DN, Decker JL, et al. Incidence of infection in systemic lupus erythematosus. Arthritis Rheum. 1974;17:1.
50. ter Borg EJ, Horst G, Limburg PC, et al. C-reactive protein levels during disease exacerbations and infections in systemic lupus erythematosus: a prospective longitudinal study. J Rheumatol. 1990;17:1642.
51. Anaya JM, Diethelm L, Ortiz LA, et al. Pulmonary involvement in rheumatoid arthritis. Semin Arthritis Rheum. 1995;24:242.
52. Calabrese LH. Vasculitis of the central nervous system. Rheum Dis Clin N Am. 1995;21:1059.
53. Feinglass EJ, Arnett FC, Dorsch CA, et al. Neuropsychiatric manifestations of systemic lupus erythematosus: diagnosis, clinical spectrum, and relationship to other features of disease. Medicine. 1976;55:323.
54. Moore PM, Cupps T. R: neurologic complications of vasculitis. Ann Neurol. 1983;14:155.
55. Sibley JT, Olszynski WP, Decoteau WE, et al. The incidence and prognosis of central nervous system disease in systemic lupus erythematosus. J Rheumatol. 1992;19:47.
56. Sigal LH. The neurologic presentation of vasculitis and rheumatologic syndromes. A review Medicine. 1987;66:157.
57. Wong KL, Woo EKW, Yu YL, et al. Neurologic manifestations of systemic lupus erythematosus: a prospective study. QJM. 1991;81:857.
58. Moore PM, Cupps T. Neurologic complications of vasculitis. Ann Neurol. 1983;14:155.
59. Clin Infect Dis 2005 Stevens-1373-406.
60. Connolly KJ, Hammer SM. Infect Dis Clin N Am. 1990;4:599.
61. Nishino H, Rubino FA, DeRemee RA, et al. Neurologic involvement in Wegener's granulomatosis: An analysis of 324 consecutive patients at the Mayo Clinic. Ann Neurol. 1993;33:4.
62. Ann Rheum Dis. 2011;70:1810–4. https://doi.org/10.1136/ard.2011.152769.
63. Navarrete MG, Brey RL. Neuropsychiatric systemic lupus erythematosus. Curr Treat Options Neurol. 2000;2:473–85.
64. Ruggieri AP. Neuropsychiatric lupus: nomenclature, classification, criteria, and other confusional states. Arthritis Rheum. 2001;45:406–9.
65. West SG. Neuropsychiatric lupus. Rheum Dis Clin N Am. 1994;20:129–58.
66. Kaandorp CJ, Van Schaardenburg D, Krijnen P, et al. Risk factors for septic arthritis in patients with joint disease. A prospective study. Arthritis Rheum. 1995;38:1819–25.
67. Doran MF, Crowson CS, Pond GR, et al. Frequency of infection in patients with rheumatoid arthritis compared with controls: a population-based study. Arthritis Rheum. 2002;46:2287–93.
68. Goldenberg DL, Red JI. Bacterial arthritis. N Engl J Med. 1985;312:764771. [PubMed]
69. Flood DA, Chan CK, Pruzanski W. Pneumocystis carinii pneumonia associated with methotrexate therapy in rheumatoid arthritis. J Rheumatol. 1991;18:1254–6.
70. Perruquet JL, Harrington TM, Davis DE. Pneumocystis carinii pneumonia following methotrexate therapy for rheumatoid arthritis. Arthritis Rheum. 1983;26:1291–2.
71. Roux N, Flipo RM, Cortet B, et al. Pneumocystis carinii pneumonia in rheumatoid arthritis patients treated with methotrexate. A report of two cases. Rev Rhum Engl Ed. 1996;63:453–6.
72. Watkin SW, Bucknall RC, Nisar M, et al. Atypical mycobacterial infection of the lung in rheumatoid arthritis. Ann Rheum Dis. 1989;48:336–8.
73. Wolfe F, Flowers N, Anderson J, et al. Tuberculosis rates are not increased in rheumatoid arthritis [abstract]. Arthritis Rheum. 2001;44:S105.
74. Lew DP, Waldvogel FA. Lancet. 2004;364:–369.
75. Korzeniowski OM. Med Clin North Am. 1991;75(2):391–404.
76. Mitchell SR, Nguyen PQ, Katz P. Increased risk of neisserial infections in systemic lupus erythematosus. Semin Arthritis Rheum. 1990;20:174–84.
77. Carratala J, Moreno R, Cabellos C, et al. Neisseria meningitis monoarthritis revealing systemic lupus erythematosus. J Rheumatol. 1988;15:532–3.
78. Feliciano R, Swedler W, Varga J. Infection with uncommon subgroup Y Neisseria meningitidis in

patients with systemic lupus erythematosus. Clin Exp Rheumatol. 1999;17:737–40.
79. Lehman TJ, Bernstein B, Hanson V, et al. Meningococcal infection complicating systemic lupus erythematosus. J Pediatr. 1981;99:94–6.
80. Tikly M, Diese M, Zannettou N, et al. Gonococcal endocarditis in a patient with systemic lupus erythematosus. Br J Rheumatol. 1997;36:270–2.
81. Gonzalez-Crespo MR, Gomez-Reino JJ. Invasive aspergillosis in systemic lupus erythematosus. Semin Arthritis Rheum. 1995;24:304–14.
82. Abramson S, Kramer SB, Radin A, et al. Salmonella bacteremia in systemic lupus erythematosus. Eight-year experience at a municipal hospital. Arthritis Rheum. 1985;28:75–9.
83. Mitchell SR, Nguyen PQ, Katz P. Increased risk of neisserial infections in systemic lupus erythematosus. Semin Arthritis Rheum. 1990;20:174–84.
84. Shahram F, Akbarian M, Davatchi F. Salmonella infection in systemic lupus erythematosus. Lupus. 1993;2:55–9.
85. Boey ML, Feng PH. Salmonella infection in systemic lupus erythematosus. Singap Med J. 1982;23:147–51.
86. Chen JY, Luo SF, Wu YJ, et al. Salmonella septic arthritis in systemic lupus erythematosus and other systemic diseases. Clin Rheumatol. 1998;17:282–7.
87. Pablos JL, Aragon A, Gomez-Reino JJ. Salmonellosis and systemic lupus erythematosus. Report of ten cases. Br J Rheumatol. 1994;33:129–32.
88. Shamiss A, Thaler M, Nussinovitch N, et al. Multiple Salmonella enteritidis leg abscesses in a patient with systemic lupus erythematosus. Postgrad Med J. 1990;66:486–8.
89. Lim E, Koh WH, Loh SF, et al. Non-typhoidal salmonellosis in patients with systemic lupus erythematosus. A study of fifty patients and a review of the literature. Lupus. 2001;10:87–92.
90. Lovy MR, Ryan PF, Hughes GR. Concurrent systemic lupus erythematosus and salmonellosis. J Rheumatol. 1981;8:605–12.
91. van de Laar MA, Meenhorst PL, van Soesbergen RM, et al. Polyarticular Salmonella bacterial arthritis in a patient with systemic lupus erythematosus. J Rheumatol. 1989;16:231–4.
92. Frayha RA, Jizi I, Saadeh G. Salmonella typhimurium bacteriuria. An increased infection rate in systemic lupus erythematosus. Arch Intern Med. 1985;145:645–7.
93. Picillo U, Italian G, Marcialis MR, et al. Bilateral femoral osteomyelitis with knee arthritis due to Salmonella enteritidis in a patient with systemic lupus erythematosus. Clin Rheumatol. 2001;20:53–6.
94. Sanchez-Guerrero J, Alarcon-Segovia D. Salmonella pericarditis with tamponade in systemic lupus erythematosus. Br J Rheumatol. 1990;29:69–71.
95. Kaandorp CJ, Dinant HJ, van de Laar MA, Moens HJ, Prins AP, Dijkmans BA. Incidence and sources of native and prosthetic joint infection: a community based prospective survey. Ann Rheum Dis. 1997;56:470–5.
96. Weston VC, Jones AC, Bradbury N, Fawthrop F, Doherty M. Clinical features and outcome of septic arthritis in a single UK health district 1982–1991. Ann Rheum Dis. 1999;58:214–9.
97. Dubost JJ, Soubrier M, De Champs C, Ristori JM, Bussiere JL, Sauvezie B. No changes in the distribution of organisms responsible for septic arthritis over a 20 year period. Ann Rheum Dis. 2002;61:267–9.
98. Edwards CJ, Cooper C, Fisher D, Field M, van Staa TP, Arden NK. The importance of the disease process and disease-modifying antirheumatic drug treatment in the development of septic arthritis in patients with rheumatoid arthritis. Arthritis Rheum. 2007;57:1151–7.
99. Ginzler E, Diamond H, Kaplan D, et al. Computer analysis of factors influencing frequency of infection in systemic lupus erythematosus. Arthritis Rheum. 1978;21:37.
100. Hellmann DB, Petri M, Whiting-O'Keefe Q. Fatal infections in systemic lupus erythematosus: The role of opportunistic infections. Medicine. 1987;66:341.
101. Hoffman GS, Kerr GS, Leavitt RY, et al. Wegener's granulomatosis: An analysis of 158 patients. Ann Intern Med. 1992;116:488.
102. (Anti-TNF therapy is associated with an increased risk of serious infections in patients with rheumatoid arthritis especially in the first 6 months of treatment: updated results from the British Society for Rheumatology Biologics Register with special emphasis on risks in the elderly.) 2011 Jan;50(1):124–31. https://doi.org/10.1093/rheumatology/keq242. Epub 2010 Jul 31.
103. Risk of infections associated with rheumatoid arthritis, with its comorbidity and treatment Rheumatology (Oxford). 2013;52(1):53–61. https://doi.org/10.1093/rheumatology/kes305. Epub 2012 Nov 28.
104. Mirise RT, Kitridou RC. Arthritis and hepatitis. West J Med. 1979;130:12–7.
105. HCV and Rheumatic Disease, American college of rheumatology.
106. Hepatitis virus arthritis, DynaMed databases.
107. Rosner I, Rozenbaum M, Toubi E, et al. The case for hepatitis C arthritis. Semin Arthritis Rheum. 2004;33:375.
108. Rivera J, García-Monforte A, Pineda A, MillánNúñez-Cortés J. Arthritis in patients with chronic hepatitis C virus infection. J Rheumatol. 1999;26:420.
109. Nesher G, Osborn TG, Moore TL. Parvovirus infection mimicking systemic lupus erythematosus. Semin Arthritis Rheum. 1995;24:297.
110. Moore TL, Bandlamudi R, Alam SM, Nesher G. Parvovirus infection mimicking systemic lupus erythematosus in a pediatric population. Semin Arthritis Rheum. 1999;28:314.
111. Török TJ. Parvovirus B19 and human disease. Adv Intern Med. 1992;37:431.
112. Moore TL. Parvovirus-associated arthritis. Curr Opin Rheumatol. 2000;12:289.

113. Reed MR, Gilliam BE, Syed RH, Moore TL. Rheumatic manifestations of parvovirus B19 in children. J Ped Infect Dis. 2009;
114. Rigau-Pérez JG. The early use of break-bone fever (Quebrantahuesos, 1771) and dengue (1801) in Spanish. Am J Trop Med Hyg. 1998;59:272.
115. Kalayanarooj S, Vaughn DW, Nimmannitya S, et al. Early clinical and laboratory indicators of acute dengue illness. J Infect Dis. 1997;176:313.
116. Mathews CJ, Weston VC, Jones A, Field M, Coakley G. Bacterial septic arthritis in adults.
117. Coakley G, Mathews C, Field M, British Society for Rheumatology Standards, Guidelines and Audit Working Group, et al. BSR & BHPR, BOA, RCGP and BSAC guidelines for management of the hot swollen joint in adults. Rheumatology (Oxford). 2006;45(8):1039–41.
118. Margaretten ME, Kohlwes J, Moore D, Bent S. Does this adult patient have septic arthritis? JAMA. 2007;297(13):1478–88, commentary can be found in JAMA 2007 Jul 4;298(1):40, Ann Emerg Med 2008 Nov;52(5):567
119. Kang SN, Sanghera T, Mangwani J, Paterson JM, Ramachandran M. The management of septic arthritis in children: systematic review of the English language literature. J Bone Joint Surg Br. 2009 Sep;91(9):1127–33.
120. Carpenter CR, Schuur JD, Everett WW, Pines JM. Evidence-based diagnostics: adult septic arthritis.
121. Poncet's disease (reactive arthritis associated with tuberculosis): retrospective case series and review of literature. Sultana Abdulaziz, Hani Almoallim, Ashraf Ibrahim, Mohammed Samannodi, Mohammed Shabrawishi, YasirMeeralam, GhadiAbdulmajeed, GhadeerBanjar, WeamQutub, HibaDowaikh , Clinical Rheumatology 2012, 31, 10, pp 1521–1528.
122. Doran MF, Crowson CS, Pond GR, O'Fallon M, Gabriel SE. Frequency of infection in patients with rheumatoid arthritis compared with controls. A population based study. Arthritis Rheum. 2002;46:2287–93.
123. Glück T, Kiefmann B, Grohmann M, Falk W, Straub RH, Schölmerich J. Immune status and risk for infection in patients receiving chronic immunosuppressive therapy. J Rheumatol. 2005;32:1473–80.
124. S van Assen, N Agmon-Levin, O Elkayam, et al. EULAR recommendations for vaccination in adult patients with autoimmune inflammatory rheumatic diseases (AIIRD)
125. Ann Rheum Dis 2011 70: 414–422 originally published online December 3, 2010: https://doi.org/10.1136/ard.2010.137216
126. Advisory Committee on Immunization Practices (ACIP) October 2011.
127. 2012 Update of the 2008 American College of Rheumatology Recommendations for the Use of Disease-Modifying Antirheumatic Drugs and Biologic Agents in the Treatment of Rheumatoid Arthritis .Arthritis Care & Research Vol. 64, No. 5, 2012, pp 625–639. https://doi.org/10.1002/acr.21641
128. An official American Thoracic Society statement. Treatment of fungal infections in adult pulmonary and critical care patients. Am J Respir Crit Care Med. 2011 Jan 1;183(1):96–128. https://doi.org/10.1164/rccm.2008-740ST.
129. Opportunistic infections in patients with and patients without Acquired Immunodeficiency Syndrome. Clin Infect Dis. 2002;34(8):1098–107. Epub 2002 Mar 21
130. An Official ATS. Workshop summary: recent advances and future directions in pneumocystis pneumonia (PCP). Proc Am Thorac Soc. 2006;3(8):655–64.
131. Pneumocystis carinii pneumonia without acquired immunodeficiency syndrome. More patients, same risk. Arch Intern Med 1995;155(11):1125–1128.
132. Pneumocystis pneumonia. N Engl J Med. 2004;350(24):2487–98.
133. Bleeker-Rovers CP, Vos FJ, de Kleijn EM, et al. A prospective multicenter study on fever of unknown origin: the yield of a structured diagnostic protocol. Medicine (Baltimore). 2007;86:26.
134. Stahl NI, Klippel JH, Decker JL. Fever in systemic lupus erythematosus. Am J Med. 1979;67:935.
135. Greenberg SB. Crit Care Clin. 2002;18:931–56.
136. National Comprehensive Cancer Network (NCCN) Clinical Practice Guidelines in Oncology. Prevention and treatment of cancer-related infections. Version 1.2012. http://www.nccn.org (Accessed on January 03, 2013).

12

Thrombosis and Autoimmune Rheumatic Disorders

Fozya Bashal

12.1 Introduction

Venous thromboembolism (VTE) is a disease of blood coagulation that occurs in the veins, most often in the calf veins first, from where it may extend and cause deep vein thrombosis (DVT) or pulmonary embolism (PE). The first described case of venous thrombosis that we know of dates back to the thirteenth century, when deep vein thrombosis was reported in the right leg of a 20-year-old man [1].

The risk of thrombosis is influenced by both genetic and environmental factors. The risk factors for venous thrombosis are immobility, major surgery, underlying medical conditions like malignancies, medication use such as hormonal therapies, obesity, and genetic predisposition. In contrast to that, the major risk factor for arterial thrombosis is atherosclerosis [2].

In 1859, a German scientist, Rudolf Virchow, elucidated the mechanism of pulmonary embolism and hence deduced the major pathogenic determinants for DVT and PE, named as Virchow's triad that comprised (1) blood stasis, (2) changes in the vessel wall, and (3) hypercoagulability. This triad still applies, with essentially all prothrombotic factors, whether systemic or molecular, influencing one of these three mechanisms [3] (Fig. 12.1).

DVT and PE are extremely common medical problems, and they are among the major cause of morbidity and death worldwide [3].

About 1–2 per 1000 individuals are affected by VTE per year with PE being the lethal complication and is associated with a high mortality rate that exceeds 15% in the first 3 months after diagnosis [4].

Although disturbance of the coagulation and anticoagulation mechanisms is a very important risk factor for VTE, several studies suggest the role of innate immunity in the development of VTE [4].

Venous thrombosis results from multiple interactions between acquired and inherited risk factors [4].

In this chapter, we discuss the association of thrombosis with autoimmune rheumatologic disorders. The pathophysiology of thrombosis, effects of inflammation, endothelial dysfunction, some novel factors on promoting thrombosis in different rheumatic disorders, diagnostic strategies for thromboembolic disease, and its treatment, management, as well as preventive measures will be addressed in detail. This chapter is useful for students, residents, fellows, and physicians interested in learning about rheumatic disease and thrombosis. The main objective of this chapter is to make the readers able to achieve the following goals:

F. Bashal (✉)
College of Medicine, Umm Al-Qura University, Makkah, Saudi Arabia
e-mail: fbbashal@uqu.edu.sa

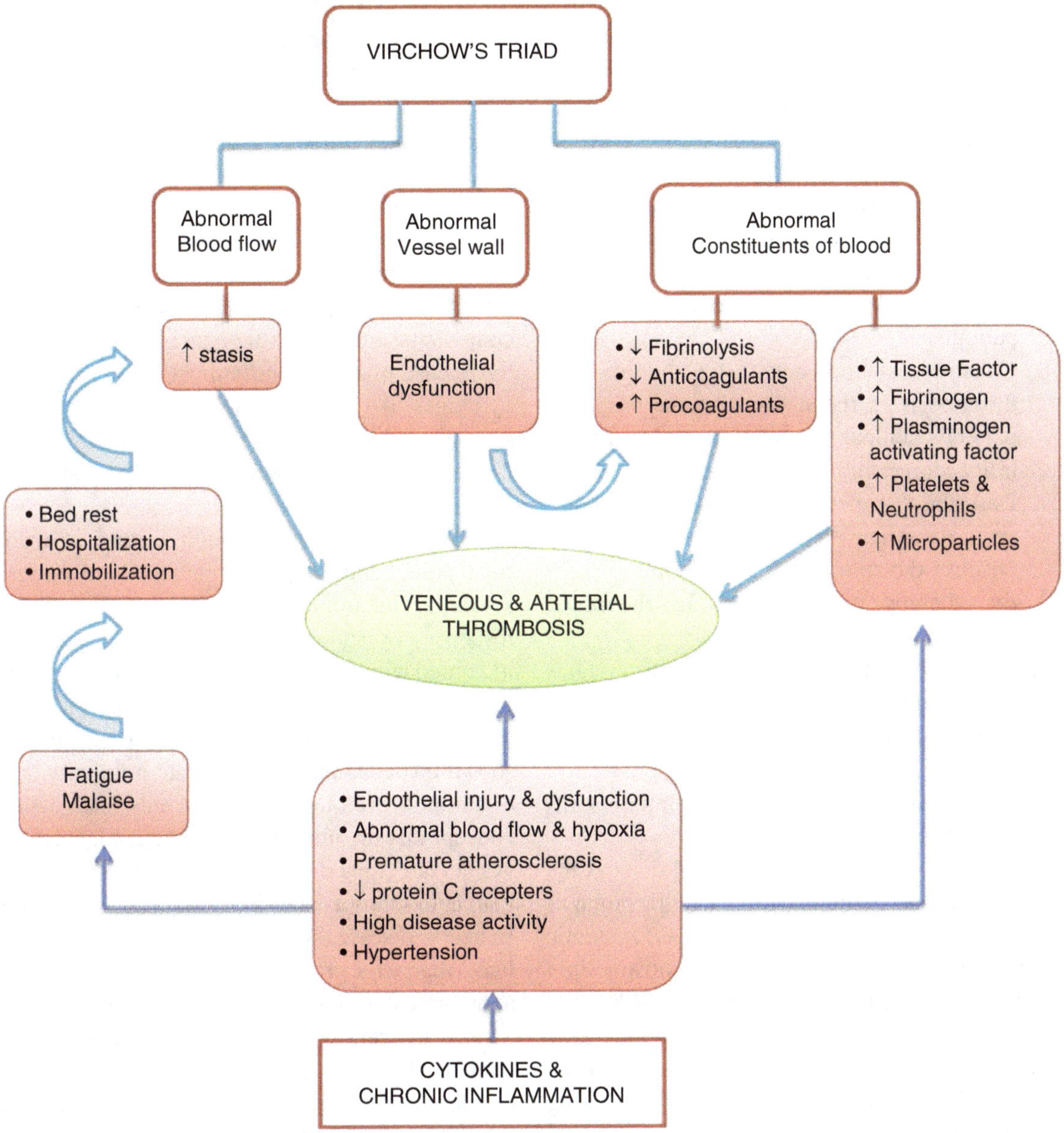

Fig. 12.1 Virchow's triad and some inflammatory changes and their association with venous and arterial thrombosis

1. Explain and discuss the pathophysiology of thrombosis in rheumatic diseases.
2. Recognize the multifactorial role of inflammation in inducing the hypercoagulable state which promote thrombosis in autoimmune rheumatic disorders.
3. Classify thrombosis in patients with rheumatologic diseases (arterial or venous) according to the presence of different risk factors and type of the disorders.
4. Identify the role of different autoantibodies in specific rheumatic diseases such as systemic lupus erythematosus and antiphospholipid syndrome that contribute to the high risk of thrombosis in these conditions.
5. Describe the effects of different therapies commonly used in patients with rheumatic disorders and their role in thrombosis promotion or prevention.

6. Recognize the clinical features of thromboembolic diseases, as well as formulate a comprehensive history of thrombosis from patients with rheumatic diseases.
7. Judge when to select specific assays for thrombophilia screening, clotting factors, autoantibodies, and other tests for thrombotic episodes in rheumatic diseases and choose the appropriate investigations necessary for the diagnosis of thrombosis in these patients.
8. Construct an approach to the diagnosis of thrombosis in rheumatic diseases based on patient's clinical presentation, pretest probability scores, and investigations.
9. Describe therapeutic regimens for thrombosis in rheumatic diseases.
10. Discuss the role of adjunctive and preventive therapy in thrombosis in rheumatic disease.
11. Identify conditions that mandate prophylaxis with antithrombotic medications in patients with rheumatic diseases.

To achieve these purposes, this chapter is written in three sections.

In Sect. 2 of this chapter, we will discuss the mechanism and pathophysiology of thrombosis in individual rheumatic disorders, i.e., systemic lupus erythematosus (SLE), antiphospholipid syndrome (APS), rheumatoid arthritis (RA), vasculitis, and Behçet's disease; this includes the effects and role of different medications used specifically in rheumatic disorders in promoting or preventing thrombosis.

In Sect. 3, we discussed in general the approach and the strategies for diagnosing VTE (DVT and PE) and arterial thrombi in different autoimmune rheumatic disorders.

In Sect. 4, we will discuss updates about the management of thrombosis in rheumatic diseases and recommendations for prophylaxis and secondary thrombosis prevention in rheumatic disorders.

12.2 Pathophysiology of Thrombosis in Rheumatic Disorders

Arterial and venous thrombosis and systemic inflammatory diseases are highly linked, and the systemic inflammation promotes an extensive cross-link to exist between inflammation and hemostasis [5]. Systemic inflammation disturbs the natural tight balance between the procoagulants and the anticoagulants in the blood by release of certain inflammatory markers and cytokines like tumor necrosis factor alpha (TNF-α) and interleukin-1 (IL-1) and interleukin-6 (IL-6) that finally promote a prothrombotic state [5] (Fig. 12.2).

Inflammation is a common feature of many rheumatic and immune-mediated disorders; systemic inflammation modulates thrombotic responses by suppressing fibrinolysis, upregulating procoagulants, and downregulating anticoagulants. Several studies indicate the role of innate immunity in promoting thrombosis as it was shown that coagulation and innate immunity have a common evolutionary origin; this leads to the concept that the immune system and coagulations system are linked [4]. These findings conclude that autoimmune disorders such as SLE, APS, Behçet's disease, RA, and vasculitis syndromes like Wegener's granulomatosis have been linked to an increased risk of venous thrombosis [4].

RA, as well as other types of arthritides and connective tissue diseases, are associated with accelerated atherosclerosis and increased cardiovascular morbidity and mortality [6].

Chronic systemic inflammation predisposes to accelerated atherosclerosis, a risk that is well-known in systemic lupus erythematosus (SLE) and in rheumatoid arthritis (RA) patients [7].

The mechanisms for an enhanced and premature atherosclerosis in autoimmune rheumatic disorders such as RA, SLE, and systemic sclerosis (SS) include chronic inflammatory process, immune dysregulation, and the classical risk fac-

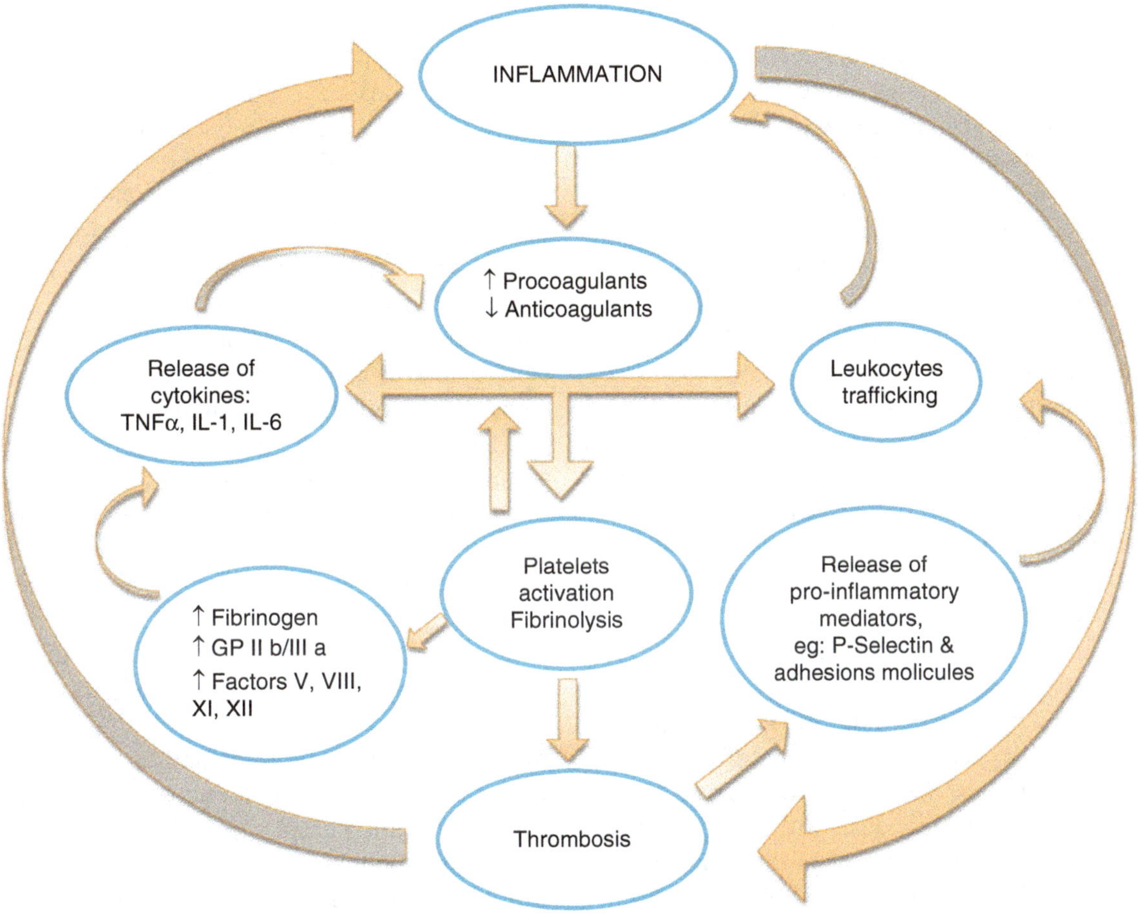

Fig. 12.2 Close relationship between mechanisms of inflammation and thrombosis in Rheumatic diseases

tors; this explains the very high risk of cardiovascular disease in patients with SLE and RA and some other autoimmune diseases [8].

The coagulation factor XII (FXII, Hageman factor) activity correlates with fibrinolysis [9]. Some studies had found the association between pulmonary embolism and decreased levels of FXII; one study was done on large cohort of patients in Japan with different rheumatic disorder reports that FXII reduction coexisted with the presence of antiphospholipid antibodies (a PL) in most thrombotic patients with rheumatic disorders; they conclude the presence of anti-FXII autoantibodies as a cause of FXII deficiency in the presence of aPL antibodies [9].

12.2.1 SLE and Thrombosis

Thrombosis in SLE is multifactorial, and hence SLE patients are at significantly increased risk of thrombosis and atherosclerosis. Arterial and/or venous thrombosis is a well-known clinical entity in SLE, with a prevalence >10%. This prevalence may even exceed 50% in high-risk patients [10]. The incidence of thrombosis in SLE patients according to two studies was 26.8 and up to 51.9 per 1000 patient-years, according to the disease duration [10]. Other study reported that the incidence of thrombosis was 36.3 per 1000 patient years [10]. In a 10-year prospective cohort study of patients with SLE, the most frequent causes of death were active SLE (26.5%), thrombosis (26.5%), and infection (25%), with thrombosis dominating the second 5-year period of follow-up [11]. Patients with SLE have thrombosis at an early age than the age of thrombosis occurrence in the general population, with the incidence being increased in the first year, which may be explained by high disease activity, circulating immune complexes, cytotoxic antibodies, or a higher inflammatory state at first year of SLE diagnosis [10].

Thrombosis is the most frequent cause of death in SLE. With its frequent manifestation in patients with SLE, thrombosis contributes significantly to high morbidity and mortality [11].

Several studies showed that atherosclerotic cardiovascular and cerebrovascular diseases are more common causes of late deaths than active SLE itself. Some studies revealed that subclinical coronary heart disease and carotid plaque were present in a significantly higher proportion of SLE patients than in control subjects of similar age and sex with similar risk factors. Compared with individuals without SLE, the risk of myocardial infarction in SLE patients is 2–50 times higher, and the risk of stroke is 2–10 times higher. The prevalence of symptomatic coronary heart disease in SLE patients has been reported to be 6–20%, depending on the characteristics of the cohort, disease duration, study design, prevalence of antiphospholipid antibodies (aPL), and ethnic composition. 3–15% of SLE patients have a nonfatal stroke [12].

12.2.1.1 Risk Factor and Etiology of Thrombosis in SLE

Inflammation and Disease Activity

Inflammation promotes thrombosis through its several effects on blood coagulation [10, 13].

Inflammation induces the expression of tissue factor (TF), which is an important factor in coagulation initiation [10, 13]. The production of plasminogen activator inhibitor (PAI) is upregulated in inflammation which leads to decreased fibrinolysis activity and increases the risk of thrombosis [10]; high levels of C-reactive protein (CRP) released in inflammatory conditions facilitate the interaction between the monocyte and the endothelial and promote plasminogen activator inhibitor-1 (PAI-1) and TF [13]. In inflammation, fibrinogen, an acute phase reactant, is secreted in higher concentrations which further increase the risk of thrombosis in patients with SLE [13]. Inflammation impairs protein C pathway and decreases protein S level, thus worsening the risk of thrombosis in SLE patients who might have thrombotic events early in the disease as compared to patients without SLE [10, 13]. It was found that SLE patients with lupus nephritis have a high disease activity and inflammation, and this is associated with increase risk of DVT and renal vein thrombosis; they also frequently have systemic hypertension and hyperlipidemia which further worsen thrombotic risk [10].

Antiphospholipid (aPL) Antibodies

aPL antibodies are type of autoantibodies that directed towards phospholipid binding proteins, anionic phospholipids, or a combination of the two [9]; they include anticardiolipin antibodies (ACA), lupus anticoagulant (LA), and anti ß2-glycoprotein I (anti-ß2-GPI) [14]. aPL antibodies induce platelet activation, interfere with coagulation inhibitors such as protein C, inhibit antithrombin and fibrinolysis, and then initiate the formation of a thrombus [10]; they are associated with an increased risk of arterial and venous thrombosis in addition to recurrent pregnancy loss in which they comprise an antiphospholipid syndrome (APS) which could occur as a primary disease (primary APS) or associated with several autoimmune disorders, most frequently in SLE patients, where it is named as secondary APS [15]. Lupus anticoagulant is considered as significant risk factor for stroke and myocardial infarction [10] as well as a strongest predictor of thrombosis [15].

There is a significant occurrence of aPL antibodies among SLE patients [16]; about one-third of patients with SLE show aPL positivity, but not all of them have the clinical presentation of thrombosis or APS [14].

In one retrospective study of 42 SLE patients, 60% were positive for one or two aPL antibodies, but only 27% of them (10 patients) had a history of APS. The most common clinical presentation was DVT/PE in eight patients. Less common was arterial thrombosis and pregnancy loss. One patient with a history of PE developed autoimmune hemolytic anemia. Another patient without history of DVT/PE presented with thrombocytopenia [16].

The risk of thrombosis in LA and ACA positive patients has been addressed by many researchers. In patients with SLE, 42% of LA-positive and 40% of ACA-positive individuals had a history of thrombosis; in contrast, the prevalence of thrombosis in LA-negative or ACA-negative SLE patients was only10–18% [10].

APS is the main cause of thrombosis and a major predictor of irreversible organ damage and death in SLE patients [15].

ACA might be transiently positive, or persistently positive, and considered significant when it tests positive on at least two occasions, 12 weeks apart. The risk of thrombosis was significantly higher in persistently positive ACA antibodies (33% risk) versus 3% risk in those with transiently positive ACA as shown in the prospective, observational cohort study by A Martinez-Berriotxoa et al. (2007) [15].

- Persistently positive ACA: patients are positive for IgG and/or IgM ACA at medium-high levels (titers ≥20 GPL and/or MPL) in whom more than two-thirds of the ACA determinations were positive; ACA were measured four or more times in all patients [15].
- Transiently positive ACA: patients are positive for IgG and/or IgM aCL in which less than two-thirds of the ACA determinations were positive; ACA were measured four or more times in all patients [15].

In all patients with SLE, even if there are no clinical manifestations, aPL antibodies should be done as they are considered part of American College of Rheumatology (ACR) classification criteria for SLE, and they have been associated with increased risk of thrombosis [10], as the first presentation can be fatal presenting with a CVA. Diagnosis allows prophylactic measures to be instituted in high-risk situations, e.g., prolonged immobility and postoperative states; increased awareness of APS should lead to earlier recognition of associated episodes and laboratory screening for all SLE patients to allow for prophylactic anticoagulation in high-risk situations [16].

Protein C and S and Antithrombin Deficiencies

They are rare but carry a higher risk for venous thrombosis [10].

Factor V Leiden

Activation of factor V leads to the formation of a cross-linked fibrin clot. Factor V Leiden (FVL) is the most common inherited risk factor for venous thrombosis in the general population and is an important factor for thrombosis in patients with SLE. FVL polymorphism is considered to be risk variant for thrombosis and confers resistance to activated protein C, thus shifting the balance towards thrombosis in the clotting cascade. FVL variant is found in 20–60% of patients with idiopathic DVT but without SLE. Patients with SLE and/or aPL positivity who have the FVL polymorphism have at least two times the odds of thrombosis compared to patients without this polymorphism. This observation places FVL to be an independent risk factor for thrombosis in SLE [11].

Hyperhomocysteinemia

Hyperhomocysteinemia is a strong and independent factor for increased risk of atherosclerosis, mainly of the carotid and coronary arteries, as well as venous thrombosis to some extent [10, 17]. 27.3% of SLE patients with thrombosis have hyperhomocysteinemia, which is significantly higher than those without thrombosis in whom it is detected at 16.9% [10]. Patients with shortened

APTT have a hypercoagulable state and were found to have high levels of homocysteine that place them at a higher risk of thrombotic events, as shown in a study done by T. M. K. Refai et al. (2002) [17]. In this study, the researchers found that 21% of SLE patients had elevated levels of homocysteine; interestingly, the level was higher in male patients more than in female ones and also those on prednisolone; they observed that lupus patients with hyperhomocysteinemia had a threefold increase in odds ratio of thrombotic episodes. This is partly because of the direct toxic effect of homocysteine on endothelium and partly indirect effects, such as induction of a vascular-endothelial-cell activator, promotion of vascular smooth muscle proliferation, and an inhibitory effect on endothelial cell growth; these findings support the hypothesis that hyperhomocysteinemia is an independent risk factor for thrombosis in young patients with SLE [17].

Traditional Risk Factors

Smoking is associated with worse outcome and mainly venous thrombosis by inducing endothelial damage; patients with SLE may have hypertension (HTN), diabetes mellitus (DM), and dyslipidemia which predispose them to thrombotic events. Older patients have more endothelial damage and vascular morbidity, and hence age is considered to be a risk factor for thrombosis in SLE [10].

12.2.1.2 Medication and Thrombosis in SLE

- Glucocorticoids have been used frequently in SLE; they mediate endothelial damage and hence lead to accelerated atherosclerosis; high doses of glucocorticoids are associated with abnormalities of the coagulation system [10]. Chronic glucocorticoid consumption has been reported to increase plasma von Willebrand factor (VWF) levels, endothelial dysfunction, increased oxidative stress, and insulin resistance. Glucocorticoids use also increases (PAI-1); it was found that secretion of t-PA levels is limited in patients receiving glucocorticoids, which further worsen the coagulation system and cause hypercoagulable state which further enhances thrombosis risk in SLE patients [18].
- Hydroxychloroquine (HCQ) is an antimalarial agent used in patients with SLE; it has anti-thrombotic effect by inhibiting platelet aggregation and adhesion and arachidonic acid release from stimulated platelets; it also decreases the thrombus size and the time of thrombus development which is dose dependent. HCQ inhibits GPIIb/IIIa receptor expression that is induced by aPL antibodies. Its role is more extended in the protection from thrombosis by lowering cholesterol level and lowering LDL; it also reduces interleukin-6 levels and decreases SLE flare episodes [10, 19].
- Aspirin (ASA) inhibits platelet aggregation through inhibition of cyclooxygenase enzyme and hence the synthesis of thromboxane A2 [10].

Table 12.1 summarizes the risk factors of thrombosis and accelerated atherosclerosis in SLE patients.

12.2.2 RA and Thrombosis

RA is a common chronic systemic inflammatory disease with worldwide distribution. There is

Table 12.1 Risk factors of thrombosis and accelerated atherosclerosis in SLE patients

1	Increased prevalence of traditional risk factors	HTN, DM, hyperlipidemia, smoking, obesity, old age.
2	Inflammation and high disease activity	↑ expression of TF, ↑ PAI, ↓ fibrinolysis, ↑CRP, lupus nephritis
3	Presence of antiphospholipid antibodies and/or APS	ACA, anti-ß2-GPI, LA in moderate to high titers
4	Hyperhomocysteinemia	
5	Genetic hypercoagulable states	Deficiency of proteins C and S, antithrombin and FVL
6	Drugs	Glucocorticoids (chronic use)

increased incidence of premature cardiovascular disease (CVD) and venous thrombosis in patients with rheumatoid arthritis and hence increased premature mortality and death on average 2.5 years earlier in community-based studies and approximately 18 years earlier in hospital-based studies than non-RA patients [20, 21]. The risk of VTE in patients with RA is increased to more than threefold than non-RA, as shown by Bacani A et al. (2012); they found that RA patients had a higher VTE cumulative incidence at 10 years than non-RA patients (6.7 in RA versus 2.8 in non-RA), and the risk of VTE was significantly higher within 90 days following hospitalization [20]. RA patients showed a higher age- and sex-adjusted increased risk of mortality (60%) and thromboembolic events (30%–50%) during a 5-year follow-up compared to non-RA patients. Similarly significant elevated risks (70% for death and 30%–40% for thromboembolic events) were seen when compared to OA patients. Several studies have shown that RA patients are 30%–60% more likely to suffer a cardiovascular event [19].

12.2.2.1 Risk Factor and Etiology of Thrombosis in RA

Lifestyle in RA

Patients with RA are physically less active due to their disease, and they may suffer from obesity, diabetes mellitus (DM), and hypertension that may result from medication use like steroids; some of RA patients are smokers as well; all these factors contribute to the accelerated atherosclerosis in RA subjects. Obesity is a time-dependent risk factor for development of VTE in RA patients, as shown by Bacani et al. in their study [20].

Inflammation

RA is characterized by a chronic inflammation that results in impaired immune system as well as persistent endothelial dysfunction, which predisposes to vascular wall damage and accelerated atherosclerosis. Such damage can be detectable by ultrasound measurement of carotid intima-media thickness (IMT) in a preclinical stage of the disease. Carotid IMT in RA patients is associated with markers of systemic inflammation and disease duration [22]. CD4+ are subsets of T cells that lack surface CD28 molecule (CD4 + CD28-) and expand when stimulated by endothelial autoantigens, in a subgroup of RA patients. Moreover, they infiltrate the atherosclerotic plaques and pose high pro-inflammatory and tissue-damaging properties which promote vascular injury. The role of these cells in contributing to early development of atherosclerosis in RA has been confirmed by recent studies which showed that RA patients with CD4 + CD28- cell expansion have a higher degree of endothelial dysfunction and a higher carotid IMT than patients without expansion of these cells [22].

High Disease Activity and High Levels of Inflammatory Markers

RA patients with high ESR and/or high CRP were found to have increased carotid artery IMT as well as increased probability of vessel plaque, which supports hypotheses of the relationship between systemic inflammation and atherosclerosis. ESR primarily reflects increased fibrinogen levels in response to systemic inflammation. The association between fibrinogen, as measured by the ESR, and increased carotid IMT suggests that inflammation-coagulation interactions may also have a role in atherogenesis. CRP is produced by the liver in response to interleukin-6, an earlier inflammation mediator, and can be found in the atheromatous lesions, suggesting its pathogenic role in atherothrombosis [23]; CRP is an independent risk factor for atherothrombotic disease [19].

Hospitalization

The relative risk factor for VTE is increased within 90 days post-hospitalization in RA patients. Orthopedic surgeries are reported to be a time-dependent cofactor risks for VTE development in RA patients that may develop within 90 days following lower extremity arthroplasty [20].

aPL Antibodies

RA patients may develop APL antibodies in 5%–75%, which increases the risk of VTE in these patients [20].

TNF-α

It causes endothelium damage and promotes blood coagulation through monocyte activation by increasing the TF levels [19].

Fibrinogen, VWF, Tissue Plasminogen Activator (t-PA) Antigen, and D-Dimer

Levels of these thrombotic variables are significantly higher in patients with RA [21].

Leukocytosis, Thrombocytosis, Increasing Platelet Activity, and Low Serum Albumin

These inflammatory markers are associated with increased cardiovascular risk and accelerated atherosclerosis in RA patients [19, 21].

High Systolic Blood Pressure (SBP) and Low Levels of High Density Lipoprotein (HDL)

High SBP in RA patients is mostly a result of a widespread use of NSAIDs and rarely can be caused by renal vasculitis and amyloidosis; HDL has a cardioprotective role against ischemia; low levels of HDL are found in RA. So, it is considered that both high SBP and low HDL are cardiovascular risk factors in patients with RA [21].

Rheumatoid Factor (RF)

RF positivity is associated with vascular injury and vasculitis, which increases plasma levels of VWF and t-PA that further enhance the thrombotic risks in RA patients [21].

Prothrombotic Condition in RA

Homocysteine (Hcy), in patients with RA the degree of inflammation is found to be correlated with Hcy levels. A positive relationship was found between the Hcy concentration and some parameters of inflammation, such as adhesion molecules and CPR [19].

Microparticles (MP) are membrane-bound vesicles that circulate in the blood and mediate inflammation and thrombosis. The most abundant MP in the blood come from platelets, and high levels of platelets MP were found in RA patients and correlated to high disease activity as measured by disease activity score (DAS 28). MP derived from granulocytes and monocytes have been found in the synovial fluid of RA patients as well; they stimulate TF and factor VII-dependent thrombin generation and lead to intra-articular inflammation and formation of fibrin clots, known as rice bodies [19].

12.2.2.2 Medications and Thrombosis in RA

- Nonsteroidal anti-inflammatory drugs (NSAIDs) are widely used for pain management in RA, associated with enhance cardiovascular events risk through rising the blood pressure, especially indomethacin and piroxicam, which rise the mean arterial BP by approximately 5 mm Hg [21].
- Glucocorticoids, through their effects on blood pressure, insulin resistance, lipid profile, body weight, coagulation, and endothelial dysfunction, might significantly increase the risk of CVD in RA patients [19].
- Disease-modifying anti-rheumatic drugs (DMARDs), methotrexate (MTX), the most common DMARDs used in RA, inhibit the homocysteine-methionine pathway which leads to hyperhomocysteinemia, but the concomitant use of folic acid reduces homocysteine level, thus decreasing the risk of CVD in AR patients; a long-term follow-up of RA patients has shown that the use of MTX is related to reduced cardiovascular mortality, probably related to a reduction of disease activity. Leflunomide and cyclosporine can cause hypertension which increases the risk of cardiovascular disease in RA patients; the suboptimal control of inflammation by both these drugs also increases the risk of thrombosis. Antimalarials, such as HCQ, have a beneficial effect in decreasing the serum cholesterol and low-density proteins [19].
- Biologic Therapy with TNF-α Blockers.

  A recent study suggested that the risk of developing any CV event in RA is lower in patients who receive TNF-α blockers. One study reported that TNF-α blockade using infliximab improves endothelial function after 12 weeks of therapy. This improvement depends on the clinical improvement of the joint manifestations and on a decrease in the

CRP and ESR levels. Other studies have shown the potential effect of short-term adalimumab therapy on endothelial function in RA patients with long-standing disease [19].

12.2.3 Vasculitis and Thrombosis

Vasculitides are a heterogeneous group of diseases characterized by the presence of vascular inflammation, which can lead to either a vessel wall destruction (leading to aneurysm or rupture) or a vessel stenosis (leads to tissue ischemia and necrosis) [24].

12.2.3.1 Large Vessel Vasculitis

They include Takayasu's (TAK) and giant cell arteritis (GCA). Chronic vascular inflammation leads to endothelial dysfunction that results in a premature atherosclerosis. The risk of arterial thrombosis is increased; strokes and transient ischemic attacks (TIA) have a similar rate of occurrence in this form of vasculitis, but there has been no clear increased risk of venous thrombosis [5].

12.2.3.2 Medium Vessel Vasculitis

Polyarteritis nodosa (PAN) is associated with increased risk of both arterial thrombi and VTE. This risk is high during active disease (3.27 events/person/year versus 0.58 in patients with inactive disease) and independent of hepatitis B status. The coronary arteries are affected mainly by arterial thrombosis, but there is no clear association between ischemic strokes and PAN [5].

12.2.3.3 Small Vessel Vasculitis

They include granulomatosis with polyangiitis (GPA), microscopic polyangiitis (MPA), and Churg-Strauss syndrome. This type of vasculitis is associated with high risk of arterial as well as venous thrombosis. The risk of a first-time symptomatic VTE has been considered by some researcher to be as seven times first symptomatic VTE risk in SLE [5]. The prevalence of cardiovascular disease is high and biphasic; the highest risk of cardiac ischemia appears either within 4 years of diagnosis or after 10 years of diagnosis. Prospective data from four European Vasculitis Study Group trials found that 14% of patients with GPA and MPA will have a cardiovascular event within 5 years of diagnosis [5]. The age-standardized annual cardiovascular mortality rate was found to be 3.7 times higher than expected in the general population. The presence of proteinase 3 (PR3) antineutrophil cytoplasmic antibodies (ANCA) was found to be protective, whereas a positive myeloperoxidase ANCA test was associated with an increased risk of cardiovascular events. There is no evidence of increased risk of ischemic stroke in small vessel vasculitis [5].

12.2.3.4 Risk Factors for Thrombosis in Vasculitis

Changes in Endothelial Function and Hypercoagulability

The endothelium loses its anti-thrombogenic activity which results from its damage and activation during inflammation. During inflammation, several cytokines are released; these cytokines along with vessel ischemia cause endothelial damage. Circulating ANCAs also cause endothelial damage, and circulating endothelial cells as a marker for endothelial damage have been detected in ANCA-associated vasculitis (AAV) patients, especially when AAV is active [25].

Hypercoagulability

Hypercoagulable state is present in patients with active AAV, and it is triggered by pro-inflammatory cytokines, such as TNF-α and IL-1. It is manifested by the presence of high levels of D-dimers and thrombin-antithrombin III complexes which reflects activated clotting system, increased expression of tissue factor, which activates factor VIII factor which in turn increases VTE risk in these patients. Increased platelet aggregation and reduced fibrinolytic capacity during active disease are among the other hypercoagulable causes of thrombosis in AAV patients [25].

Hypereosinophilia in Churg-Strauss

Eosinophils contain preformed protein-containing granules which are released when activated. Some of these proteins have prothrombotic effects through releasing tissue factor and several other proteins and enzymes which result in decrease fibrinolysis and block the anticoagulant effects of endothelial bound and exogenous heparin, stimulate the production of platelet factor 4 from platelets, and inhibit protein C activation [5].

aPL Autoantibodies

They are well-known cause of VTE, and they are detectable in some patients with vasculitis (especially AAV); aPL antibodies were detected in 19% in patients with GPA (formerly known as Wegener's granulomatosis) according to one study [25].

12.2.3.5 Medications and Thrombosis in Vasculitis

- Cyclophosphamide, the most commonly drug used in the treatment of vasculitis, is associated with an increased risk of VTE in patients with AAV, through induction of vascular endothelial damage, endothelial cells apoptosis, platelet activation, and cytokines release [5].
- Corticosteroids, particularly in high doses, can be thrombogenic through induction of high levels of factor VIII and lower fibrinolytic activity [25].
- Low-dose ASA is proven to be beneficial in the prevention of cerebrovascular insults and visual loss in GCA and thus is recommended to use for same purpose in TAK [5].

12.2.4 Behçet's Disease (BD)

BD is a chronic inflammatory disorder of unknown cause; its manifestations are considered to be caused by an underlying vasculitis [26], characterized by recurrent oral aphthous ulcers, genital ulcers, and uveitis, followed by involvement of other systems causing thrombophlebitis, arthritis, pulmonary and neurological involvement, erythema nodosum, and gastrointestinal disease [27]. Vascular involvement is common in BD; it affects up to 40% of patients resulting in arterial and venous thrombosis and aneurysms particularly of pulmonary arteries [5, 27]; vessels of all sizes are involved, both in the arterial and venous systems [28]. Venous thrombi are more common with involvement of DVT and superficial thrombophlebitis [27]. Asymptomatic DVT of the extremities in patients with BD with no history of vascular thrombosis is reported to be 6% which is higher than that seen in a healthy population [5]. BD is associated with low rate of pulmonary thrombosis (between 4 and 10%); this is because of tight adhesions of the peripheral thrombosis to the venous walls [5]. Other sites of venous thrombi in BD are vena cava thrombosis, Budd-Chiari syndrome (which coexists with inferior vena cava and portal vein thrombosis), and cerebral venous sinus thrombosis. BD complicated with Budd-Chiari syndrome is associated with poor and mean survival of 10 months compared with 16 months in patients affected with Budd-Chiari syndrome without BD. Cerebral venous sinus thrombosis (CVT) is estimated to occur in 8% of BD patients and in about 13% of BD with neurologic involvement. CVT most commonly manifests as intracranial hypertension. CVT in BD more likely affects male gender, presents at a younger age, and less likely develops venous infarcts [5]. The mortality rate is higher in patients with BD who had venous thrombosis, especially if large vessel is involved (mortality rate reached 12.1%) than in those without VTE [28].

12.2.4.1 Risk Factors for Thrombosis in BD

Endothelial Cell Dysfunction

Inflammation and resultant endothelial dysfunction suppresses nitric oxide (NO) secretion in patients with active BD, thereby impairing its normal function of vasodilation and inhibition of platelet aggregation, which in turn increases the risk of thrombosis in BD [5].

Low Protein C

BD is associated with a significant reduction in activated protein C, lower endothelial protein C receptor levels, and increased resistance to activated protein C, leading to significant impairment of anticoagulation as well as anti-inflammatory properties of protein C. Lower levels of activated protein C is found in patients with a history of VTE as compared to those without VTE history, which increase the risk of recurrent thrombi further [5].

Activated Platelets and Microparticles (MP)

MP are small membrane particles derived from platelets, monocytes, and leukocytes; they are secreted in higher levels during active inflammation and lead to the expression of TF tissue factor and anionic phospholipids which trigger the coagulation cascade and increase the risk of thrombosis in patients with BD [5].

Vascular Endothelial Growth Factor (VEGF)

VEGF levels in BD patients with acute thrombosis were higher than those of BD patients in chronic stage. Also, higher levels of MCP-1 were found in BD patients with acute thrombosis as compared with healthy controls. The positive correlation of the elevated levels of various factors with venous thrombosis can be a useful marker to predict the likelihood of thrombosis in BD [29].

HLA-B51 and HLA-B35 Positivity

BD patient positive for HLA-B51 are at increased risk of VTE, while those with HLA-B35 are protective from VTE [55].

12.2.4.2 Medications and Thrombosis in BD

- Azathioprine, immunosuppression with azathioprine 2.5 mg/kg per day, decreased the rate of DVT according to one control trial [5].
- Glucocorticoids, cyclophosphamide, one large study had found that immunosuppressives and glucocorticoids significantly decreased the risk of recurrent DVT in 807 patients with BD [5]. The European League Against Rheumatism (EULAR) in 2008 recommended the use of immunosuppressants (glucocorticoids, azathioprine, cyclophosphamide, and cyclosporine A) in the management of acute DVT in patients with BD disease [5]. Immunosuppressive agents improve prognosis in patients with BD by decreasing the odds of venous thrombosis relapse in BD by fourfold; immunosuppression in Budd-Chiari syndrome is associated with a significant improvement in prognosis as shown in a study done by Desbois et al. [28]. A retrospective study of 37 patients with venous thrombosis in BD compared immunosuppressive agents, anticoagulation treatment, and the combination of immunosuppressive agents and anticoagulation treatment; 3 of the 4 patients in the anticoagulant-treated group (75%) developed new thromboses, compared to 2 of 16 patients in the immunosuppressive agent-treated group (12.5%) and 1 of 17 patients in the combination-treated group (5.9%) [28].

12.2.5 Antiphospholipid Syndrome (APS) and Thrombosis

APS is characterized by recurrent venous and arterial thrombosis and/or fetal loss in combination with the persistent presence of circulating aPL antibodies, which comprise LA, ACA, and/or anti β2GPI antibodies [30].

DVT is the most frequent clinical manifestation of APS. Larger veins like subclavian, iliofemoral, upper abdomen, portal, and axillary veins may be affected as well. Thrombosis of almost every organ has been described in APS, which result in different clinical conditions and syndromes, such as superficial thrombophlebitis; superior vena cava syndrome; renal vein thrombosis; adrenal infarction; Addison's syndrome; Budd-Chiari syndrome; pulmonary hypertension, due to recurrent pulmonary embolism; and diffuse pulmonary hemorrhage, due to microthromboses [31].

Arterial thrombosis consists a main clinical feature of APS, but appears less frequently than Venous, the most common site of arterial thrombosis is the cerebral circulation, leading to stroke or transient ischemic attack (TIA), CVT, coronary, renal and mesenteric arteries thrombosis has been observed also. In women under 50 years, LA is considered to be a major risk factor for arterial thrombosis as shown in RATIO study (Risk of Arterial Thrombosis In Relation to Oral Contraceptives). CNS involvement in APS mainly strokes and TIAs is associated with high morbidity and mortality [31].

Other manifestations of hypercoagulopathy and thrombosis in APS include thrombocytopenia, hemolytic anemia, pregnancy loss, eclampsia, livedo reticularis, purpura, Libman-Sacks valvulopathy, amaurosis fugax, retinal vessels thrombosis, and avascular necrosis of the bones [32].

Table 12.2 Determinants of high- and low-risk factors for thrombosis in patients with APS

Patient's characteristics		Thrombosis risk level
1	Isolated (LA) positivity	High
2	Triple positivity (LA + aCL + anti-β2GPI)	High
3	Isolated persistent positivity of aCL (medium-high titers)	High
4	Isolated, intermittent positivity of aCL or anti-β2GPI (low and medium titers)	Low
5	Concomitant SLE	High
6	Presence of hypertension, hypercholesterolemia	High
7	Smoking, use of oral contraceptive pills	High

12.2.5.1 Risk Factors for Thrombosis in APS

aPL Autoantibodies

aPL antibodies are a heterogeneous group of different autoantibodies with distinct specificity for cardiolipin or for plasma proteins with affinity for anionic phospholipids such as β2 GPI, prothrombin, or annexin A5 [33]. Oxidized β2 GPI is able to bind to and activate dendritic cells which results in autoantibodies production [32]. aPL antibodies are highly thrombotic. The ACA are directed against cardiolipin and b2GPI, the anti-β2GPI antibody is directed against β2GPI, while the LA measures functional anti-β2GPI antibodies and antiprothrombin antibodies. β2GPI antibodies are responsible for the increased risk of thromboembolic complications; patients positive for all three aPL antibodies have a significant increased risk of recurrence of thromboembolic disease, while patients positive for only one of the three aPL antibodies hardly have a significant increase in recurrence compared to patients with thrombosis but without aPL antibodies as shown by Pengo et al. (2011) [34].

The presence of LA, triple positivity (combination of LA, aCL and β2GPI antibodies), isolated, but, persistently positive aCL at medium–high levels are conditions considered as a high risk serological aPL profile for thrombosis. Patients with triple positivity have aPL levels much higher than others, thus making thrombosis highest risk of thrombosis in this group. Patients with isolated aCL or β2GPI at low-medium titers, particularly if intermittently positive, are considered to have a low-risk profile for thrombosis [30] (Table 12.2).

LA positivity increased the risk of stroke 48-fold and the risk of myocardial infarction 11-fold, while β2GPI antibodies are associated with double risk for stroke as shown by Urbanus RT et al. in the RATIO study [30].

The Effects of aPL Antibodies on Endothelial Cells

Anti-β2GPI antibodies result in increased expression of adhesion molecules (ICAM-1, VCAM-1, E-selectin); aPL autoantibodies increase the synthesis and secretion of pro-inflammatory cytokines IL-1, IL-6, and IL-8 and increase TF expression and upregulation of tissue factor messenger RNA (mRNA) as well as enhancement of endothelin-1 levels [32]. aPL antibodies cause defective apoptosis of endothelial cells, which exposes membrane phospholipids to the binding of various plasma proteins [31, 32].

Hypercoagulable Effect of aPL Antibodies

Production of antibodies against coagulation factors, including prothrombin, protein C, protein S, and annexins, platelets activation to enhance endothelial adherence, activation of vascular endothelium, which, facilitates the binding of platelets and monocytes that result in a hypercoagulable state. aPL antibodies react with oxidized LDL and predispose to atherosclerosis. Moreover, complement activation by aPL has been recognized as a possible significant cause in APS pathogenesis. Emerging evidence from murine models suggests that APL-mediated complement activation may be a primary event in pregnancy loss [32].

Platelet Activation and Aggregation by aPL

β2GPI antibodies activate platelets aggregation and release of platelets factor 4 (PF4) and thromboxane B2; aPL cannot bind to the surface of "intact" platelets, while they have the ability to bind to platelets with exposed negatively charged phospholipids in their membranes [31]. Bleeding time is prolonged in about 40% of patients with APS, without accompanying bleeding tendency, which indicates impaired platelet function in APS as a result of platelet activation by aPL. The expression of platelet membrane glycoproteins, particularly GPIIb-IIIa (fibrinogen receptor, critical in platelet aggregation) and GPIIIa, is also increased that enhance platelets aggregation further [31]. Another mechanism of platelets activation is the production of high plasma levels of active VWF in patients with β2GPI antibodies. In the normal conditions, binding of β2GPI to VWF results in inhibiting its ability to promote adhesion and platelet aggregation, but in the presence of anti-β2GPI antibodies, this anticoagulant effect is blocked [31]. β2GPI antibodies and LA induce the formation of stable thrombi and large aggregates, as shown by Jankowski et al. in animal model [31].

β2GPI Binding with Platelet Factor 4 (PF4)

PF4 is recognized recently as the dominant β2GPI-binding protein. PF4 binds in vitro, with high-affinity, recombinant β2GPI; PF4 tetramers can bind two β2GPI molecules simultaneously. Anti-β2GPI antibodies selectively interact with complexes composed of (β2GPI)2-(PF4)4. This reaction is higher against PF4-β2GPI complex than against β2GPI alone. Anti-β2GPI-β2GPI-PF4 complex significantly induced platelet p38 MAPK phosphorylation and thromboxane A_2 production [37]. p38 MAPK is mitogen-activated protein (MAP) kinase that controls many cellular responses, such as proliferation, migration, differentiation, and apoptosis. In platelets, p38 MAPK regulates platelet adhesion to collagen and aggregation [37]. β2GPI antibodies form stable complexes with PF4, leading to the stabilization of β2GPI, which facilitates antibody recognition. This interaction is found to be involved in the procoagulant tendency of APS [36].

Activation of Monocytes by aPL Antibodies

This will result in increased TF expression and activity as well as increased production of proinflammatory cytokines, which increases the risk of thrombosis in APS patients; many researchers had found high levels of soluble TF (sTF) in the peripheral blood of patients with a history of thrombosis and aPL [31, 35].

Other Risk Factors for Thrombosis in APS

Hypertension, smoking, hypercholestrolemia or estrogen use: the coexistent presence of these factors is associated with thrombosis. The interaction between aPL, smoking, and oral contraceptive pills (OCP) has been identified and clarified in the case-control study; the risk for suffering a stroke doubled among smoking LA-positive women, as compared with non-smokers; the risk of stroke among OCP users is increased to sevenfold. One study showed that all smoker women who had LA suffered a myocardial infarction [29]. Concomitant SLE in APS (SAPS) increases the risk of thrombosis further in these patients (see SLE and thrombosis in this chapter) [29].

12.3 Approach and Diagnosis of Thrombosis in Rheumatic Diseases

The clinical features of thrombosis in patients with rheumatic diseases are similar to that in patients with other diseases and the general population; therefore it is very important for the physician who attends such patients to take a careful detailed history, perform a thorough physical examination, and do an appropriate workup (laboratory and imaging).

Unprovoked (idiopathic) venous thrombotic events are defined as venous thrombosis that occurs in the absence of any of the known risk factors; about 50% of patients presenting with a first idiopathic venous thrombosis have an underlying thrombophilia [38]; therefore special attention is needed to consider thrombophilia in the history and the workup of thrombosis.

12.3.1 History Taking

Symptoms of PE and DVT are not specific, so it is important to ask about the risk factors such as the age, previous history of VTE, recent long-distance travelling for active malignancy, coagulation disorders, hormone replacement therapy (HRT) in postmenopausal women, use of an oral contraceptive pills (OCP) in a female of child-bearing age, abdominal/pelvic surgery/knee joint replacement, and diseases or conditions that lead to limited mobility [39–42], as well as a comprehensive history of rheumatic disorders that associated with increased risk of thrombosis, especially if VTE is recurrent, or unusual presentation in the absence of the known risk factors, or if the patient is a young one with no known predisposing factors for thrombosis, or if the patient presents with multiple thrombi at different sites or had both arterial and venous thrombosis.

Detailed history of medications must be taken in patients with rheumatic disorders, as some of them have thrombotic risks, while others have a protective role (see details of thrombosis and medications in individual disorder in Sect. 1).

Inquire about the constitutional symptoms in rheumatic disorders, this includes fever, sweats, loss of appetite and weight.

History of skin rashes, such as malar rash, photosensitivity, raynaud's phenomenon if SLE is considered in the differential diagnosis of VTE. Mouth and genital ulcers and visual complaints may provide a clue to the presence of BD or other rheumatic diseases.

A careful obstetrical history is mandatory if APS (either primary or secondary) is suspected to be the cause of thrombosis in a young female in the absence of the traditional risk factors.

Inquiries about the renal complications must be included in the history in patients with SLE who presents with thrombotic episodes.

Patients with PE present to the emergency room (ER) and may complain of sudden dyspnea, pleuritic and non-pleuritic chest pain, cough or hemoptysis, fever, and diaphoresis; they may have cyanosis or syncope especially if massive PE [41, 43, 44]. Patients may have DVT at the same time which can be asymptomatic, since less than 25% of PE patients presented with symptoms and signs of DVT [41].

Patients suffering from DVT may complain of sudden ipsilateral leg swelling, redness, intermittent cramps, and pain in the calf or leg [45–47]. Presence of risk factors will increase suspicious of DVT which include prior history of DVT or PE, recent surgery, active cancer, trauma, hospitalization, immobility, co morbidities, family history of VTE, advanced age, current pregnancy, hormonal contraceptives and hormonal replacement therapy, and obesity [42, 45, 47, 48].

DVT and PE are considered combined emergency problem; 70% of patients diagnosed with PE have DVT in their leg and 50% of DVT patients established asymptomatic PE [47]. For that, we must diagnose DVT to prevent PE by history, physical examination, and investigations [48].

12.3.2 Physical Examination

The physical examination of patients with PE reveals some signs, of which tachypnea is the most common [43, 49]; other signs such as hypotension and cardiogenic shock may present in massive PE. Signs of right ventricular failure (RVF) such as tachycardia, distended neck veins, and tricuspid regurgitation may be there; wheezes, loud pulmonary component of second heart sound (loud P_2), and pleural rub may also be heard sometimes [44]. Signs of DVT must be looked for [43]; they include leg redness, edema, warmth, tenderness, superficial dilation of veins,

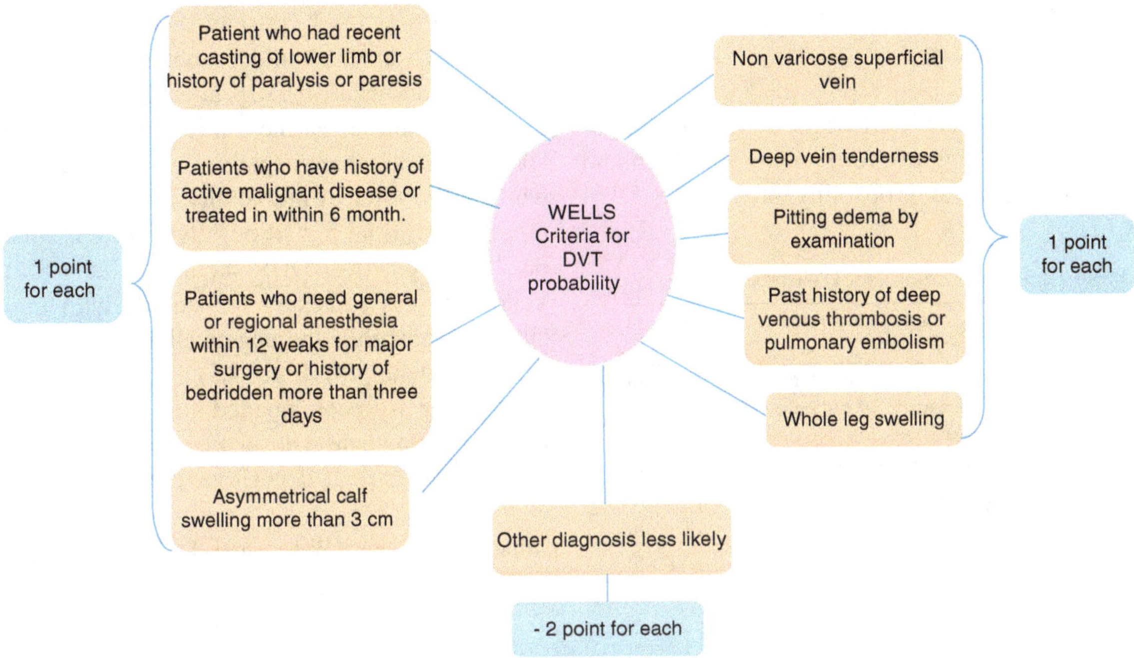

Fig. 12.3 Wells Criteria for DVT Probability

and fever; tachycardia and sign of pulmonary embolism should be looked for as well even in the absence of symptoms [47, 50].

Rheumatic disorders should be considered as the top most differential diagnosis in unusual presentation of different forms of thromboembolic diseases such as young patients with no known risk factors, or thrombosis in unusual sites, or in case of multiple or mixed arterial and venous thrombi; thus, a careful examination should be done.

Many diseases mimic the sign and symptoms of DVT and PE, rendering the physical examination to be not enough for diagnosis, although very essential to perform [47, 50]. Therefore, another methods need to be used before going further to work up these patients.

12.3.3 Clinical Pretest Probability (CPTP) for VTE

CPTP includes Wells and modified Wells criteria [44, 51]; it is a useful and important method to determine the probability of DVT and PE, respectively, and to classify the risk as low, medium, and high and is helpful in selecting the proper test for workup [41].

Wells criteria is based on history and physical examination and classifies the patient as high risk if score is between 3 and 8 points, moderate risk if 1–2 points, and low risk if 0 to −2 points [44, 45, 48, 50, 52]. For details see Fig. 12.3 and Table 12.3.

In modified Wells criteria, the total point is 12, based on symptoms and signs and risk to get the disease. Patients are considered low risk if less than 2 points, intermediate risk if 2 to 6 points, and high risk if more than 6 points [8, 16]; the probability of PE is also categorized as likely and less likely; if it was more than 4 points, the patients are likely to have PE [44]. Clinical sign and symptoms of DVT (3points), other diagnosis less likely than pulmonary embolism (3 points), heart rate (HR) > 100/min (1.5 points), immobilization >3 days or surgery in previous 4 weeks (1.5 points), previous PE or DVT (1.5 point), hemoptysis (1 point) and malignancy (1 point) [44, 51]. Figure 12.4 and Table 12.4.

12.3.4 Laboratory and Radiology Workup

Duplex ultrasound (DUS) is recommended as an initial imaging test for patients with high and moderate clinical probability of DVT, if DUS is positive then DVT is established, but if negative then D-dimer should be obtained, positive D-dimer and negative DUS after that follow up the patient and repeat the ultrasound, but if both DUS and D dimer are negative, DVT is ruled out, while a low clinical probability of DVT require D-dimer as initial test, if negative, DVT is ruled out, but if positive, DUS should be done [44]. Venography is indicated in patients with high clinical probability and negative DUS or if DUS cannot be done [48] (Fig. 12.5).

D-dimer is recommended for patients with low or intermediate risk for PE, and, if negative, PE is ruled out, but if positive, then CT pulmo-

Table 12.3 Wells criteria for DVT probability

1	Active cancer or cancer treated within 6 month	1 point
2	Calf swelling 3 cm greater than the other leg (measured 10 cm below the tibial tuberosity)	1 point
3	Prominent superficial veins (non-varicose)	1 point
4	Pitting edema in symptomatic leg	1 point
5	Paralysis, paresis, or recent orthopedic casting of a lower extremity	1 point
6	Localized tenderness in the deep vein system	1 point
7	Recent bed rest for >3 days or major surgery requiring regional or general anesthetic within past 12 weeks	1 point
8	Previous history of DVT or PE	1 point
9	Swelling of entire leg	1 point
10	Alternative diagnosis at least as probable	-2 point

Table 12.4 Modified Wells criteria for PE probability

1	Clinical sign and symptoms of DVT	3 points
2	Alternative diagnosis less likely than PE	3 points
3	Heart rate > 100/min.	1.5 points
4	Immobilization >3 days or surgery in previous 4 weeks	1.5 points
5	Previous PE or DVT	1.5 points
6	Hemoptysis	1 points
7	Malignancy	1 points

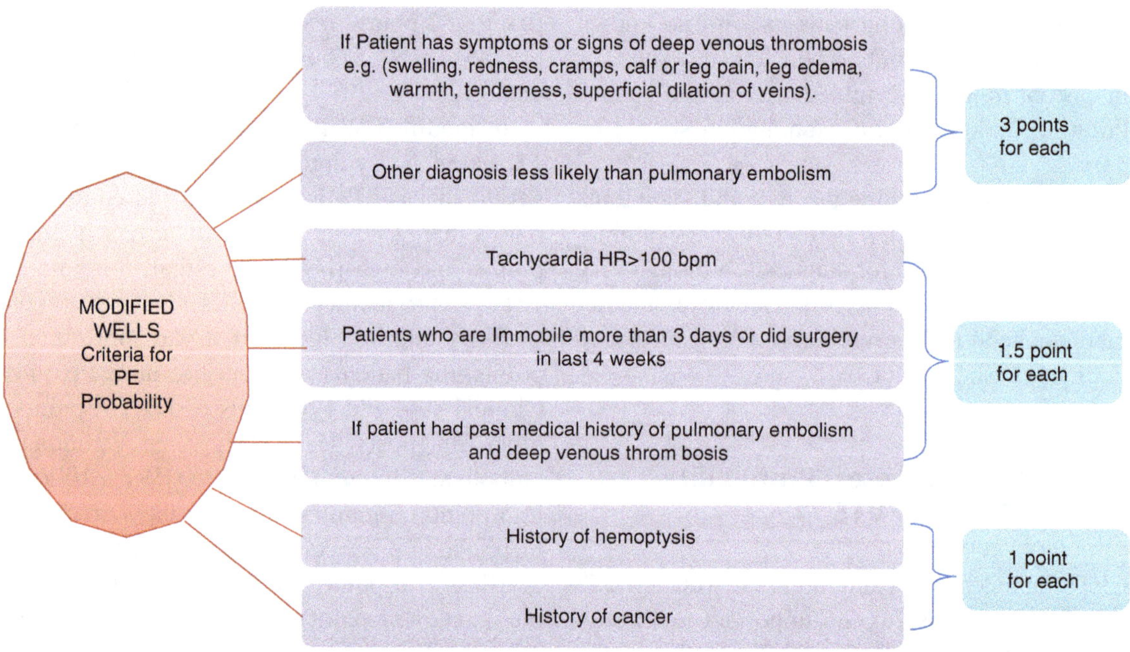

Fig. 12.4 Modified Wells Criteria for PE Probability

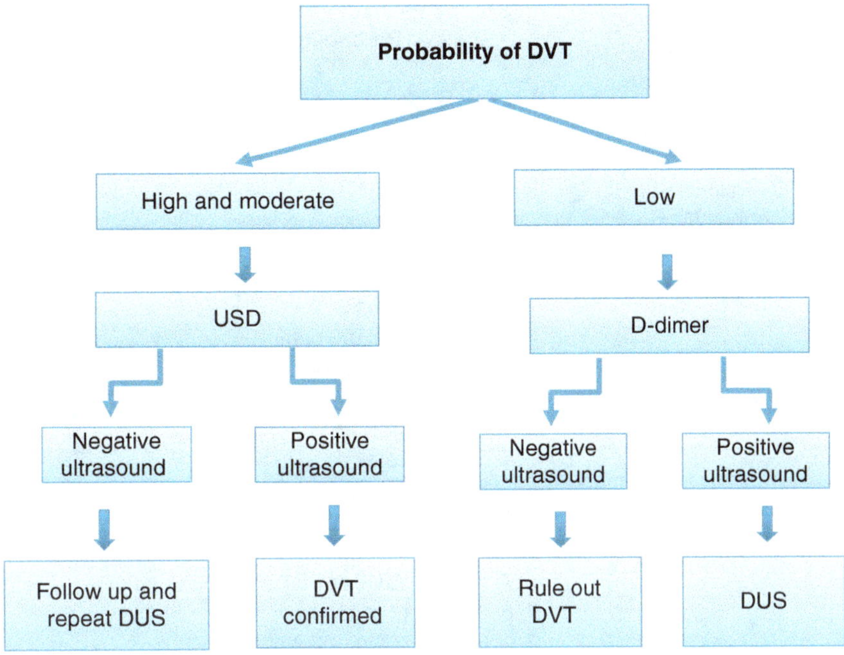

Fig. 12.5 Probability of DVT algorithm

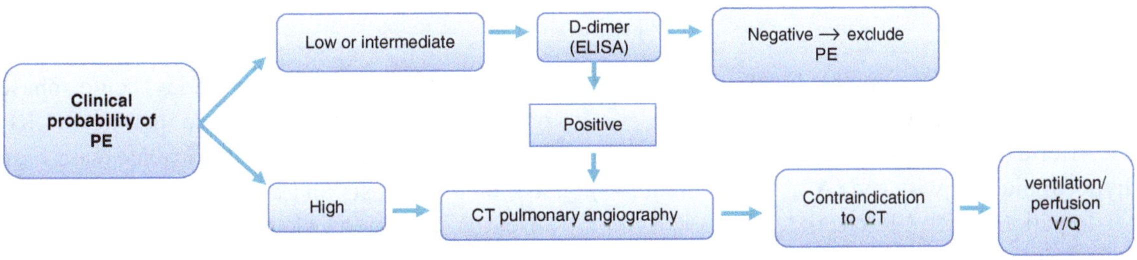

Fig. 12.6 Clinical probability of PE

nary angiography (the gold standard) [39] is required. If patient's risk for PE is high, CT pulmonary angiography should be done, but in situation where contraindication for contrast is used in CT angiogram such as in patients with renal failure, ventilation/perfusion (V/Q) scan can be done [43, 51, 53] (Fig. 12.6).

Pulmonary embolism rule out criteria (PERC) is used in patients who are less likely to have PE (4 points or less); factors of PERC are age < 50 years, HR < 100/min, oxygen saturation >94%, no unilateral leg swelling, no hemoptysis, no surgery or trauma within 4 weeks, no prior DVT or PE, and no estrogens or progestin use. If patients met these criteria, they are regarded as negative for PE, and no further investigations are needed, but if PERC is not met, they are considered positive for PE, and D-dimer should be tested; if it is negative, PE is ruled out [44, 54] (Fig. 12.7).

Other imaging such as chest X-ray may be required to confirm the diagnosis; chest X-ray is usually normal in PE, but it is important to exclude other diseases. Signs of PE on chest radiograph are atelectasis, pleural-based infiltrates, or effusions, there may be a wedge shaped opacity and oligemia - cut off - of arteries, and right descending enlargement of the pulmonary artery) [39, 43, 44].

In PE, ECG may show supraventricular arrhythmia, signs of right ventricular (RV) strains, right axis derivation, T-wave inversion in

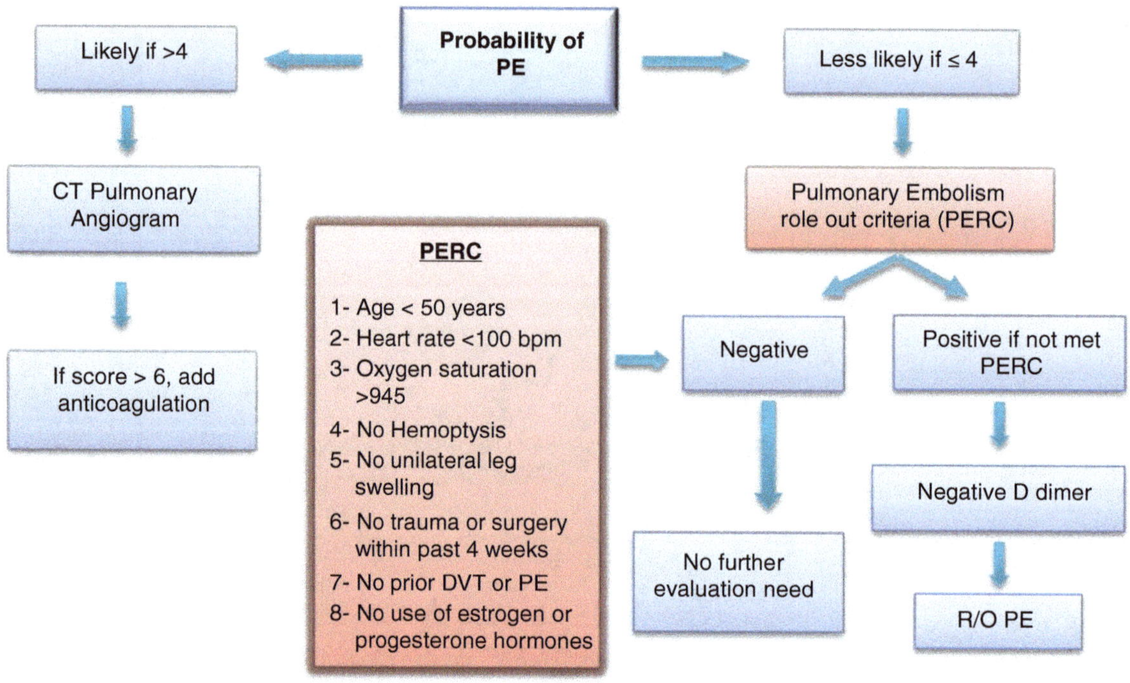

Fig. 12.7 Probability of Pulmonary Embolism algorithm

V_1–V_4, right bundle branch block, $S_1Q_3T_3$, and QR in V_1 or P pulmonale [39, 43, 44].

Arterial blood gases can show hypoxemia, hypocapnia, and widened (A-a) O2 gradient [44].

In patients with PE, check troponin and brain natriuretic peptide (BNP) levels, since their high levels are associated with RV strain and linked to increased mortality in PE [44].

Laboratory investigations include general and specific workup. Generally, for all patients with thrombosis, full blood count, renal and liver function, and coagulation profile need to be done. Specific workup for thrombophilia and hereditary hypercoagulable disorders, this includes: Factor V Leiden, Prothrombin 20210A, Protein C and S, Antithrombin III [38], as they also can present in autoimmune rheumatic disorders such as SLE. Acquired hypercoagulable states includes anti- aPL antibodies (LA, ACA, β2GP1) should be done in idiopathic thrombosis or if there multiple thrombi, HLA-B51 test for BD if thrombosis is at an usual site (Bud Chairi syndrome) or both arterial and venous thrombi or idiopathic CVT should be considered [55].

Other blood workup includes acute phase reactants that measure disease activity (CRP, ESR), since their high levels correlate with high risk of thrombosis and atherosclerosis in certain diseases such as RA [19].

12.4 Management of Thrombosis in Rheumatic Diseases, Prophylaxis, and Secondary Prevention of Thrombosis

12.4.1 Management of Thrombosis in Rheumatic Diseases

There are no specific recommendations for the management of thrombosis in patients with rheumatic disorders, the same plan of treatment as of patients with other diseases and general population. Anticoagulation with intravenous unfractionated heparin (UFH) or subcutaneous low molecular weight heparin (LMWH), followed by warfarin, is the initial treatment strategy for cases with acute thrombosis [57].

Treatment of patients with PE depends on clinical probability of pulmonary embolism and hemodynamic stability of patients, initial treatment with anticoagulant if clinical probability is high or intermediate and cannot get the investigation within 4 h and in case of low probability and investigation deferred for 24 hours, anticoagulant therapy include LMWH, or fondaparinux, both are administered subcutaneously, do not require monitoring of PT and APTT, and not to be used in renal failure, UFH is administered intravenously and it is preferred in massive PE. If there is contraindication to anticoagulant, then inferior vena cava filter should be considered. Thrombolytic therapy is used in patients who have hemodynamic instability [40, 41] (Fig. 12.8).

In patients with DVT, LMWH is recommended, as it is superior to UFH especially in pregnant and patient with cancer, but it should not be used in patient with renal failure; they should be treated with unfractionated heparin (Fig. 12.9); warfarin should be started together with LMWH until targeted INR is reached; inferior vena cava filter is indicated in patient with contraindication to anticoagulation therapy [45, 48, 56] (Fig. 12.10).

Compression stocking is used within 1 month of DVT diagnosis to prevent post-thrombotic syndrome and for at least 1 year after diagnosis [45, 56].

Anticoagulation with warfarin had been associated with several disadvantages related to the drug itself such as slow onset of action, variable pharmacologic effects, food-drug interactions, prolonged half-life, and the need for close monitoring of INR [65]. However, several large studies have been done in this field, and researchers had found that the NOACs are now emerging as the alternative anticoagulation therapy to conventional therapy for patients with acute VTE; the advantages of these novel anticoagulant therapy are many and overcome the troubles of warfarin therapy, such as the fixed therapeutic dose, without the need of dose adjustment; they do not require routine laboratory monitoring of PT and INR. They reach their peak efficacy within 1 to 4 h after ingestion; thus a prolonged period of bridging therapy is not required when switching from initial treatment with UFH or LMWH to

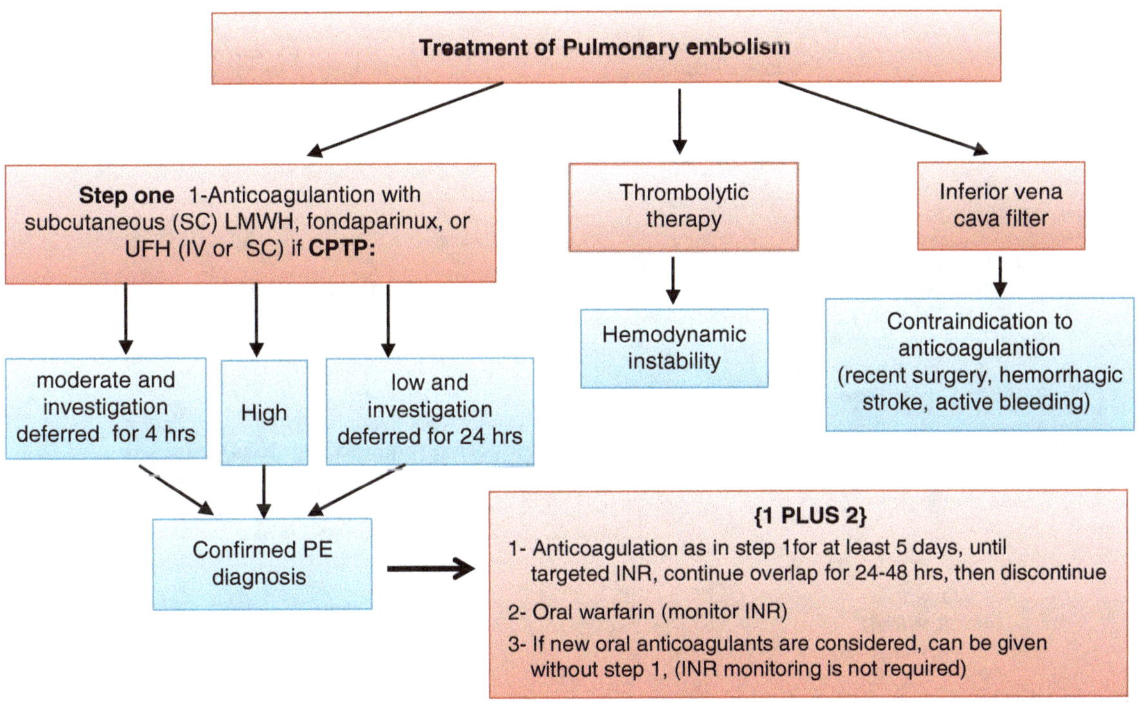

Fig. 12.8 Treatment of PE

Fig. 12.9 Characteristics of special population and types of heparin

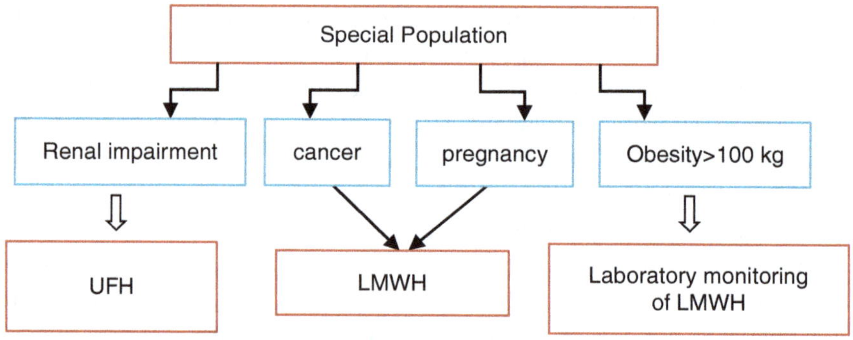

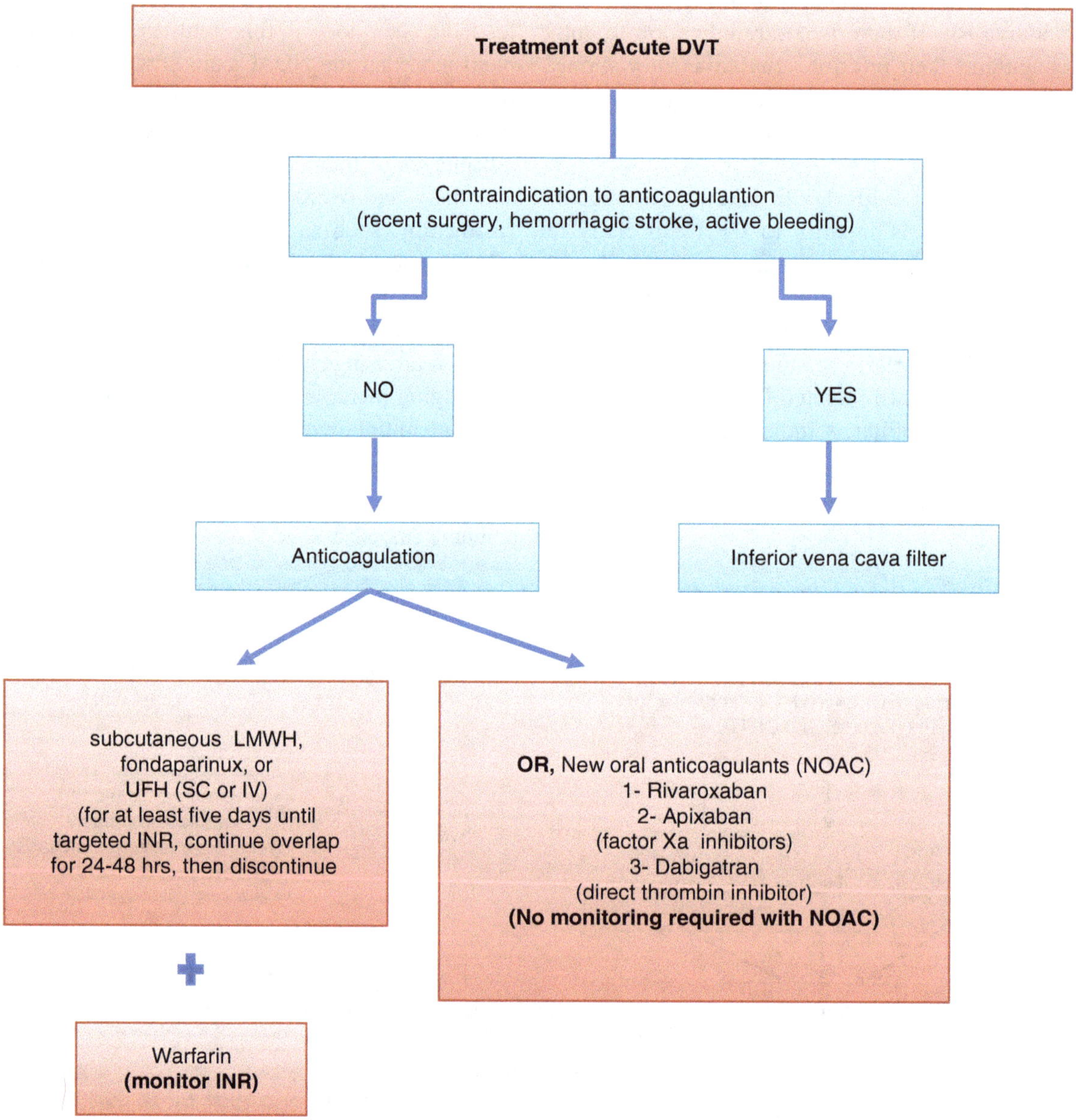

Fig. 12.10 Management of DVT algorithm.

these novel agents and less risks of major bleeding. Unfortunately, the antidote for bleeding events is not available yet [64,65,66]. No data is available regarding the safety of NOACs in pregnancy, for which it should be avoided in a pregnant patient and also in some other conditions such as patients with mechanical heart valves and in severe renal insufficiency [65].

Two groups of NOACs are available, factor Xa inhibitors (rivaroxaban, apixaban) and direct thrombin inhibitors (dabigatran). The safety and efficacy of these agents for the treatment and prevention of recurrent VTE have been studied by large randomized prospective trials [64].

Apixaban has a rapid onset of action and is approved for use in the prevention of stroke and systemic embolism in adult patients with nonvalvular atrial fibrillation (AF) and in the primary prevention of VTE in adult patients who have undergone elective total hip or total knee arthroplasty [65].

Apixaban is effective for the prevention of recurrent VTE if patients complete 6 to 12 months of anticoagulant therapy for acute VTE, with major bleeding risk similar to those for placebo.

Therapy with apixaban was compared with conventional anticoagulant therapy in patients with acute symptomatic VTE in the AMPLIFY trial (Apixaban for the Initial Management of Pulmonary Embolism and Deep-Vein Thrombosis as First-Line Therapy) [66]. The AMPLIFY study has very impressive results and concluded that a fixed-dose oral apixaban alone was as effective as conventional treatment which consists of enoxaparin followed by warfarin and was associated with a clinically relevant reduction of 69% in major bleeding, and its efficacy in patients with PE was similar to that in the patients with DVT. Moreover, the efficacy and the reduction in major bleeding with apixaban were consistent with that of warfarin, but clinically relevant non-major bleeding were less. Interestingly, The efficacy and safety of apixaban were consistent in all patients participated in the trial including patients older than 75 years, obese patients of more than 100 kg, use of parenteral anticoagulant treatment before randomization, and treatment duration. AMPLIFY trial results are very promising and encouraging to consider apixaban a safe and effective regimen for the initial and long-term VTE treatment [66].

12.4.1.1 Special Consideration for Thrombosis in Rheumatic Disorders

- Patients with rheumatic diseases and thrombosis need a long-term management (indefinite) for thrombosis especially those with aPL autoantibodies to prevent recurrent thrombosis, that is, secondary thrombosis prevention; they require the optimal intensity of anticoagulation with warfarin [30, 57].
- Several studies had proven that high-intensity treatment with warfarin to maintain INR = 3.0 with or without low-dose aspirin was more effective than moderate-intensity warfarin or low-dose aspirin for the prevention of recurrent thrombosis in aPL-positive patients, but, recently, some trials demonstrated that high-intensity anticoagulation (INR 3.1–4.0) was no better than moderate intensity (INR 2.0–3.0). So, moderate-intensity anticoagulation is the current standard of treatment of first venous thrombosis [57–60] (Fig. 12.9).
- For the management of acute DVT in BD immunosuppressive agents such as corticosteroids, azathioprine, cyclophosphamide, and cyclosporine A are recommended, but there is no evidence of benefit from, and uncontrolled experience with anticoagulation, use of antiplatelet or antifibrinolytic agents in the management of DVT or for the use of anticoagulation in arterial thrombosis in patients with BD, in patients with CVT (dural sinus thrombosis) treatment with is corticosteroids is recommended (modified EULAR 2008 recommendation) [59]. Anticoagulant therapy must be used cautiously and only after systemic immunosuppressant, and if thrombi are not extensive, antiplatelet treatment with low-dose aspirin is probably sufficient [61].
- • In patients with a low-risk aPL profile, who had first venous thrombosis in the presence of a known transient risk factor, anticoagulation could be limited to 3–6 months [30].

12.4.2 Prophylaxis and Secondary Thrombosis Prevention in Rheumatic Disorders

- Daily ASA in doses of 75–325 mg are suitable for inhibition of platelet aggregation for prophylaxis against cardiovascular events in RA patients [19].
- Prophylaxis use of LMWH to prevent venous thrombosis during periods of immobilization, as immobilization in RA patients is related to disease activity and inflammation [19].
- ASA (75–150 mg/day) is recommended for the prevention of cerebrovascular events and vision loss in GCA, and it should be also considered for the primary prevention of cardiovascular events in TAK [5].

12.4.2.1 Primary Prophylaxis in SLE Patients

- HCQ reduces thrombotic risk and disease-related morbidity and mortality in SLE and is recommended for all patients unless it is contraindicated [10].
- HCQ plus low-dose ASA is recommended for SLE patients with positive LA or ACA (medium-high titers) [30].

12.4.2.2 Primary Prophylaxis in APS Patients

- In asymptomatic individuals, aPL antibodies positivity is an incidental finding; thus, primary prophylaxis can be considered with ASA 81 mg per day [59, 60].
- Healthy individuals, with positive aPL antibodies in high titers and with no thrombotic manifestations, should be advised for a primary prophylaxis with ASA 325 mg orally daily [60].
- HCQ 400 mg orally daily decreases aPL antibody titers and thus protects from further thrombotic episode; that is based on trials in animal models and an indirect evidence from human studies, so more studies are needed to prove this effect of HCQ for standard recommendation in healthy aPL-positive patients [60] (Fig. 12.11).

12.4.2.3 Primary Prophylaxis in High-Risk Situations

All patients with aPL positivity should receive usual doses of LMWH in high-risk situations, such as surgery, prolonged immobilization, and puerperium [30]; the same is applied for all patients with other rheumatic disorders.

12.4.2.4 Secondary Prophylaxis in Patients with Positive aPL Antibodies

- Patient who suffered from either arterial or venous thrombosis and aPL who do not fulfill criteria for APS should be managed in the same manner as aPL-negative patients with similar thrombotic events [30].
- Recurrent venous thrombosis has been reported in patients with APS at 3% to 24%. Secondary prophylaxis with high-intensity warfarin (INR = 3–4), or moderate-intensity warfarin (INR = 2–3) plus ASA is recommended [60].
- Treatment of APS patients with arterial thrombosis is controversial, and only ASA 325 mg/day can be given or moderate-intensity warfarin (INR = 2–3) alone or combined low-dose ASA or high-intensity warfarin (INR > 3) [30, 60].
- In pregnant women, with recurrent fetal loss, a combination of ASA and heparin is recommended. ASA 81 mg/day should be started when attempting conception, and when the pregnancy is confirmed, heparin subcutaneously should be started as LMW (enoxaparin 1 mg/kg/day, dalteparin 5000 units/day, or nadroparin 3800 units/day) or as unfractionated (5000–10,000 units 12 hourly) [60].
- In catastrophic APS, a combination therapy is required with (1) anticoagulation with intravenous (IV) heparin for 7–10 days, (2) steroids in high doses with (IV) methylprednisolone 1 g daily for 3 or more days, (3) IV immune globulin (IVIG) 0.4 mg/kg/body weight/day for 4–5 days, and/or (4) plasmapheresis for 3–5 days at least with fresh frozen plasma replacement [60].

(See Fig. 12.11 for treatment and secondary prophylaxis of thrombosis in APS)

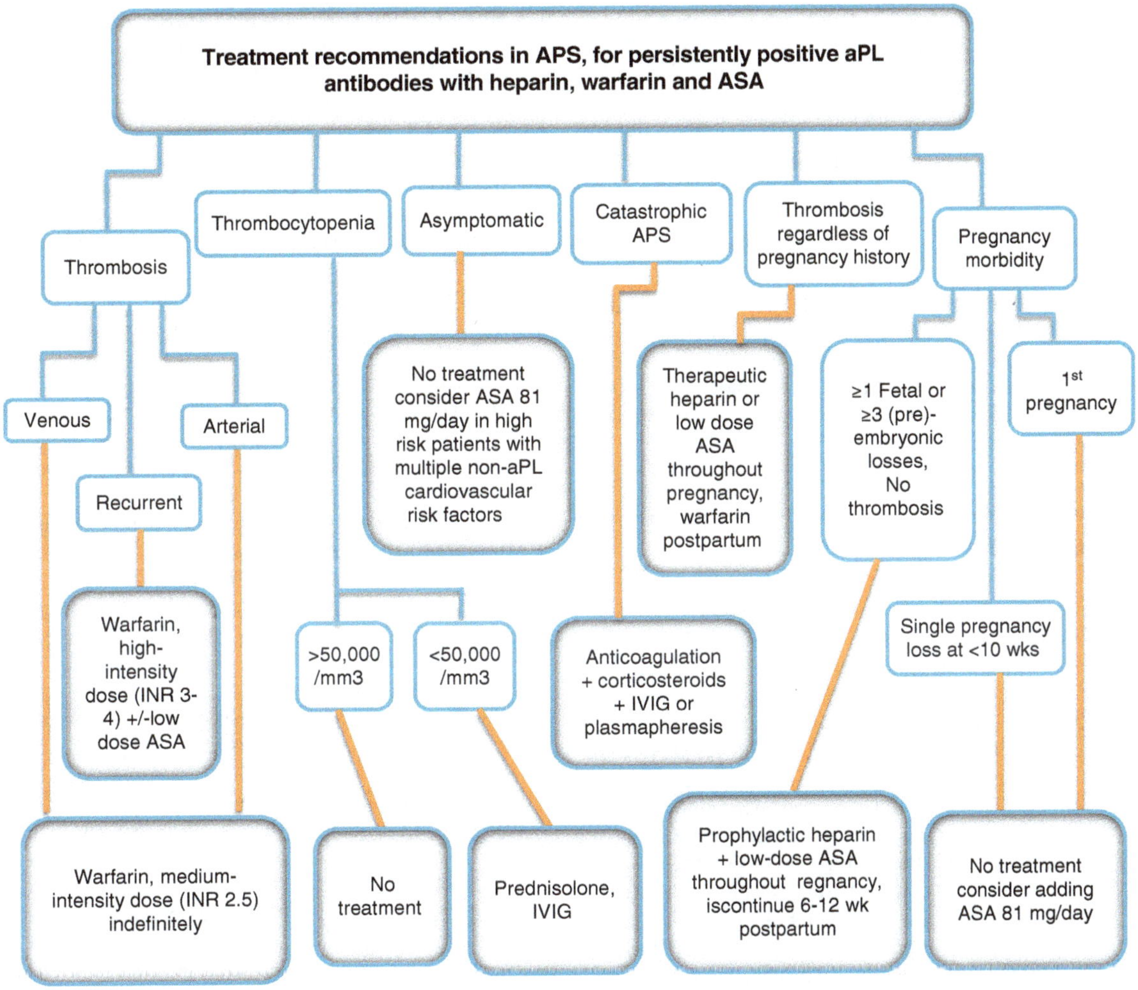

Fig. 12.11 Recommendation for treatment and prevention of thrombosis in patients with APS

- In patients with a low-risk aPL profile without SLE, who have first non-cardioembolic cerebral arterial event due to one of the reversible risk factors, antiplatelet agents are considered for the secondary prophylaxis [30].

12.4.2.5 Refractory and Difficult Situations in aPL-Positive Patients

In patients with difficult management due to recurrent thrombosis, fluctuating INR levels, major bleeding, or a high risk for major alternative therapies with a long-term low LMWH, HCQ or statins are needed for the management of acute thrombosis as well as the secondary prophylaxis [30].

12.4.2.6 Statin Role for the Prophylaxis against Thrombosis in Rheumatic Diseases

Statins have pleiotropic effect (anti-inflammatory, antioxidant, and potent antithrombotic) in addition to a lipid-lowering effect. Thus, by inhibition of atherosclerosis progression, statin decreases the cardiovascular risk for arterial thrombosis in rheumatic and other diseases [62]. Several studies revealed that the use of statins is associated with decrease levels of inflammatory markers such as IL-6, IL-8, MCP-1, and CRP which cause endothelial dysfunction. In addition to that, statins were found to exert an antioxidant function by increasing nitric oxide synthase level. In the JUPITER trial, use of rosuvastatin in patients with elevated CRP levels results in a significant reduction of DVT [63]. Knowing these advantageous effects of statin, it is advised to consider it for prophylaxis of venous thrombosis in rheumatic diseases, but further trials are needed in this field [63].

Acknowledgments The author gratefully acknowledges Dr. Albatool Algailani (medical intern graduated from Umm Al-Qura University, Makkah, KSA) for her help in the preparation of this chapter. The authors also would like to thank Dr. Waleed Hafiz for his assistance in the development of this chapter.

References

1. Lijfering WM, Rosendaal FR, Cannegieter SC. Risk factors for venous thrombosis – current understanding from an epidemiological point of view. Br J Haematol. 2010;149:824–33.
2. Konkle B. Part 2. Cardinal manifestations and presentation of diseases. Section 10, hematologic alterations. In: Online, Harrison's principles of internal medicine. 18th ed. Chapter 58, Bleeding and Thrombosis.
3. López JA, Kearon C, Lee AYY. Deep venous thrombosis. Journal of Hematology. 2004:439–56.
4. Zöller B, Li X, Sundquist J, Sundquist K. Autoimmune diseases and venous thromboembolism: a review of the literature. Am J Cardiovasc Dis. 2012;2(3):171–83.
5. Springera J, Villa-Forteb A. Thrombosis in vasculitis. Curr Opin Rheumatol. 2013;25(1):19–25.
6. Kerekes G, et al. Validated methods for assessment of subclinical atherosclerosis in rheumatology. Nat Rev Rheumatol. 2012;8:224–34.
7. Santos MJ, et al. Early vascular alterations in SLE and RA patients—a step towards understanding the associated cardiovascular risk. 2012;7(9):1–6.
8. Cojocaru M, Cojocaru IM, Silosi I, Vrabie CD. Accelerated atherosclerosis in autoimmune rheumatic diseases. J Clin Exp Invest. 2010;1(3):232–4.
9. Takeishi M, Mimori A, Nakajima K, Mimura T, Suzuki T. 2003. Reduction of factor XII in antiphospholipid antibody-positive patients with thrombotic events in the rheumatology clinic. Clin Rheumatol. 2003;22:40–4.
10. Al-Homood IA. Thrombosis in Systemic Lupus Erythematosus: A Review Article. ISRN Rheumatology. 2012;428269:6. https://doi.org/10.5402/2012/428269. ISSN 2090-5467
11. Kaiser R, et al. Factor V Leiden and thrombosis in patients with systemic lupus erythematosus: a meta-analysis. Genes Immun. 2009;10:495–502.
12. Mok CC, Tang SSK, Chi Hung To, Petri M. Incidence and risk factors of thromboembolism in systemic lupus Erythematosus. Arthritis & Rheumatism. 2005;52(9):2774–82.
13. Esmon CT. The interactions between inflammation and coagulation. Br J Haematol. 2005;131:417–30.
14. Hakim A, Clunie G, Haq I. Antiphospholipid (antibody) syndrome and systemic lupus erythematosus. Third ed: Oxford Handbook of Rheumatology; 2011. p. 329.
15. Martinez-Berriotxoa A, et al. Transiently positive anticardiolipin antibodies and risk of thrombosis in patients with systemic lupus erythematosus. Lupus. 2007;16:810–6.
16. McMahon MA, Keogan M, O'Connell P, Kearns G. The prevalence of antiphospholipid antibody syndrome among systemic lupus erythematosus patients. Ir Med J Nov-Dec. 2006;99(10):296–8.
17. Refai TMK, et al. Hyperhomocysteinaemia and risk of thrombosis in systemic lupus Erythematosus patients. Clin Rheumatol. 2002;21:457–61.
18. van Zaane B, et al. Systematic review on the effect of glucocorticoid use on procoagulant, anti-coagulant and fibrinolytic factors. J Thromb Haemost. 2010;8:2483–93.
19. Mameli A, Barcellona D, Marongiu F. Review: rheumatoid arthritis and thrombosis. Clin Exp Rheumatol. 2009;27:846–55.
20. Kirstin Bacani A, et al. Noncardiac vascular disease in rheumatoid arthritis. Increase in venous thromboembolic events? Arthritis & Rheumatism. 2012;64(1):53–61.
21. McEntegart A, et al. Cardiovascular risk factors including thrombotic variables, in a population with rheumatoid arthritis. Rheumatology. 2001;40:640–4.
22. Shoenfeld, et al. Accelerated Atherosclerosis in Autoimmune Rheumatic Diseases. Circulation. 2005:3337–47.
23. Del R'n, et al. Association between carotid atherosclerosis and markers of inflammation in rheumatoid arthritis patients and healthy subjects. Arthritis & Rheumatism. 2003;48(7):1833–40.
24. Hakim A, Clunie G, Haq I. Primary vasculitides. Third ed: Oxford Handbook of Rheumatology; 2011. p. 406.
25. Stassen PM, et al. Venous thromboembolism in ANCA-associated vasculitis—incidence and risk factors. Rheumatology. 2008;47:530–4.
26. John H. Klippel. 2008. Vasculitides, E. Miscellaneous Vasculitis. Primer on the Rheumatic Diseases. 13, chapter 21, p 435.
27. Ames PRJ, et al. Thrombosis in Behçet's disease: a retrospective survey from a single UK centre. Rheumatology. 2001;40:652–5.
28. Desbois, et al. Immunosuppressants reduce venous thrombosis relapse in Behçet's disease. Arthritis & Rheumatism. 2012;64(8):2753–60.

29. Shankar S, Gill S. Predicting thrombosis in Behçet's disease with novel biomarkers. Indian J Rheumatol. 2011;6(4):166–7.
30. Ruiz-Irastorza G, et al. Evidence-based recommendations for the prevention and long-term management of thrombosis in antiphospholipid antibody-positive patients: report of a task force at the 13th international congress on Antiphospholipid antibodies. Lupus. 2011;20:206–18.
31. Marina P. Sikara, Eleftheria P. Grika and Panayiotis G. Vlachoyiannopoulos. 2011. Pathogenic Mechanisms of Thrombosis in Antiphospholipid Syndrome (APS). ISBN: 978-953-307-872-4, Thrombophilia book http://www.intechopen.com/books/thrombophilia/pathogenicmechanisms-of-thrombosis-in-antiphospholipid-syndrome-aps.
32. http://emedicine.medscape.com/article/333221-overview#a0104. Date of citation Feb 05, 2014.
33. de Groot PG, et al. Pathophysiology of thrombotic APS: where do we stand? Lupus. 2012;21:704–7.
34. Groot PGDE, Meijers JCM, Urbanus RT. Recent development in understanding of APS. Int J Lab Hematol. 2012;34:223–231.nternational.
35. Zhou, et al. Characterization of monocyte tissue factor activity induced by IgG antiphospholipid antibodies and inhibition by dilazep. Blood. 2004;104(8):2353–8.
36. Sikara, et al. β2 glycoprotein I (β2GPI) binds platelet factor 4 (PF4): implications for the pathogenesis of antiphospholipid syndrome. Blood. 2010;115(3):713–23.
37. N Rukoyatkina et al. 2013. p38 MAPK in platelet apoptosis. Online citation from: Cell Death and Disease (2013) 4, e931. https://doi.org/10.1038/cddis.2013.159. www.nature.com/cddis. Date of cita tion Feb 22, 2014 G.
38. Paul Schick. Updated: Feb 19, 2013. Hypercoagulability - Hereditary Thrombophilia and Lupus Anticoagulants Associated With Venous Thrombosis and Emboli. http://emedicine.medscape.com/article/211039-overview. Date of citation March 3, 2014.
39. Bělohlávek J, Dytrych V, Linhart A. Pulmonary embolism, part I: epidemiology, risk factors and risk stratification, pathophysiology, clinical presentation, diagnosis and nonthrombotic pulmonary embolism, experimental and clinical cardiology journal, PubMed. NCBI. 2013;18(2):129–38.
40. Campbell IA, Fennerty A, Miller AC. Guidelines for the management of suspected acute pulmonary embolism. British Thoracic Society Thorax. 2003;58(6):470–84.
41. Takach Lapner S, Kearon C. Diagnosis and management of pulmonary embolism. BMJ. 2013;346:f757.
42. Goldhaber SZ. Risk factors for venous thromboembolism. J Am Coll Cardiol. 2010;56(1):1–7.
43. Gregory Piazza, Samuel Z, Goldhaber. 2006. Acute Pulmonary Embolism Part I: Epidemiology and Diagnosis, American heart association,114: e28-e32. Date of citation 5June 2013.
44. Dupras D et al., 2013, Venous Thromboembolism Diagnosis and Treatment. Thirteenth Edition. N. Institute for Clinical Systems Improvement. http://bit.ly/VTE0113
45. Goodacre S. In the clinic deep venous thrombosis. Annal of Intern Med. 2008;149(5):ITC3–1.
46. Strijkers RHW, ten Cate-Hoek AJ, Bukkems SFFW, Wittens CHA. Management of deep vein thrombosis and prevention of post-thrombotic syndrome. BMJ. 2011;343:d5916.
47. Saeed M. Deep vein thrombosis and its diagnosis. Techniques in Orthopaedics, Lippincott Williams & Wilkins, Inc. 2008;23(3):273–85.
48. Kyrle PA, Eichinger S. Deep vein thrombosis. Lancet. 2005;365:1163–74.
49. B Taylor Thompson, Charles A Hales. 2013. Overview of acute pulmonary embolism, up to date. Date of citation 5 June 2013.
50. Brydon JB Grant. 2013. Diagnosis of suspected deep vein thrombosis of the lower extremity, up to date. Date of citation June 9, 2013.
51. Wells PS, et al. Derivation of a simple clinical model to categorize patients probability of pulmonary embolism: increasing the models utility with the SimpliRED D-dimer. J Thromb Haemost. 2000;83(3):358–519.
52. Fancher TL, White RH, Kravitz RL. Combined use of rapid D-dimer testing and estimation of clinical probability in the diagnosis of deep vein thrombosis: systematic review. BMJ. 2004;329:821.
53. BMJ Publishing Group. Pulmonary embolism, best practice. BMJ. 2013;
54. Hugli O, et al. The pulmonary embolism rule-out criteria (PERC) rule does not safely exclude pulmonary embolism. J Thromb Haemost. 2011;9(2):300–4.
55. Rocha, et al. Risk-assessment algorithm and recom mendations for venous thromboembolism prophylaxis in medical patients. Vascular Health and Risk Management. 2007;3(4):533–53.
56. Snow V, et al. Management of Venous Thromboembolism: a clinical practice guideline from the American College of Physicians and the American Academy of family physicians. ACP. 2007;146(3):204–10.
57. Michael H. Weisman et al. 2010. **Targeted Treatment of the Rheumatic Diseases.** 1st edition. Chapter 11. Management of acute thrombosis and secondary thrombosis prevention in APS. ISBN 978-1-4160-9993-2. Date of online citation March 05, 2014.
58. Khamashta MA. Management of Thrombosis in the Antiphospholipid-antibody syndrome. N Engl J Med. 1995;332(15):993–7.
59. Kelley's text book of Rheumatology, ninth edition. Antiphospholipid Syndrome, chapter 82, pages 1331–1341, and Behçet's Disease, chapter 93, pages 1525–1532.
60. Leslie Kahl.2012. Antiphospholipid syndrome. The Washington manual rheumatology subspecialty consult, second edition, chapter 39, pages 333–334.
61. Emad Y, Abdel-Razek N, Gheita T, El-Wakd M, El Gohary T, Samadoni A. Multislice CT pulmo-

nary findings in Behçet's disease. Clin Rheumatol. 2007;26:879–84.
62. Bielinska A, Gluszko P. Statins – are they potentially useful in rheumatology? Pol Arch Med Wewn. 2007;117(9):420–5.
63. Rodriguez, et al. Statins, inflammation and deep vein thrombosis: a systematic review. J Thromb Thrombolysis. 2012;33(4):371–82.
64. Gregory YH Lip, Russell D Hull. 2014. Treatment of lower extremity deep vein thrombosis. UpTodate. www.uptodate.com/contents/treatment-of-lower-extremity-deep-vein-thrombosis#H32722067. Date of citation March 13, 2014.
65. Gonsalves WI, Pruthi RK, Patnaik MM. The new Oral anticoagulants in clinical practice. Mayo Clin Proc. 2013;88(5):495–511.
66. Agnelli G, et al. Oral Apixaban for the treatment of acute venous thromboembolism. NEJM. 2013;369(9):799–808.

13

Rheumatology and Hematological Abnormalities

Nahid Janoudi and Ammar AlDabbagh

13.1 Introduction

Hematologic disorders including anemia, white blood cells abnormalities, platelet abnormalities, coagulopathy, and hematologic malignancies can be manifested in many autoimmune rheumatic diseases [1].

This chapter discusses the most common hematological abnormalities in rheumatoid arthritis (RA) and systemic lupus erythematosus (SLE). It also provides a simple approach to evaluate hematological abnormalities in patients with RA or SLE. This approach includes the most common causes, differential diagnosis, treatment, and prevention, with a special emphasis on ruling out life-threatening and urgent conditions.

13.2 Objectives

- Describe hematological manifestations of rheumatic diseases including different types of anemia, white blood cells, and platelets abnormalities, with brief about malignancies in rheumatoid arthritis.
- Construct a diagnostic approach to anemia in rheumatoid arthritis.
- Describe hematological manifestations of systemic lupus erythematosus including different types of anemia, white blood cells, and platelets abnormalities, with brief about lymphadenopathy, splenomegaly, and antibodies to clotting factors and antiphospholipids.
- Construct a diagnostic approach to anemia in systemic lupus erythematosus.
- Describe macrophage activation syndrome (MAS), and construct a diagnostic approach to it.

13.3 Hematological Manifestations of Rheumatoid Arthritis (RA)

13.3.1 Introduction

A review of hematologic involvement in RA is presented here, with an algorithm constructing a simple approach to RA patients with hematological manifestations (causes, diagnosis, and treatment) which is shown in Fig. 13.1.

13.3.1.1 Anemia

Anemia of chronic disease (ACD) and iron deficiency anemia (IDA) are considered the most common hematologic manifestations in patients with rheumatic diseases [2], with an estimated

N. Janoudi
Doctor Soliman Fakeeh Hospital,
Jeddah, Saudi Arabia

A. AlDabbagh (✉)
Internal Medicine, Gastroenterology and Hepatology
Consultant, Jeddah, Saudi Arabia
e-mail: aaldabbagh@fakeeh.care

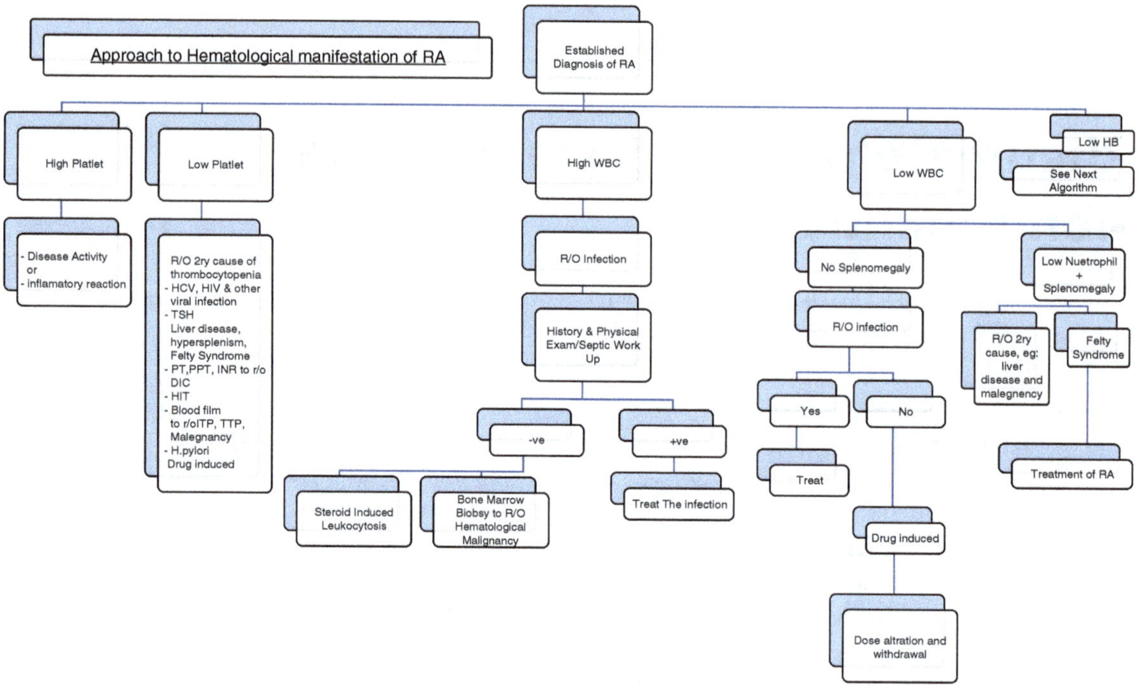

Fig. 13.1 Algorithmic approach for hematological manifestations of rheumatoid arthritis (RA). Classified by the affected component of the blood (platelets, HB, or WBC), in this approach; the authors suggest to broaden the differential diagnosis and to rule out non-rheumatological causes of mentioned abnormalities, including systemic diseases, infections, and drug-induced and primary hematological diseases. The evidence to support this approach is based on cumulative literature, current guidelines, and the author's experience (Abbreviations: *RA* rheumatoid arthritis, *R/O* rule out, *HCV* hepatitis C virus, *HIV* human immunodeficiency virus, *TSH* thyroid stimulating hormone, *PT* prothrombin time, *PTT* partial thromboplastin time, *INR* international normalization ratio, *DIC* disseminated intravascular coagulation, *HIT* heparin-induced thrombocytopenia, *ITP* immune thrombocytopenic purpura, *TTP* thrombotic thrombocytopenic purpura, *H. pylori Helicobacter pylori*, *WBC* white blood cell, *HB* hemoglobin, *2ry* secondary, *-ve* negative, *+ve* positive)

prevalence in RA (30%–70%) in different studies [3, 4].

Anemia of Chronic Disease (ACD)

The ACD is associated with the following laboratory abnormalities:

- Mean corpuscular volume (MCV) and mean corpuscular hemoglobin concentration (MCHC) are usually normal (normocytic and normochromic) but may decrease due to concurrent iron deficiency, often to values characteristic of microcytic hypochromic anemia.
- The ferritin level is usually high with low serum levels of transferrin and iron [5].
- Bone marrow biopsy usually shows the presence of hemosiderin and normal cellularity, with increased numbers (in most cases) of plasma cells that are associated with lymphoid aggregates. However, these findings are unpredictable and usually represent the various etiologies of cytopenias in RA patients.

The pathogenesis of the ACD is not entirely known. There are two major reasons seem to be of significant: defect in hemoglobin synthesis due to the diminished available iron secondary to iron trapping in macrophages and difficulty in bone marrow to produce more red blood cells in response to the anemia [6]. Immune mediators, such as tumor necrosis factor-alpha (TNF-alpha), interleukin-1, interleukin-6, interleukin-10, and interferon gamma, have great impact on these changes [6, 7]. Hepcidin, that is produced by the liver in response to inflammation, may have a great role in ACD, as it decreases iron absorption in the intestines and iron release from macrophages.

Low levels of erythropoietin and decreased response to erythropoietin may lead to the anemia in RA; these findings led to using erythropoietin in such patients which resulted in some increase in hemoglobin levels in few patients with improvement in arthritis symptoms [2, 8, 9].

Since the anemia may correlate with RA activity, patients may need higher doses of erythropoietin, which a medication with a high cost [10]. Hence, it should be considered only for patients with severe symptomatic anemia [11].

In the algorithm provided, if RA patient presents with normocytic normochromic anemia without hemolytic manifestations (normal levels of LDH and reticulocyte and negative Coombs' test) and no other obvious inflammatory causes, patient should be treated with iron supplement and disease modifying anti-rheumatic drugs (DMARDs), and consider erythropoietin for symptomatic anemia (Fig. 13.2).

Iron Deficiency Anemia (IDA)

Iron deficiency anemia can be seen in up to 50% to 75% of RA patients who have chronic active disease [12].

It is mostly caused by chronic blood loss from gastritis (induced by prednisone [13] and/or non-steroidal anti-inflammatory drugs), peptic ulcer, or gastro esophageal reflux.

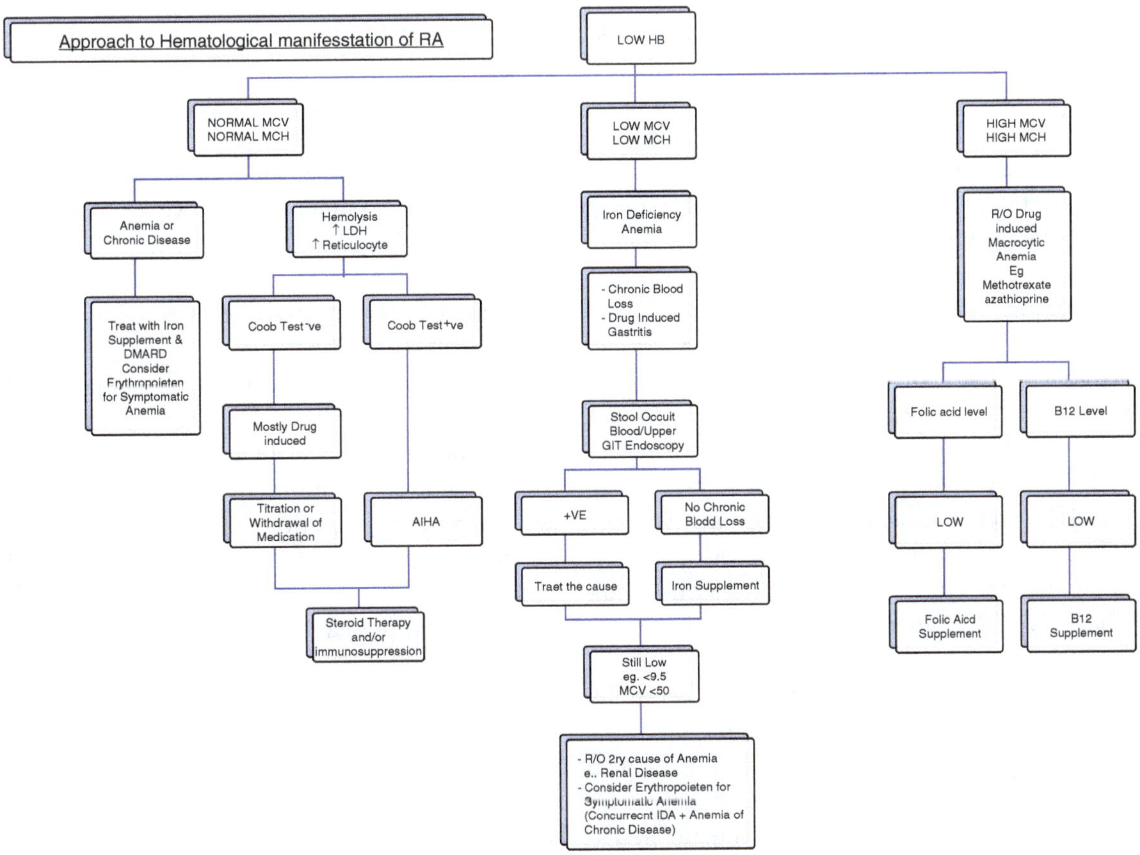

Fig. 13.2 Algorithmic approach for anemia in RA patients. In this approach the authors classified the anemia according to MCV and MCH, aiming to widen the differential diagnosis and to include non-rheumatological causes and co-factors. The evidence to support this approach is based on cumulative literature, current guidelines, and the author's experience (Abbreviations: *HB* hemoglobin, *MCV* mean corpuscular volume, *MCH* mean corpuscular hemoglobin, *LDH* lactate dehydrogenate, *−ve* negative, *+ve* positive, *DMARD* disease-modifying anti-rheumatic drugs, *AIHA* autoimmune hemolytic anemia, *2ry* secondary)

As with all patients, occult blood in stool should not be neglected. All RA patients with IDA, epigastric pain, and/or occult blood in the stool should undergo upper gastrointestinal endoscopic examination.

Making the diagnosis of IDA among RA patients could be challenging, since the routine laboratory indices with mild to moderate iron deficiency may overlap with the ACD [14.15]. Thus, if iron deficiency is suspected, it may be most reliably verified by the absence of iron stores on bone marrow examination [14]. However, pursuing for bone marrow biopsy may be unnecessary if clear signs of iron deficiency such as a mean cell volume below 85, serum ferritin concentration below 40 mcg/L, and transferrin saturation ≤ 7% are present [15].

RA patients frequently may have both IDA and ACD. In such case, the hemoglobin level usually decreases to below 9.5 g/dL, and the mean corpuscular volume is usually less than 80.

Measurement of serum soluble transferrin receptor (TfR) may be useful in differentiating IDA from anemia of chronic disease. [16].

Macrocytic Anemia

Less frequently, a megaloblastic anemia secondary to deficiency of folic acid or vitamin B12, methotrexate, or azathioprine is found in RA patients [2].

One study of 25 patients with RA noted vitamin B12 and folic acid deficiency in 29% and 21% of patients, respectively [2]. It was found that more than one type of anemia can present simultaneously in RA patients with anemia. Identifying each type could be masked by another.

Folic acid deficiency anemia in RA is usually due to the combination of increased requirements and reduced intake (e.g., pregnancy in a patient on a restricted diet) or to concurrent iron deficiency. On the other hand, there may be a genetic predisposition to develop macrocytosis and bone marrow toxicity with azathioprine. Approximately 0.3% of normal subjects have very low levels of thiopurine methyltransferase, one of the enzymes responsible for azathioprine metabolism. This abnormality is genetically determined and is linked to a higher risk of myelosuppression and macrocytic anemia [5].

The diagnosis is established by demonstrating a reduced folate level or vitamin B12 level, ; however, blood film is recommended to suggest the diagnosis and to rule out malignancies.

Hemolytic Anemia

Hemolytic anemia is not a typical feature of RA, although antibody-mediated, Coombs' positive hemolytic anemia has been described, primarily in Felty's syndrome [17].

Drug-induced hemolysis may also occur and is usually reversible when the offending drug is withdrawn, but most patients require corticosteroid therapy.

Bone Marrow Hypoplasia with Anemia

One of the serious hematologic complication of RA is bone marrow hypoplasia, ; luckily it is not frequently seen in RA patients. When present, it is mostly observed in association with Felty's syndrome, renal failure, and the administration of gold, penicillamine, azathioprine, cyclophosphamide, or other immunosuppressive agents.

Pure Red Cell Aplasia

This uncommon hematologic abnormality among RA patient should be suspected if the patient has severe normocytic normochromic anemia with very low absolute reticulocyte count without evidences of blood loss or hemolysis. Autoimmune suppression of erythroid stem cells, DMARDs, and parvovirus infection have been implicated in this complication [18], although single case report suggests that pure red cell aplasia could be an extraarticular manifestation of RA [19]. Isolated case reports have noted improvement in patients treated with corticosteroids, cyclophosphamide, azathioprine, or cyclosporine [20].

Treatment of Anemia in RA

Effective therapy of patient with RA and anemia is based upon an accurate determination of the cause of the anemia. As a result:

- Vitamin deficiencies leading to anemia should be corrected by the administration of folic acid or vitamin B12.
- Iron should not be given unless iron deficiency has been documented. It is recommended to

start with a combination of oral ferrous sulfate, which is usually given with 250 to 325 mg of ascorbic acid and on an empty stomach to enhance iron absorption. Alternatively, ferrous gluconate 300 mg three times daily may be used.

- Patients with persistent gastric intolerance to iron tablets may tolerate elixir of ferosol.
- If oral therapy fails, it is switched to intramuscular iron, and only very rarely parenteral iron as a slow IV infusion can be used.
- **Hemolysis** can be managed with corticosteroids (prednisone 60 mg/day).
- If no response is observed after 1 to 2 weeks, an immunosuppressive agent may be administered, such as azathioprine (50 to 150 mg/day).
- **DMARD-induced bone marrow suppression** should be treated by dose alteration or complete withdrawal of the suspected drug.
- **The ACD** often responds to therapy directed against RA, including DMARDs, and/or corticosteroids (prednisone at a dose of 0.5 to 1.0 mg/kg per day) [2].
- Several interventional studies have demonstrated the efficacy of erythropoietin in treating the anemia of RA [11]; however, only a limited number of patients with RA and ACD may require this treatment. High doses (300 to 800 units/kg/week given subcutaneously once or twice a week) are required, making this an expensive form of therapy. One specific role for erythropoietin among patients with RA is in the peri-operative management of anemia. Treating anemia in this setting may prevent the need for transfusion [2].

13.3.1.2 White Blood Cell (WBC) Count Abnormalities

Neutropenia and Felty's Syndrome

The principal leukopenic disorder among patients with RA is Felty's syndrome, which is defined as a triad of RA, splenomegaly, and neutropenia.

- Splenomegaly is not necessarily present [21].
- This disorder occurs in about 1% of patients with RA. Patients with this syndrome often has an advanced form of nodular RA, with high levels of rheumatoid factor.
- This disorder may be accompanied by severe infections, vasculitis, ulcers, neuropathic symptoms, interstitial lung disease, secondary Sjögren's syndrome, hepatomegaly, and lower extremity hyperpigmentation. These manifestations are rare in the current era of early aggressive therapy with DMARDs.

Although leukopenia is a common consequence of many rheumatic diseases, it is most frequently caused by the administration of DMARDs, including azathioprine, methotrexate, gold salts, sulfasalazine, and penicillamine [22, 23]. In addition, viral infections are another important differential diagnosis and should be excluded before considering the diagnosis of Felty's syndrome.

Management of Felty's syndrome is aimed at suppressing the inflammatory rheumatoid disease. There are several reports on the good outcome with use of gold salts, methotrexate, and biological therapy in these patients. In one retrospective review of all Felty's syndrome cases (1979 to 2003), it was concluded that Felty's syndrome is considered a mild disease and is not commonly linked to infectious complications. Gold is an effective treatment of Felty's syndrome [21].

Leukocytosis

Leukocytosis can occur during an inflammatory flare of RA. However, an associated bacterial infection must be considered and should excluded in such patients.

Eosinophilia

Significant eosinophilia occurs in some patients with RA. It usually correlates with the presence of vasculitis, pleuropericarditis, pulmonary fibrosis, subcutaneous nodules, or gold-induced skin rashes [23].

13.3.1.3 Platelet Abnormalities

Thrombocytosis is common in RA, and a positive correlation has been found between the platelet count and disease activity. Extreme thrombocytosis has been noticed with extraarticular manifestations of the disease, particularly pulmonary involvement, peripheral neuropathy, and vasculitis [24]. The mechanism of thrombocytosis is unclear yet.

Thrombocytopenia is rare in RA, mostly induced by drug treatment such as gold, penicillamine, methotrexate, azathioprine, and TNF antagonists [25, 26]. Felty's syndrome, is another cause of thrombocytopenia in RA patients.

13.3.1.4 Hematological Malignancies in RA

Several studies have noted a higher risk of hematologic malignancy among RA patients contributing significantly to a higher morbidity and mortality of the disease [27–30]. Most large registries noted a higher risk for the development of lymphoproliferative diseases, particularly non-Hodgkin lymphoma (NHL). A study of nearly 18, 000 RA patients noted a higher risk of lymphoma in patients with RA in comparison to the general population (the standardized incidence ratio or SIR) (SIR of1.9) [31]. Although the risk in those treated with anti-tumor necrosis factor-alpha agents was greater than that for patients treated with methotrexate (SIRs of 2.9 and 1.7, respectively), the authors of the study noted that this difference could result if patients with active RA, who have a higher increased risk of developing lymphoma, were more often managed with anti-TNF therapy than those with less active RA.

The results of studies that have addressed the question of whether TNF inhibitor use is associated with increased cancer risk are mixed, and large observational studies were unable to demonstrate a significant increase in either hematologic malignancies or solid tumors for patients taking biologic DMARDs compared with those taking methotrexate [32, 33].

13.4 Hematological Manifestations of Systemic Lupus Erythematosus (SLE)

13.4.1 Introduction

Hematological involvement is commonly seen in (SLE) and could be the presenting manifestations of SLE in many patients. Also, it could mimic many primary hematological disorders.

The most common forms of hematologic manifestations in patients with SLE are anemia, leukopenia, thrombocytopenia, and the antiphospholipid syndrome (APS). Further details about APS and thrombosis are found in Chap. 12 (Thrombosis in Rheumatological diseases).

In this chapter; an overview of the hematologic manifestations of SLE will be discussed, with an algorithm at the end constructing a simple approach to hematological manifestations in SLE patients (Fig. 13.3).

13.4.1.1 Anemia

Many patients with SLE may have anemia at some point of time; the most common types of anemia in such patients are anemia of chronic disease, IDA, autoimmune hemolytic anemia (AIHA), drug-induced myelosuppression, and anemia associated with chronic renal failure which is uncommon [34]. There are different mechanisms which may explain the development of anemia in patients with SLE; at the end of this chapter, you will find a simple approach regarding common differential diagnosis, causes, and investigations. Figure 13.4 shows an algorithmic approach for Anemia in SLE patients.

Anemia of Chronic Disease

In a single-center prospective study of 132 SLE patients with anemia, ACD found as the most common type, representing 37% of all patients [34]. ACD is classified as normocytic and normochromic anemia and may be associated with a low reticulocyte count and a low serum iron, ; however bone marrow iron stores are adequate, and ferritin concentration is usually high.

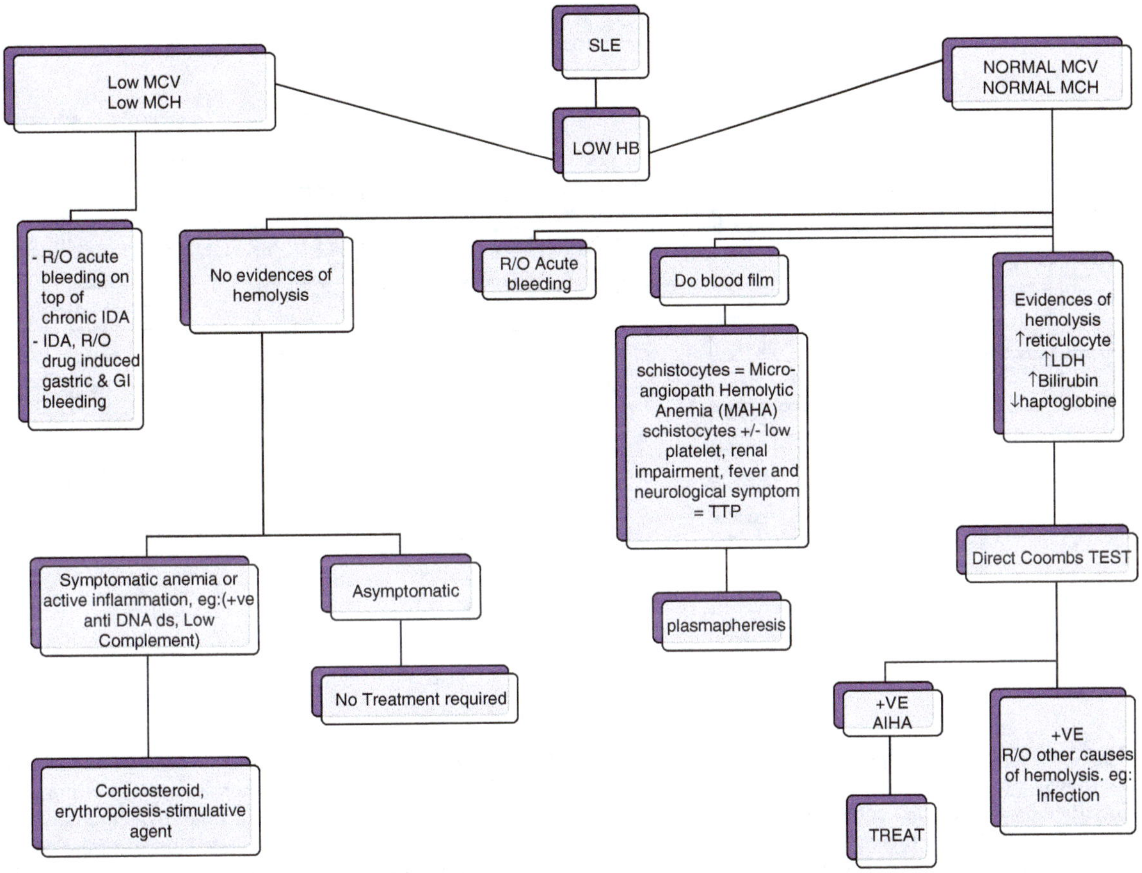

Fig. 13.3 Algorithmic approach for anemia in SLE patients. In this approach the authors classified the anemia according to MCV and MCH, aiming to widen the differential diagnosis and to include non-rheumatological causes, life-threatening causes, and co-factors. The evidence to support this approach is based on cumulative literature, current guidelines, and the author's experience (Abbreviations: *HB* hemoglobin, *MCV* mean corpuscular volume, *MCH* mean corpuscular hemoglobin, *LDH* lactate dehydrogenate, *–ve* negative, *+ve* positive, *IDA* iron deficiency anemia, *AIHA* autoimmune hemolytic anemia, *TTP* thrombotic thrombocytopenic purpura, *2ry* secondary)

13.4.2 Treatment

Usually the treatment is not indicated unless the patient has symptomatic anemia or renal impairment.

Patients with symptomatic anemia secondary to ACD and with no indication for corticosteroid or other immunosuppressant agents may be offered a therapy to enhance erythropoiesis, e.g., epoetin alfa (recombinant human erythropoietin). It should be started at 80 to 120 units/kg per week (usually as 2 to 3 injections per week). The patient should be reassessed after one month, and the dose should be increased monthly until the hemoglobin level is maintained at ≥11 g/dL.

Darbepoetin alfa; a unique molecule that stimulates erythropoiesis with a longer half-life than recombinant human erythropoietin. A typical dose of darbepoetin alfa for adults is 0.45 mcg/kg once a week.

Erythropoietin was evaluated in patients with SLE and ACD; it was found that 58% of patients in one study had an adequate response to erythropoietin supplementation [35].

Patients with symptomatic anemia secondary to ACD who had insufficient response to erythro-

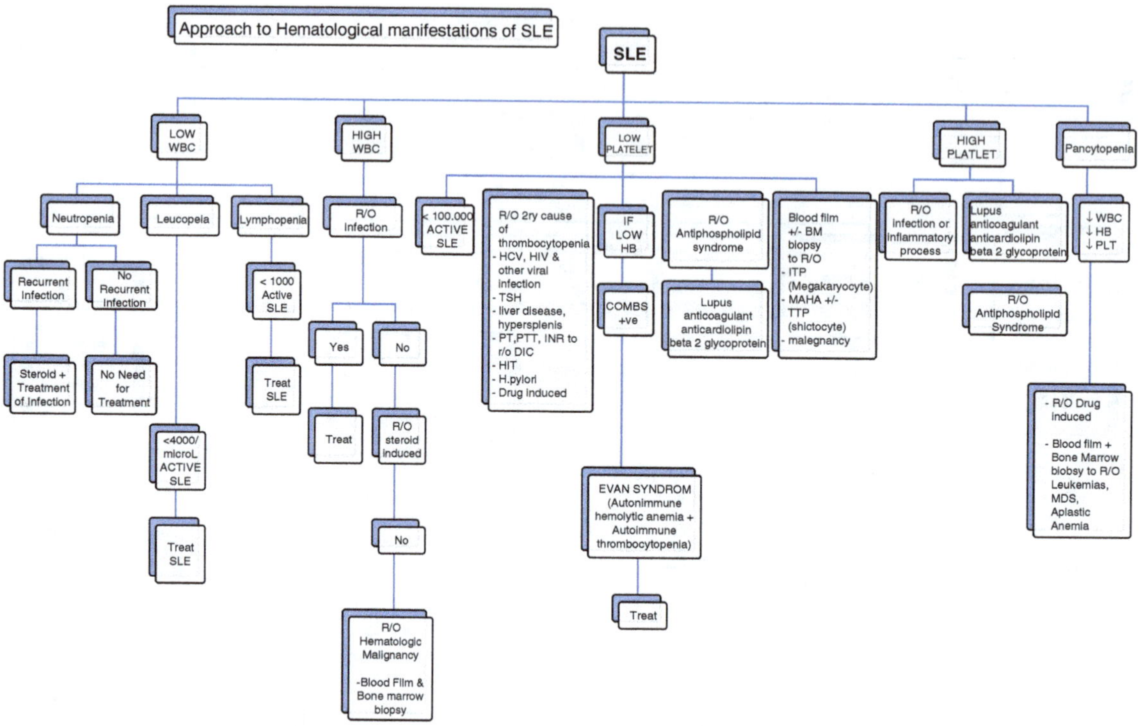

Fig. 13.4 Algorithmic approach for hematological manifestations of systemic lupus erythematosus (SLE). Classified by the affected component of the blood (platelets, HB, or WBC), in this approach, the authors suggest to broaden the differential diagnosis and to rule out non-rheumatological causes of mentioned abnormalities, including systemic diseases, infections, and drug-induced and primary hematological diseases. The evidence to support this approach is based on cumulative literature, current guidelines, and the author's experience (Abbreviations: *RA* rheumatoid arthritis, *R/O* rule out, *HCV* hepatitis C virus, *HIV* human immunodeficiency virus, *TSH* thyroid stimulating hormone, *PT* prothrombin time, *PTT* partial thromboplastin time, *INR* international normalization ratio, *DIC* disseminated intravascular coagulation, *HIT* heparin-induced thrombocytopenia, *ITP* immune thrombocytopenic purpura, *TTP* thrombotic thrombocytopenic purpura, *MAHA* microangiopathic hemolytic anemia, *H. pylori Helicobacter pylori*, *WBC* white blood cell, *HB* hemoglobin, *Plt* platelets, *2ry* secondary, *-ve* negative, *+ve* positive, *BM* bone marrow, *MDS* myelodysplastic syndrome)

poietin supplementation, often improve on glucocorticoids at high doses (1 mg/kg/day) which is usually the next step in their management.

After 1 month of being on steroid, if the response is insufficient (e.g., hemoglobin still <11 g/dL), glucocorticoids dose should be tapered down rapidly and stopped.

If there is a response, the dose should be tapered as rapidly as to possible to the lowest dose that maintains the improvement.

13.4.2.1 Iron Deficiency Anemia (IDA)

IDA is the second most prevalent type of anemia in patients with SLE [36]; in female, it could be secondary to menorrhagia, or it may represent an acute or chronic blood loss from gastrointestinal tract usually as a result of chronic administration of NSAIDs and corticosteroids. It can exacerbate and/or coexist with ACD.

Long-standing anemia of chronic inflammation can also result in to IDA.

Diffused pulmonary hemorrhage is an uncommon cause of anemia in patients with SLE.

13.4.2.2 Autoimmune Hemolytic Anemia (AIHA)

AIHA is an antibody-mediated erythrocyte destruction, and it may found in 5% to 14% of SLE patients [35].

(AIHA) is characterized by:

- High reticulocyte count,
- Reduced haptoglobin levels,
- High indirect bilirubin concentration,
- Positive direct Coombs' test,
- Found in up to 10% of SLE patients [37, 38].

Approximately 2/3 of patients with SLE-associated AIHA have symptoms at the onset of SLE [26]. The presence of hemolytic anemia could be associated with other sever SLE features including lupus nephritis, neuropsychiatric manifestations, and serositis. Some patients may have a positive Coombs' test without evidence of hemolysis. [36, 37]. The antibodies are divided into IgG-mediated "warm, ", and IgM-mediated "cold" agglutinin.

Treatment: AIHA usually improves on corticosteroids (1 mg/kg/day of prednisone) in 75 to 96% of patients [39].

Once the hematocrit starts to increase and the reticulocyte count decreases, prednisone can be quickly tapered down.

If the patient didn't achieve response, pulse steroid can be considered (e.g., 1 g methylprednisolone intravenously daily for 3 days) [39], azathioprine (up to 2 mg/kg per day) [40], cyclophosphamide (up to 2 mg/kg) [40], or splenectomy [41, 42].

Response rates for splenectomy in AIHA can reach up to 60% [41], ; however, other study has contradictory result [30]. In case of refractory AIHA, one can consider intravenous immune globulin [30], danazol (in doses of 600 to 800 mg/day) [42], mycophenolate mofetil [44], and rituximab [45].

Anemia due to chronic kidney disease:

An inappropriately low level of erythropoietin is the major feature of anemia due to chronic kidney disease. In this setting, typically decreased production of erythropoietin by the impaired kidneys plays a major role in the pathogenesis of this type of anemia. In such patients, specially patients with no other evidence of inflammation, prescribing erythropoiesis-stimulating agents could be indicated in symptomatic anemia or if the hemoglobin is less than 11 g/dL.

13.4.2.3 Red Cell Aplasia

In SLE, red cell aplasia may occur secondary to antibody-mediated injury to erythropoietin or erythroblast in the bone marrow, although it is uncommon, but it has been reported [46, 47]. This type of anemia usually improves on corticosteroid, ; in refractory cases cyclophosphamide and cyclosporine have been successfully used.

13.4.2.4 Microangiopathic Hemolytic Anemia (MAHA)

SLE is one of many causes of thrombotic microangiopathic hemolytic anemia [48]. It usually presents with schistocytes in peripheral blood smear and high serum lactate dehydrogenase (LDH) levels as well as high indirect bilirubin concentration.

As you will see in the algorithm at the end of this chapter, it is essential to consider MAHA in any SLE patient who present with normocytic normochromic anemia, MAHA is manifested by schistocytes in peripheral film which necessitate urgent treatment with plasmapheresis and corticosteroid .

Thrombotic thrombocytopenic purpura (TTP), which is life-threatening condition, is typically manifested by a pentad of thrombocytopenia, fever, microangiopathic hemolytic anemia (MAHA), neurologic manifestations, and renal impairment.

Other patients with MAHA may not manifest with fever or neurologic abnormalities, presenting a condition called hemolytic-uremic syndrome (HUS). The pathogenesis of this syndrome isn't entirely known [49].

Treatment: In MAHA and TTP, plasmapheresis is considered the most important acute intervention. Because of the adverse outcome which associated with delay in its initiation, it should be started immediately in all patients with suspected TTP [50, 51].

In a review study, 28 patients with TTP managed with plasmapheresis, glucocorticoids alone, or no therapy. The mortality rate was 25% in those treated with plasmapheresis, 50% in glucocorticoids alone group, and 100% in those who received no therapy [53].

The current recommendations suggest that plasma exchange should be immediately in the patients diagnosed to have TTP; it should be carried on at least for 5 days, along with pulse steroid (methylprednisolone 1 g intravenously daily for 3 days) with the first dose usually given immediately after the first plasmapheresis session [50]. Recently, in some cases of TTP anti-CD20 antibody, rituximab has been used, however more data are needed [52].

TTP-HUS is often associated with reduced activity of ADAMTS13 (<10%), usually due to an inhibitor of ADAMTS13 activity. However, results of ADAMTS13 activity measurement should not influence the decision to initiate plasma exchange, and plasmapheresis shouldn't be delayed while awaiting its result [50, 53].

13.4.3 WBC Abnormalities

At the end of this chapter, the reader will find an algorithm which constructing an approach to SLE patients who present with WBC abnormalities; including leukocytosis, leucopenia, neutropenia, lymphocytopenia, and other abnormalities. This approach emphasizes rolling out serious conditions as well as considering SLE related WBC disorders.

13.4.3.1 Leucopenia and Neutropenia

Leucopenia is a characteristic feature of SLE and can include lymphopenia, neutropenia, or both. It defined as less than 4000 cells/mL of white blood cell (WBC) count, and it usually represents an active disease. According to the American College of Rheumatology (ACR, leucopenia is considered as one of the criteria to diagnose SLE [54]. It can be seen in up to 50% to 60% of SLE patients [55, 56].

Other comparative retrospective study which was done in Saudi Arabia showed that the most common hematologic presentation among SLE patients was leukopenia which was found in 58.7% of the patients [57].

In some cases, leukopenia becomes challenging specially if the patients require a medication that can cause bone marrow suppression, e.g., cyclophosphamide, azathioprine, methotrexate, and, rarely, cyclosporine, mycophenolate mofetil, or HCQ. If a patient developed a rapid leucopenia, hemophagocytic syndrome should be considered, and proper workup should be perused [55].

Neutropenia may reflect primary hematological disease, infection, or treatment side effects (e.g., cyclophosphamide or azathioprine); however, all those causes should be considered in correlation with history and clinical finding. In SLE, neutropenia which attributed to an active disease usually respond to steroids.

13.4.3.2 Lymphocytopenia

Lymphopenia is considered one of the most prevalent hematological features of SLE, and although it was noted to be contributory to leucopenia, yet it can be independent to total white blood cell count. Reduced absolute lymphocytic count can correlate with SLE activity, and those with absolute lymphocytic count less than 1500/μL at diagnosis may have a higher frequency of fever, musculoskeletal manifestations, and neuropsychiatric manifestations [55].

13.4.3.3 Decreased Eosinophils and Basophils

Generally, corticosteroids may contribute to a low absolute eosinophil and monocyte counts.

Basophil count can be reduced as well in SLE, especially during lupus flare, basophil degranulation usually occurs which result in the release of platelet activating factor and as well as other mediators which can play a role in vascular permeability and immune complex deposition [31].

13.4.3.4 Treatment of Leukopenia

Not all SLE patients with leucopenia need to be treated, unless the patient has neutropenia with recurrent infections. On other hand, side effects of the treatment may complicate the situations, ; prednisone (10 to 60 mg/day) may increase the leucocyte count but may result in high risk of infections as well; immunosuppressive therapies like azathioprine or cyclophosphamide may contribute toward the worsening of the leukopenia through their effect on bone marrow suppression [31]. In such cases, these medications should be used with caution and frequent monitoring of white blood cell count and for signs of infections.

Treating leukopenia in SLE in other settings may result in unfavorable outcomes. As an example, recombinant granulocyte colony-stimulating factor (G-CSF) studied in the treatment of sever neutropenia associated with refractory infections, although it was effective in increasing neutrophilic count, yet it was associated SLE flare in three out of the nine patients in this study [32].

13.4.3.5 Leukocytosis

Leukocytosis can be found in patients with SLE. Two contributing factors include underlying infectious process or leukocytosis associated with high dose of steroids [31]. It also can be found during SLE flare. In case of leukocytosis secondary to infections, shifting of granulocytes to more immature forms (a left shift) is usually seen.

13.4.4 Platelet Abnormalities

Both qualitative and quantitative disorders of platelets are not uncommon in SLE patients; at the end of this chapter, you will find a simple approach to platelets disorders, considering the life-threatening conditions, disease activity, and other associated diseases. It has been found that almost in 25% to 50% of SLE patients may have a mild thrombocytopenia with platelet counts ranging between 100, 000 and 150, 000/microL, and 10% of SLE patients may have more severe form in which the counts become less than 50, 000/microL [1].

In a cohort study of 632 patients with SLE, the percentage of patients with platelet counts ranging between 50, 000 to 100, 000/μL was 54%, while those with counts between 20, 000 and 50, 000/μL represent 18%, and patients with counts less than 20, 000/μL represent 28% of the cohort [58].

There are many potential causes of thrombocytopenia in SLE patients. Among them, immune-mediated platelet destruction is considered the most common cause, but platelet consumption is another factor specially in association with MAHA or may be due to reduced platelet production secondary to cytotoxic medications.

Pathogenesis—the main mechanism is binding of immunoglobulin to the surface of the platelets which later get involved in the phagocytosis inside the spleen, similar to idiopathic thrombocytopenic purpura (ITP) [51]. Another mechanism in some patients involves bone marrow suppression by cytotoxic medications, increased consumption due to a thrombotic microangiopathy (e.g., TTP), the antiphospholipid syndrome, or antibodies against the thrombopoietin receptor on megakaryocytes or their precursors.

Patients with SLE can present initially with ITP followed by other manifestations later on.

In patients with isolated ITP, it has been found that 3–15% may develop SLE [59]. Evans syndrome, which is defined as the presence of both autoimmune thrombocytopenia and autoimmune hemolytic anemia, can also precede the onset of SLE.

Thrombocytopenia is uncommonly severe, and complications related to bleeding are generally low as a minority of patients only experiences severe bleeding. However, it is well-known that thrombocytopenia in patients with SLE considered poor prognostic factor and put the patient at risk of other organ involvement such as cardiac involvement, nephritis, or neuropsychiatric manifestation [38, 48].

Our algorithm at the end of this chapter simplified the approach to thrombocytopenia in SLE patients;, we suggest to do peripheral blood smear to rule out serious conditions such as MAHA, TTP, and malignancies; to order lupus anticouagulant and anticardiolipin to rule out APS; to do hemolysis workup and direct Coombs' test to rule out AIHA and Evans syndrome;, and to consider disease activity as well as secondary thrombocytopenia causes in your differential diagnosis.

Treatment: In patients with thrombocytopenia with counts ranging between 20, 000/microL and 50, 000/microL, usually they have prolonged bleeding time; however bleeding is rarely seen with this range, while counts of less than 20, 000/ microL can be associated with petechiae, purpura, ecchymoses, epistaxis, gingival, and other clinical bleeding. Treatment is usually indicated for patients with symptoms and counts of less than 50, 000/microL and for those with counts of less than 20, 000/microL. Glucocorticoid therapy is the main treatment, prednisone (1 mg/kg per day in divided doses) [47]. Dexamethasone also can be used as 40 mg/day dose for 4 days, with repeating the doses every 2–4 weeks, an intervals of 2–4 weeks may have similar remission rates and better long-term responses than those treated with daily prednisone [39]. The majority of patients improve on glucocorticoid within 1–8 weeks; in case of no response within 1–3 weeks or intolerance to steroids, other lines of therapy should be considered. The choice of second medication depends on the severity of the thrombocytopenia and the presence of other SLE manifestations.

- **Azathioprine** (0.5 to 2 mg/kg per day) [60].
- **Cyclophosphamide**, given as daily oral doses or intravenous pulse therapy. Intravenous pulse cyclophosphamide is usually preferred in patients with concurrent active lupus nephritis [40].
- **Intravenous immune globulin**, which is an effective and usually considered a first choice in conditions when a quick increase in platelets is needed, e.g., active bleeding or in case of emergency surgery [43].
- **Mycophenolate mofetil**, usually considered in patients who failed other medications [41].
- **Rituximab**—It is a chimeric monoclonal antibody which has been used as well to treat primary ITP (without SLE) refractory to previously mentioned therapies. It is given as once weekly dose for 4 consecutive weeks at doses of 375 mg/m^2 [42].
- **Splenectomy**—Splenectomy may increase the platelet count, but it does not reliably make a consistent remission of thrombocytopenia. After splenectomy, relapse may happen and has been reported at varying times from 1 to 54 months following surgery.
- **Thrombocytopenia following splenectomy—**Some patients may have persistent thrombocytopenia following splenectomy;, those patients may respond to azathioprine, cyclophosphamide, rituximab, intravenous immunoglobulin, or danazol [44]. Patient who underwent splenectomy is at high risk of pneumococcal infections;, that's why it is highly recommended for patients to receive immunization with pneumococcal vaccine before splenectomy if possible.
- **Danazol** (400 to 800 mg/day) [45]—May be considered for patients who failed other therapies. In a series of 34 patients, excellent long-term results were achieved with danazol [46].
- **Vincristine—**Successful use of vincristine has been reported [46].

13.4.4.1 Thrombocytosis

Thrombocytosis is unfrequently seen in patients with SLE.

We suggest to ruling out secondary causes such as infection or other inflammatory process, or APS.

As an example, among 465 patients with SLE, 17 (3.7%) were found to have thrombocytosis (platelet ≥400, 000/mm3). Three of these patients had one or more of the following features on peripheral blood film: Howell-Jolly bodies, spherocytes, and target cells.

Ultrasound, CT, and liver-spleen scintigraphy failed to demonstrate a spleen. All three patients had aPL [69]. These observations suggest that autosplenectomy may occur in patients with SLE, perhaps mediated by aPL.

13.4.5 Pancytopenia

Destruction of all three cell line (red blood cells, white blood cells, and platelets) may occur peripherally;, it also may suggest bone marrow failure, as in the case in aplastic anemia. Hence, bone marrow biopsy is the most significant diagnostic test to do. In a study published in 2012, concluded that among SLE patients with peripheral cytopenia, the incidence of bone marrow abnormalities is high. Bone marrow may be one of the common affected organs by immune dysregulation in active SLE. Peripheral cytopenia can be consequently improved after treatment of disease activity; hence, bone marrow biopsy should be recommended in patients with refractory cytopenia to conventional treatment [61].

There are many causes of bone marrow failure which include drugs and coexisting diseases such as acute leukemias, myelodysplastic syndromes, severe megaloblastic anemia, paroxysmal nocturnal hemoglobinuria (PNH), and infections. Furthermore, unexplained cytopenia can be associated with bone marrow necrosis, dysplasia, and distortion of the bone marrow architecture [62, 63].

13.4.6 Lymphadenopathy and Splenomegaly

Patients with SLE may present with lymphadenopathy, which could be regional or peripheral lymphadenopathy. The common sites involved in SLE lymphadenopathy are cervical and axillary nodes. In a cohort of 698 patients with SLE, lymphadenopathy was found in 59% of the study group. Patients who presented with lymphadenopathy as initial presentation represented 1% of the cohort. Furthermore, the lymph nodes' size ranged from 3 to 4 centimeter in diameter, most of them were not tender and soft. [64].

The typical histological finding in SLE lymphadenopathy includes reactive lymphoid follicular hyperplasia with variable levels of coagulative necrosis. A usual finding, yet highly associated with SLE, is the presence of hematoxylin bodies [1].

SLE lymphadenopathy is present usually initially at the diagnosis and during SLE flares in most of the cases. When SLE patient presents with an enlarged lymph node, other etiologies should be considered such as infection and lymphoproliferative disorders (e.g., angioimmunoblastic T-cell lymphoma); both of these diseases are relatively common in SLE compared to normal population. In case of infectious lymphadenopathy, lymph nodes are usually tender.

Splenomegaly may present in 10–46% of SLE patients, especially during SLE flares, and it should not necessarily be linked to cytopenia.

Based on the fact that splenomegaly and lymphadenopathy are common among SLE patients, physicians should consider lymphoproliferative disorders in those patients, especially because patients with SLE have up to fivefold higher risk of non-Hodgkin lymphoma [65].

Kikuchi-Fujimoto disease (KFD), also known as histiocytic necrotizing lymphadenitis, is a disease characterized by the presence of fever, lymphadenopathy commonly in cervical nodes, and constitutional symptoms [67].

KFD is usually self-limited, and sometimes confused with SLE or lymphoma. Typically, it is present in young women, and preceded by flu-like illness. The etiology of KFD remains unknown. No specific laboratory tests are associated with this disease, ; however, 50% of the patients may develop mild leucopenia. Histological finding of hematoxylin bodies and plasma cells and the DNA deposition in the blood vessels are highly associated with SLE lymphadenitis and help differentiating between the two diseases. It is always recommended to exclude SLE with proper serological testing before making the diagnosis of KFD. There have been few reports of SLE with coexisting KFD [55, 64, 66].

Castleman disease, also known as angiofollicular lymph node hyperplasia, is one of the rare lymphoproliferative diseases which manifested as enlarged lymph node that may or may not be associated with constitutional symptoms and could be confused with SLE or lymphoma. Its etiology remains unknown.

13.4.7 Antibodies to Clotting Factor and Phospholipids

Hematologic manifestations of SLE may involve coagulation system in some patients. SLE patients may have antibodies directed against the following factors VIII, IX, XI, XII, and XIII [1].

These antibodies can cause a biochemical abnormality (in vitro), but it also can cause some clinical abnormalities manifested as overt bleeding.

Antiphospholipid antibodies (aPL) are commonly seen in SLE patients. They can cause a prolonged partial thromboplastin time through lupus anticoagulant activity. Clinically, these antibodies have well-recognized risks of arterial as well as venous thrombosis and thrombocytopenia. Additionally, female in childbearing age with aPL is at high risk fetal loss [68].

Moderate to high titers of aPL and other antibodies to binding proteins such anticardiolipin antibodies can be associated with certain clinical features. If aPL is present with certain clinical features, it may suggest the presence of antiphospholipid syndrome (APS) (see Chap. 12, , Thrombosis in Rheumatological diseases).

High prevalence of aPL in SLE patients following treatment with cyclophosphamide was noted in a single retrospective study that compared 177 cyclophosphamide-treated SLE patients to 203 patients with SLE never treated with this alkylating agent [52]. Sero-conversion occurred at a higher rate in the cyclophosphamide-treated patients (19 versus 1%, respectively).

13.5 Macrophage Activation Syndrome (MAS)

13.5.1 Introduction

The macrophage activation syndrome (MAS), also known as hemophagocytic lymphohistiocytosis (HLH), is a condition that requires urgent attention and treatment. It is classically associated with systemic juvenile idiopathic arthritis in children and adult onset Still's disease [69], but can occur in any rheumatic disease including SLE, RA, vasculitis, Sjögren's syndrome, mixed connective tissue disease, systemic sclerosis, and inflammatory myopathies [70]. MAS can develop anytime during rheumatologic disease. It can be the first manifestation of the rheumatologic disease or may occur while patient is on treatment. It may also be associated with infection.

Hematological manifestation of MAS includes pancytopenia, hepatosplenomegaly, hyperferritinemia, and coagulopathy.

An overview of MAS is presented here, with an algorithm at the end constructing a simple approach to diagnose MAS/HLH in a patient with rheumatologic disorder.

13.5.1.1 Pancytopenia

Together, anemia and thrombocytopenia are present in more than 80% of patients [71–73]. The median hemoglobin level is 7.2 g/dl, and platelet count is 69, 000/microL [71]. Neutropenia with absolute counts below 1000/microL is not uncommon.

Patients with juvenile idiopathic arthritis and adult onset Still's disease may develop cytopenia later in the course of disease as they tend to have elevated blood counts prior developing MAS.

13.5.1.2 Hepatosplenomegaly

Reticuloendothelial system is commonly affected in MAS/HLH. In retrospective study including 249 patients of HLH, hepatomegaly was observed in 95% and lymphadenopathy in 33% of the patients. Another European registry includes 122 patients, 97% of them were found to have splenomegaly [74].

13.5.1.3 Hyperferritinemia

Severe hyperferritinemia is associated with MAS/HLH;, a level above 10, 000 ng/mL is 90% sensitive and 96% specific for MAS/HLH [75].

In HLH-94 study, it was found that ferritin greater than 10,000, 5000, and 500 ng/mL were seen in 25, 42, and 93%, respectively [72]. It is very rare to have MAS/HLH with ferritin levels below 500, ; however, low ferritin does not totally exclude MAS.

13.5.1.4 Coagulopathy

High partial thrombin time and high prothrombin time due to liver involvement and impaired liver synthetic function in association with disseminated intravascular coagulopathy are seen in MAS/HLH [70].

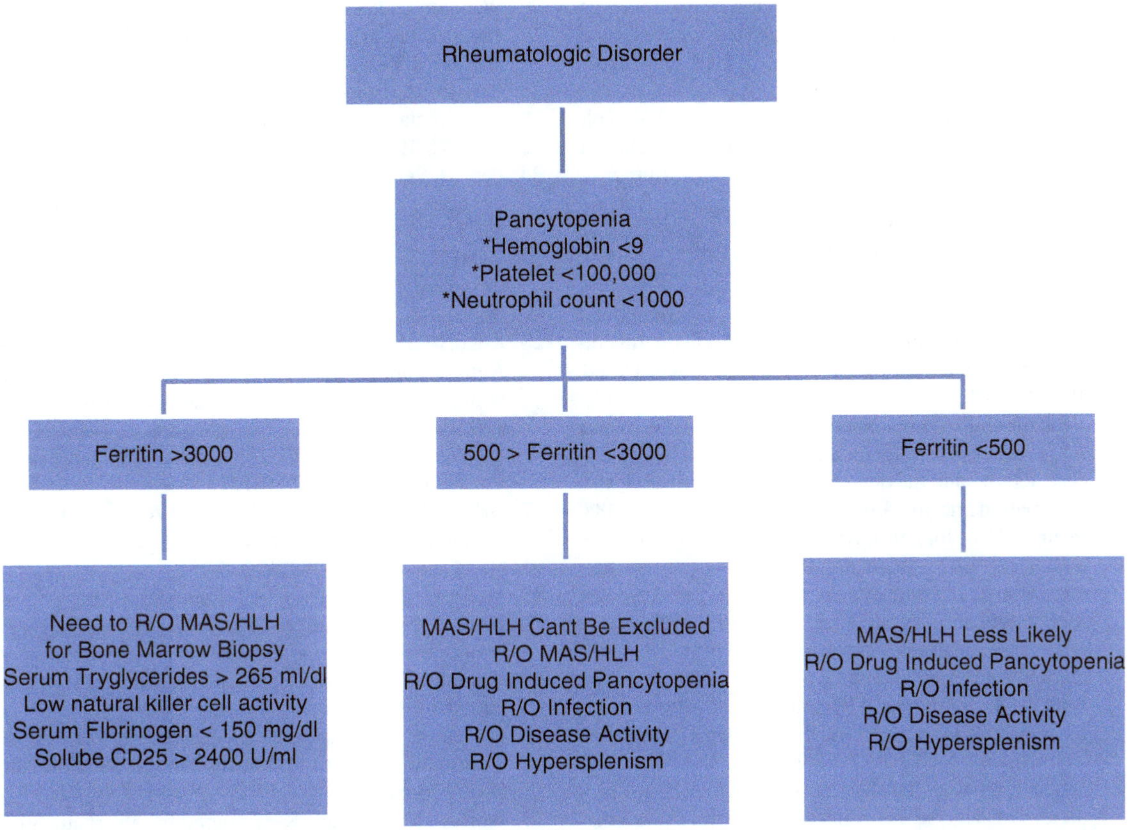

Fig. 13.5 Algorithmic approach for hyperferritinemia with pancytopenia in rheumatological diseases patients. This approach is based on ferritin level; the authors suggest to broaden the differential diagnosis and to rule out disease activity and non-rheumatological causes, including systemic diseases, infections, and drug-induced and primary hematological diseases. The evidence to support this approach is based on cumulative literature, current guidelines, and the author's experience. (Abbreviations: *R/O* rule out, *MAS* macrophage activation syndrome, *HLH* hemophagocyticlymphohistiocytosis)

The HLH-2004 revised diagnostic criteria are used to diagnose MAS/HLH. Five out of the eight criteria as shown in Fig. 13.5 are required for the diagnosis.

13.5.2 Treatment

Salvage treatment for adults with refractory/relapsing HLH usually requires intensification using combined chemotherapy and consolidation with allogenic stem cell transplantation. Novel agents are providing promising therapeutic alternatives including those incorporating ruxolitinib (JAK1/2 inhibitor), anakinra (IL-1 blockade), alemtuzumab, and emapalumab [76].

References

1. Yukawa N. Hematologic, biochemical and immunological tests in clinical practice of rheumatoid arthritis; Nihon rinsho. Japanese Journal of Clinical Medicine. 2013;71(7):1178–82.
2. Baer AN, Dessypris EN, Krantz SB. The pathogenesis of anemia in rheumatoid arthritis: a clinical and laboratory analysis. Semin Arthritis Rheum. 1990;19:209.
3. Hansen NE. The anaemia of chronic disorders. A bag of unsolved questions. Scand J Haematol. 1983;31:397.
4. Rajapakse CN, Holt PJ, Perera B. Diagnosis of true iron deficiency in rheumatoid arthritis. Ann Rheum Dis. 1980;39:596.
5. Porter DR, Sturrock RD, Capell HA. The use of serum ferritin estimation in the investigation of anaemia in patients with rheumatoid arthritis. Clin Exp Rheumatol. 1994;12:179.

6. Swaak A. Anemia of chronic disease in patients with rheumatoid arthritis: aspects of prevalence, outcome, diagnosis, and the effect of treatment on disease activity. J Rheumatol. 2006;33:1467.
7. Voulgari PV, Kolios G, Papadopoulos GK, et al. Role of cytokines in the pathogenesis of anemia of chronic disease in rheumatoid arthritis. Clin Immunol. 1999;92:153.
8. Boyd HK, Lappin TR. Erythropoietin deficiency in the anaemia of chronic disorders. Eur J Haematol. 1991;46:198.
9. Pincus T, Olsen NJ, Russell IJ, et al. Multicenter study of recombinant human erythropoietin in correction of anemia in rheumatoid arthritis. Am J Med. 1990;89:161.
10. Vreugdenhil G, Löwenberg B, Van Eijk HG, Swaak AJ. Tumor necrosis factor alpha is associated with disease activity and the degree of anemia in patients with rheumatoid arthritis. Eur J Clin Investig. 1992;22:488.
11. Peeters HR, Jongen-Lavrencic M, Vreugdenhil G, Swaak AJ. Effect of recombinant human erythropoietin on anaemia and disease activity in patients with rheumatoid arthritis and anaemia of chronic disease: a randomised placebo controlled double blind 52 weeks clinical trial. Ann Rheum Dis. 1996;55:739.
12. Bari MA, Sutradhar SR, Sarker CN, Assessment of anaemia in patients with rheumatoid arthritis, Mymensingh Med J 2013;22(2):248–254.
13. Wolfe F, Hawley DJ. The comparative risk and predictors of adverse gastrointestinal events in rheumatoid arthritis and osteoarthritis: a prospective 13 year study of 2131 patients. J Rheumatol. 2000;27:1668.
14. Doube A, Davis M, Smith JG, et al. Structured approach to the investigation of anaemia in patients with rheumatoid arthritis. Ann Rheum Dis. 1992;51:469.
15. Mulherin D, Skelly M, Saunders A, et al. The diagnosis of iron deficiency in patients with rheumatoid arthritis and anemia: an algorithm using simple laboratory measures. J Rheumatol. 1996;23:237.
16. Fitzsimons EJ, Houston T, Munro R, et al. Erythroblast iron metabolism and serum soluble transferrin receptor values in the anemia of rheumatoid arthritis. Arthritis Rheum. 2002;47:166.
17. Hansen OP, Hansen TM, Jans H, Hippe E. Red blood cell membrane-bound IgG: demonstration of antibodies in patients with autoimmune haemolytic anaemia and immune complexes in patients with rheumatic diseases. Clin Lab Haematol. 1984;6:341.
18. Rodrigues JF, Harth M, Barr RM. Pure red cell aplasia in rheumatoid arthritis. J Rheumatol. 1988;15:1159.
19. Martini A, Ravelli A, Di Fuccia G, et al. Intravenous iron therapy for severe anaemia in systemic-onset juvenile chronic arthritis. Lancet. 1994;344:1052.
20. Dessypris EN, Baer MR, Sergent JS, Krantz SB. Rheumatoid arthritis and pure red cell aplasia. Ann Intern Med. 1984;100:202.
21. Almoallim H, Klinkhoff A. Longterm outcome of treatment of Felty's syndrome with intramuscular gold: case reports and recommendations for management. J Rheumatol. 2005 Jan;32(1):20–6.
22. Wenham C, Gadsby K, Deighton C. Three significant cases of neutropenia with etanercept. Rheumatology (Oxford). 2008;47:376.
23. Panush RS, Franco AE, Schur PH. Rheumatoid arthritis associated with eosinophilia. Ann Intern Med. 1971;75:199.
24. Farr M, Scott DL, Constable TJ, et al. Thrombocytosis of active rheumatoid disease. Ann Rheum Dis. 1983;42:545.
25. Vidal F, Fontova R, Richart C. Severe neutropenia and thrombocytopenia associated with infliximab. Ann Intern Med. 2003:139:W.
26. Kokori SI, Ioannidis JP, Voulgarelis M, et al. Autoimmune hemolytic anemia in patients with systemic lupus erythematosus. Am J Med. 2005;108(3):108–204. Mellemkjaer L, Linet MS, Gridley G, et al. Rheumatoid arthritis and cancer risk. Eur J Cancer 1996; 32A:1753
27. Gridley G, McLaughlin JK, Ekbom A, et al. Incidence of cancer among patients with rheumatoid arthritis. J Natl Cancer Inst. 1993;85:307.
28. Askling J, Fored CM, Baecklund E, et al. Haematopoietic malignancies in rheumatoid arthritis: lymphoma risk and characteristics after exposure to tumour necrosis factor antagonists. Ann Rheum Dis. 2005;64:1414.
29. Baecklund E, Askling J, Rosenquist R, et al. Rheumatoid arthritis and malignant lymphomas. Curr Opin Rheumatol. 2004;16:254.
30. Wolfe F, Michaud K. Lymphoma in rheumatoid arthritis: the effect of methotrexate and anti-tumor necrosis factor therapy in 18, 572 patients. Arthritis Rheum. 2004;50:1740.
31. Hepburn AL, Narat S, Mason JC. The management of peripheral blood cytopenias in systemic lupus erythematosus. Rheumatology (Oxford). 2010;49(12):2243–54.
32. Carmona L, Abasolo L, Descalzo MA, et al. Cancer in patients with rheumatic diseases exposed to TNF antagonists. Semin Arthritis Rheum. 2011;41:71.
33. Laurence J, Wong JE, Nachman R. The cellular hematology of systemic lupus erythematosus. In: Systemic lupus Erythematosus, 2nd, Lahita RG (Ed). New York: Churchill Livingstone; 1992.
34. Manadan AM, Harris C, Schwartz MM, Block JA. The frequency of thrombotic thrombocytopenic purpura in patients with systemic lupus erythematosus undergoing kidney biopsy. J Rheumatol. 2003;30:1227.
35. Giannouli S, Voulgarelis M, Ziakas PD, Tzioufas AG. Anaemia in systemic lupus erythematosus: from pathophysiology to clinical assessment. Ann Rheum Dis. 2006;65:144.
36. Daniel J , Bevra H : Lupus erythematosus and related syndromes 8th edition 2013 , hematological and lymphoid abnormalities chapter.. 2013;34:438.
37. Pereira A, Mazzara R, Monteagudo J, et al. Thrombotic thrombocytopenic purpura/hemolytic uremic syndrome: a multivariate analysis of factors predicting the response to plasma exchange. Ann Hematol. 1995;70(6):319–23.

38. Hara A, Wada T, Kitajima S, et al. Combined pure red cell aplasia and autoimmune hemolytic anemia in systemic lupus erythematosus with anti-erythropoietin autoantibodies. Am J Hematol. 2008;83:750.
39. Gomard-Mennesson E, Ruivard M, Koenig M, et al. Treatment of isolated severe immune hemolytic anaemia associated with systemic lupus erythematosus: 26 cases. Lupus. 2006;15:223.
40. Murphy S, LoBuglio AF. Drug therapy of autoimmune hemolytic anemia. Semin Hematol. 1976;13:323.
41. Rivero SJ, Alger M, Alarcón-Segovia D. Splenectomy for hemocytopenia in. 139:773.
42. Chan AC, Sack K. Danazol therapy in autoimmune hemolytic anemia associated with systemic lupus erythematosus. J Rheumatol. 1991;18:280.
43. Coon WW. Splenectomy for cytopenias associated with systemic lupus erythematosus. Am J Surg. 1988;155:391.
44. Alba P, Karim MY, Hunt BJ. Mycophenolate mofetil as a treatment for autoimmune haemolytic anaemia in patients with systemic lupus erythematosus and antiphospholipid syndrome. Lupus. 2003;12:633.
45. Nesher G, Hanna VE, Moore TL, et al. Thrombotic microangiographic hemolytic anemia in systemic lupus erythematosus. Semin Arthritis Rheum. 1994;24:165.
46. Voulgarelis M, Kokori SI, Ioannidis JP, et al. Anaemia in systemic lupus erythematosus: aetiological profile and the role of erythropoietin. Ann Rheum Dis. 2000;59:217.
47. Jeffries M, Hamadeh F, Aberle T, et al. Haemolyticanaemia in a multi-ethnic cohort of lupus patients: a clinical and serological perspective. Lupus. 2008;17:739.
48. Voulgarelis M, Kokori SI, Ioannidis JP, et al. Autoimmune hemolytic anemia in patients with systemic lupus erythematosus. Am J Med. 2000;108(3):198–204.
49. Budman DR, Steinberg AD. Hematologic aspects of systemic lupus erythematosus. Current concepts. Ann Intern Med. 1977;86:220.
50. Blombery P, Scully M. Management of thrombotic thrombocytopenic purpura: current perspectives. J Blood Med. 2014;5:15–23. eCollection 2014
51. Pereira A, Mazzara R, Monteagudo J, et al. Thrombotic thrombocytopenic purpura/hemolytic uremic syndrome: a multivariate analysis of factors predicting the response to plasma exchange. Ann Hematol. 1995;70(6):319–23.
52. cully M, McDonald V, Cavenagh J, et al. A phase 2 study of the safety and efficacy of rituximab with plasma exchange in acute acquired thrombotic thrombocytopenic purpura. Blood. 2011;118(7):1746–53.
53. Tsai HM. Advances in the pathogenesis, diagnosis, and treatment of thrombotic thrombocytopenic purpura. J Am Soc Nephrol. 2003;14(4):1072.
54. Hochberg MC. Updating the American College of Rheumatology revised criteria for the classification of systemic lupus erythematosus. Arthritis Rheum. 1997;40(9):1725.
55. Daniel J , Bevra H : Lupus erythtomatous and related syndromes 8th edition 2013, hematological and lymphoid abnormalities chapter.. 2013;34:452.
56. Michael SR, Vural IL, Bassen FA, et al. The hematologic aspects of disseminated (systemic) lupus erythematosus. Blood. 1951;6(11):1059–72.
57. Abid N, Khan AS. Systemic lupus erythematosus (SLE) in the eastern region of Saudi Arabia. A comparative study. Lupus. 2013 Dec;22(14):1529–33.
58. Ziakas PD, Giannouli S, Zintzaras E, et al. Lupus thrombocytopenia: implications and prognostic significance. Ann Rheum Dis. 2005;64(9):1366–9.
59. Habib GS, Saliba WR, Froom P. Pure red cell aplasia and lupus. Semin Arthritis Rheum. 2002;31:279.
60. Corley CC Jr, Lessner HE, Larsen WE. Azathioprine therapy of "autoimmune" diseases. Am J Med. 1966;41:404.
61. Wanitpongpun C, Teawtrakul N. Bone marrow abnormalities in systemic lupus erythematosus with peripheral cytopenia. Clin Exp Rheumatol. 2012;30(6):825.
62. Sultan SM, Begum S, Isenberg DA. Prevalence, patterns of disease and outcome in patients with systemic lupus erythematosus who develop severe haematological problems. Rheumatology (Oxford). 2003;42:230.
63. Dold S, Singh R, Sarwar H, et al. Frequency of microangiopathic hemolytic anemia in patients with systemic lupus erythematosus exacerbation: distinction from thrombotic thrombocytopenic purpura, prognosis, and outcome. Arthritis Rheum. 2005;53:982.
64. Quismorio F. Hematologic and lymphoid manifestations of SLE. In: Wallace DJ, Hahn BH, editors. Dubois' lupus erythematosus, ed 7. Baltimore: Lippincott Williams & Wilkins; 2007.
65. Gayed M, Bernatsky S. Lupus and cancer. Lupus. 2009;18(6):479.
66. Kucukardali Y, Solmazgul E, Kunter E, Oncul O, Yildirim S, Kaplan M. Kikuchi–Fujimoto disease: analysis of 244 cases. Clin Rheumatol. 2007;26:50–4.
67. Santana A, Lessa B, Galrao L, Lima I, Santiago M. Kikuchi-Fujimoto's disease associated with systemic lupus erythematosus: case report and review of the literature. Clin Rheumatol. 2005;24:60–3.
68. Martínez-Baños D, Crispín JC, Lazo-Langner A, Sánchez-Guerrero J. Moderate and severe neutropenia in patients with systemic lupus erythematosus. Rheumatology (Oxford). 2006;45:994.
69. Davì S, Minoia F, Pistorio A, et al. Performance of current guidelines for diagnosis of macrophage activation syndrome complicating systemic juvenile idiopathic arthritis. Arthritis Rheumatol. 2014;66(10):2871 80.
70. Fukaya S, Yasuda S, Hashimoto T, et al. Clinical features of haemophagocytic syndrome in patients with systemic autoimmune diseases: analysis of 30 cases. Rheumatology (Oxford). 2008;47(11):1686–91.
71. Niece JA, Rogers ZR, Ahmad N, Langevin AM, Mcclain KL. Hemophagocytic lymphohistiocytosis in Texas: observations on ethnicity and race. Pediatr Blood Cancer. 2010;54(3):424–8.
72. Trottestam H, Horne A, Aricò M, et al. Chemoimmunotherapy for hemophagocyticlympho-

histiocytosis: long-term results of the HLH-94 treatment protocol. Blood. 2011;118(17):4577–84.
73. Palazzi DL, Mcclain KL, Kaplan SL. Hemophagocytic syndrome in children: an important diagnostic consideration in fever of unknown origin. Clin Infect Dis. 2003;36(3):306–12.
74. Aricò M, Janka G, Fischer A, et al. Hemophagocyticlymphohistiocytosis. Report of 122 children from the international registry. FHL study group of the Histiocyte society. Leukemia. 1996;10(2):197–203.
75. Allen CE, Yu X, Kozinetz CA, Mcclain KL. Highly elevated ferritin levels and the diagnosis of hemophagocyticlymphohistiocytosis. Pediatr Blood Cancer. 2008;50(6):1227–35.
76. La rosée P, Horne A, Hines M, et al. Recommendations for the management of hemophagocytic lymphohistiocytosis in adults. Blood. 2019;133(23):2465–77.

Permissions

All chapters in this book were first published by Springer; hereby published with permission under the Creative Commons Attribution License or equivalent. Every chapter published in this book has been scrutinized by our experts. Their significance has been extensively debated. The topics covered herein carry significant information for a comprehensive understanding. They may even be implemented as practical applications or may be referred to as a beginning point for further studies.

The contributors of this book come from diverse backgrounds, making this book a truly international effort. We would like to thank all the contributing authors for lending their expertise to make the book truly unique. They have played a crucial role in the development of this book. Without their invaluable contributions this book wouldn't have been possible. They have made vital efforts to compile up to date information on the varied aspects of this subject to make this book a valuable addition to the collection of many professionals and students.

This book was conceptualized with the vision of imparting up-to-date and integrated information in this field. To ensure the same, a matchless editorial board was set up. Every individual on the board went through rigorous rounds of assessment to prove their worth. After which they invested a large part of their time researching and compiling the most relevant data for our readers.

The editorial board has been involved in producing this book since its inception. They have spent rigorous hours researching and exploring the diverse topics which have resulted in the successful publishing of this book. They have passed on their knowledge of decades through this book. To expedite this challenging task, the publisher supported the team at every step. A small team of assistant editors was also appointed to further simplify the editing procedure and attain best results for the readers.

Apart from the editorial board, the designing team has also invested a significant amount of their time in understanding the subject and creating the most relevant covers. They scrutinized every image to scout for the most suitable representation of the subject and create an appropriate cover for the book.

The publishing team has been an ardent support to the editorial, designing and production team. Their endless efforts to recruit the best for this project, has resulted in the accomplishment of this book. They are a veteran in the field of academics and their pool of knowledge is as vast as their experience in printing. Their expertise and guidance has proved useful at every step. Their uncompromising quality standards have made this book an exceptional effort. Their encouragement from time to time has been an inspiration for everyone.

The publisher and the editorial board hope that this book will prove to be a valuable piece of knowledge for students, practitioners and scholars across the globe.

Index

www.ingramcontent.com/pod-product-compliance
Lightning Source LLC
LaVergne TN
LVHW062130200926
848484LV00007B/1796